THE NEW AMERICAN ENCYCLOPEDIA OF CHILDREN'S HEALTH

by
Robert Hoekelman, M.D., Noni MacDonald, M.D., and David Baum, M.D.

NAL BOOKS

NEW AMERICAN LIBRARY

A DIVISION OF PENGUIN BOOKS USA INC., NEW YORK

NOTE TO THE READER
The ideas, procedures and suggestions contained in this book
are not intended as a substitute for consulting with your
physician. All matters regarding your children's health require
medical supervision.

Conceived, edited, designed and produced by
Duncan Petersen Publishing Ltd,
5 Botts Mews, Chepstow Road
London, W2 5AG.

NAL BOOKS TRADEMARK REG U.S. PAT. OFF. AND
FOREIGN COUNTRIES
REGISTERED TRADEMARK – MARCA REGISTRADA
HECHO EN ESTELLA, SPAIN

SIGNET, SIGNET CLASSIC, MENTOR, ONYX, PLUME,
MERIDIAN and NAL BOOKS are published by New
American Library, a division of Penguin Books USA Inc.,
1633 Broadway, New York, NY 10019.

First Printing, November, 1989

1   2   3   4   5   6   7   8   9

PRINTED IN SPAIN

First and last, this is a book designed for easy reference. Just look up the topic that concerns you – all the entries are in alphabetical order and they feature not only illnesses but symptoms and general problems. There is no index.

Whenever, in the course of an entry, you see a word in *LARGE ITALIC CAPITALS*, this means that there is a full entry on the topic elsewhere in the book which it is advisable to look up in order to complete your understanding of the topic.

Cross-references in SMALL CAPITALS mean the entry is well worth looking up, but not essential.

Occasionally you will find a word in capitals that does not correspond exactly to the title of the entry itself. The reason for this discrepancy is simply convenience of expression.

Entries are generally of three types:

Main entries, usually divided into multiple sub-headings, cover the illnesses, diseases and other problems of childhood and adolescence.

Background entries, usually with few sub-headings, cover general topics such as major symptoms, typically COUGH, ABDOMINAL PAIN, CHEST PAIN: having read such an entry, you will almost certainly wish to look up further, specific entries to which you will have been referred. Background entries also cover important general topics such as ACCIDENTS IN THE HOME, ADDITIVES IN FOOD and first-aid procedures.

'Signpost' entries direct to you the main entry where the topic is fully covered. They often feature colloquial terms for symptoms (for example NITS See *LICE*) but they may also cover technical terms or names for diseases which are covered under the other headings (for example HYPERVENTILATION see *OVERBREATHING, STRESS SYMPTOMS*).

Remember that the book features not only physical illness but mental problems too – indeed the coverage of psychological disorders is particularly full. Also covered are many peripheral, but essential topics such as FAMILY PROBLEMS, GIFTED CHILD, JEALOUSY, LIES AND FIBS, and SEAT BELTS.

Except for the extraordinarily rare disorders – those which most doctors see perhaps once in a lifetime – the book covers everything that could possibly have a bearing on your child's physical and mental well-being.

INTRODUCTION

I have been a doctor for almost 40 years. During that time, I have practiced as a pediatrician and have directed the care of infants, children, and adolescents in a large university medical center. The most memorable moments during these years have been those during which parents whose children were seriously ill or who had died lamented, 'If we had only known what was wrong'; 'If we had only known what to do', or 'If we had only known enough to have come to the doctor sooner.'

In any medical care system for children, the parents are the most important members of the team, because they must recognize when things are not right with their child. They must decide, sometimes in a matter of moments, what to do to avoid disaster and when to seek medical care. That is a heavy burden for them to bare, particularly when they have not been taught how to recognize the signs and symptoms of serious childhood illnesses. They usually seek the advice of their own parents or their friends or neighbors, who are no better informed about what should be done.

The rest of the child health-care team – the doctors, nurses, and other health professionals – are very well trained. They know what to do for a sick child and when to do it, and what proper measures to take to prevent illnesses from occuring, and when to take them. But their expertise is of no use if the parents do not seek help from them soon enough.

The New American Encyclopedia of Child Health was written solely for the purpose of teaching parents what they need to know about preventing childhood illnesses, how to recognize childhood illnesses early on, what to do in emergencies, when to seek help from other members of the child-health team, and what to expect once that help is obtained.

I have written and edited many textbooks for doctors and nurses – textbooks that are designed to teach them how to prevent and treat childhood illnesses. These books and many others are available in some hospitals and in some public libraries for parents to read. But such books are very technical and are not written for parents. And when parents do read them and gain some knowledge of why their child is ill and what to do when their child becomes ill, it is often too late to make a difference.

The New American Encyclopedia of Child Health is a book that provides all of the information parents, as the first-contact members of the child health-care team, need to have to do their job well. It is written in non-technical language, and can be read from cover to cover at one's leisure, or used as a quick reference during an emergency or when there is any concern, major or minor, about a child's health.

I consider my contribution to this book to be far more important than those I have made to any of the other child-health books I have written or edited: for this book will do more to improve the health of our children than will any of the others.

Robert A. Hoekelman, M.D.
Consulting editor
Professor and Chairman, Department of Pediatrics
University of Rochester School of Medicine and Dentistry
Pediatrician-in-Chief
Strong Memorial Hospital, Rochester, New York

The illustrations on the following pages are designed as a complement to the textual entries in the body of the book. They identify the major organs and systems of the body, and explain some of the key terms associated with them.

THE SKELETON

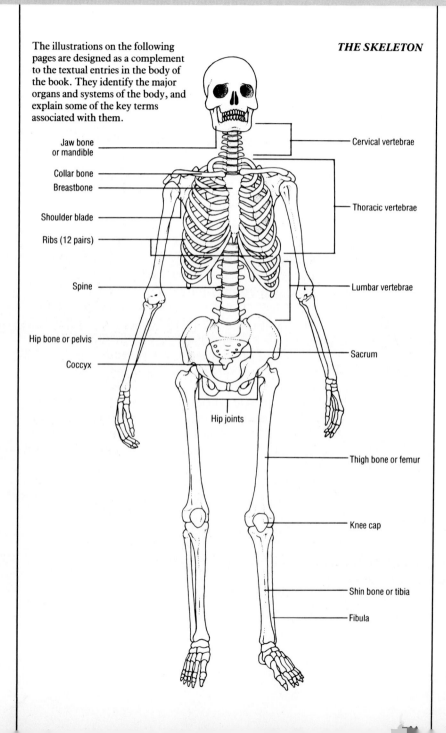

Jaw bone or mandible

Collar bone

Breastbone

Shoulder blade

Ribs (12 pairs)

Spine

Hip bone or pelvis

Coccyx

Hip joints

Cervical vertebrae

Thoracic vertebrae

Lumbar vertebrae

Sacrum

Thigh bone or femur

Knee cap

Shin bone or tibia

Fibula

THE HEAD AND NECK

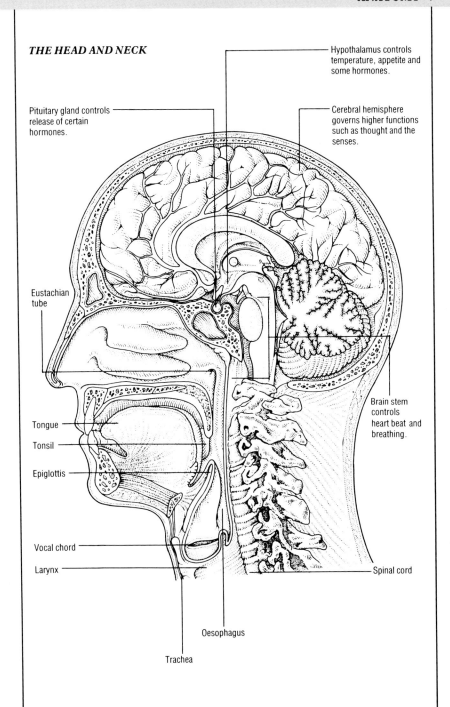

Hypothalamus controls temperature, appetite and some hormones.

Pituitary gland controls release of certain hormones.

Cerebral hemisphere governs higher functions such as thought and the senses.

Eustachian tube

Tongue

Tonsil

Epiglottis

Brain stem controls heart beat and breathing.

Vocal chord

Larynx

Spinal cord

Oesophagus

Trachea

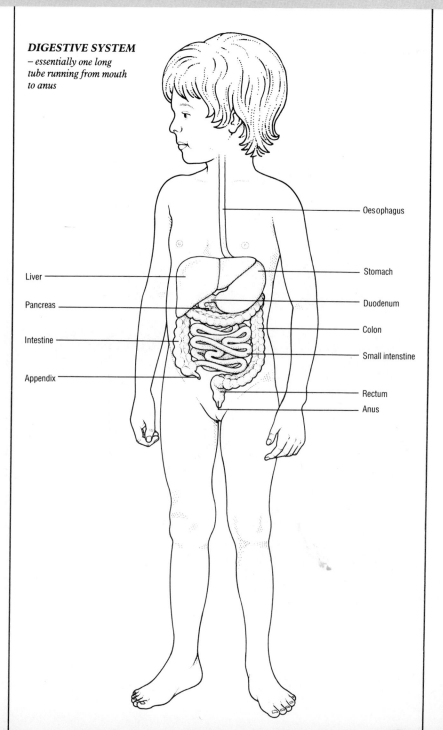

DIGESTIVE SYSTEM
– essentially one long tube running from mouth to anus

Oesophagus

Liver

Stomach

Pancreas

Duodenum

Colon

Intestine

Small intenstine

Appendix

Rectum

Anus

THE HEART AND LUNGS

– work in harness: the heart is a muscular pump, driving blood to the lungs for re-oxygenization and to the rest of the body via the aorta; the lungs are a gas exchange system, enabling oxygen breathed in to pass to the bloodstream.

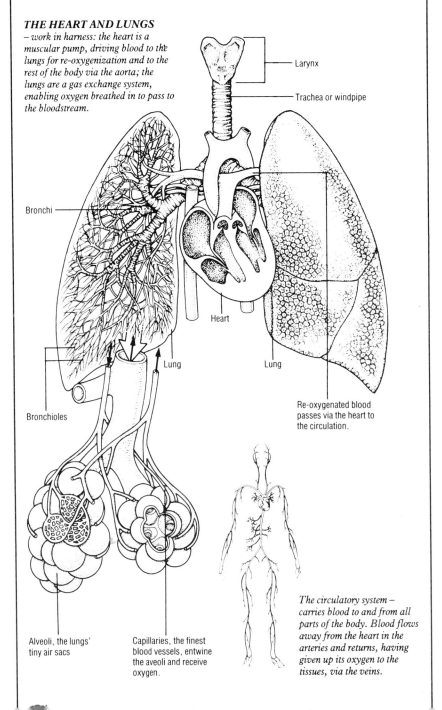

Larynx

Trachea or windpipe

Bronchi

Heart

Lung

Lung

Re-oxygenated blood passes via the heart to the circulation.

Bronchioles

Alveoli, the lungs' tiny air sacs

Capillaries, the finest blood vessels, entwine the aveoli and receive oxygen.

The circulatory system – carries blood to and from all parts of the body. Blood flows away from the heart in the arteries and returns, having given up its oxygen to the tissues, via the veins.

THE EYE

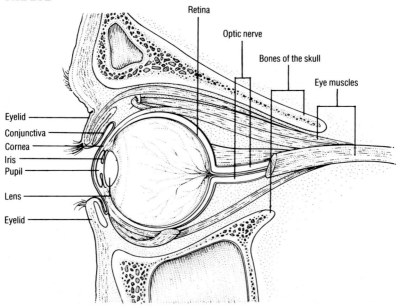

Retina

Optic nerve

Bones of the skull

Eye muscles

Eyelid

Conjunctiva

Cornea

Iris

Pupil

Lens

Eyelid

THE EAR

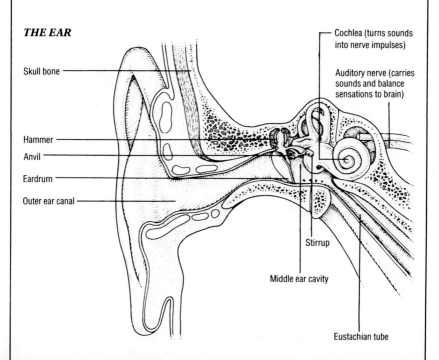

Cochlea (turns sounds into nerve impulses)

Auditory nerve (carries sounds and balance sensations to brain)

Skull bone

Hammer

Anvil

Eardrum

Outer ear canal

Stirrup

Middle ear cavity

Eustachian tube

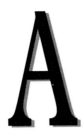

ABDOMINAL PAIN

Caused by different problems at different ages.

■ IN GENERAL If the child is otherwise well and can be distracted from the pain, the problem is probably a minor one due to excess intestinal gas or indigestion. If the cause is serious, as with anything that may lead to PERITONITIS, the child looks ill and cannot be distracted from the misery of the pain. There may also be other symptoms, such as loss of APPETITE, CONSTIPATION or DIARRHEA, FEVER or VOMITING.

■ IN BABIES Crying babies are often thought to have COLIC. The symptoms are thought to be due to swallowed air getting trapped in the intestine as an 'air bubble' causing distension and discomfort. However, the problem with a crying baby is not always a matter of excess intestinal gas, and it is generally not helpful to burp babies obsessively during and after every feeding.

■ ACTION Try to identify other reasons why your baby is crying. Does he look ill? Is he thriving? (See *FAILURE TO THRIVE*.) Is he in pain? The problem of an unsettled baby is common. A simple cause or explanation is rare. But if the problem persists or you think the baby is ill or has acute pain – see *VOLVULUS* and *INTUSSUSCEPTION* – then get medical advice.

■ IN TODDLERS See *GASTROENTERITIS*, a common cause of episodes of diarrhea, vomiting and abdominal pain. Many illnesses associated with fever, such as sore throat or ear infection, may also cause a small child to complain of tummy-ache – see *MESENTERIC ADENITIS* for explanation. URINARY TRACT INFECTION is a cause of special importance, particularly in girls.

■ IN OLDER CHILDREN The child can describe the pain and separate it from other symptoms. Acute episodes of abdominal pain are usually clearly associated with other symptoms, such as those that occur with gastroenteritis or a urinary tract infection. However, recurrent or low-grade persistent abdominal pain in the absence of other symptoms is often less obviously explained – see also *RECURRENT ABDOMINAL PAIN*.

If you or your child are worried about the pain, get medical advice. In the child who is otherwise in good health, increasing the fiber in the diet may sometimes alleviate the pain. In others, the origins may be psychological (such as teasing or stress at school; or tension at home) – nevertheless, the pains are real for the child. If the child is ill, then many different possible causes need to be considered. You should therefore get medical advice.

■ ACTION Try to get the child to tell you, calmly, as much as possible about the pain. What action you should take depends upon the severity, persistence and tempo of the complaint. Watch out for other symptoms: appetite, bowel habit. If the child does not seem ill and can move about normally, you might want to discuss the problem with your doctor at your convenience. If your child appears ill or develops any of the signs of peritonitis, get urgent medical help.

ABDOMINAL SWELLING

Toddlers often look pot-bellied at the age when they are learning to walk and run. Between the ages of two and five years, the abdomen becomes less prominent, flatter and more muscular. This is related to the natural straightening of the lower spine, together with strengthening of the abdominal muscles as the upright posture is established.

Other causes of generalized abdominal swelling are rare, but include a range of serious conditions including INTESTINAL OBSTRUCTION and enlargement of abdominal organs, symptomatic of many diseases.

ABRASIONS

See *CUTS AND GRAZES*.

ACCIDENT-PRONE CHILD

See *CLUMSINESS*.

ACCIDENTS IN THE HOME, PREVENTION

All new parents need to survey their house or apartment to see what changes are needed to protect a child from accidents, above all when he is left unattended. Common-sense measures *do* save lives. As your child grows, yet more safety measures will be needed.

Wide-ranging specific measures are suggested on the opposite page, and also on pages 16 and 17.

ACHONDROPLASIA

A dominant INHERITED DISORDER diagnosed at birth: the baby is found to have short arms and legs – see *SHORT STATURE*. Males and females are equally affected. Adult height usually turns out to be less than 4½ ft (1.4 m). The back has a rather exaggerated curve and the head is large. Most such children enjoy good health and have normal intelligence. Some may have difficulties with HYDROCEPHALUS and/or pressure on the spinal cord in the neck area. Occasionally surgical treatment is necessary.

ACNE

The combination of blackheads and whiteheads on the face and upper trunk – a problem of puberty and adolescence.

■ CAUSE The underlying cause is the effect of the male sex hormones on the oil-producing glands in the skin. Both boys and girls produce these hormones as they approach puberty. They stimulate the activity of the sebaceous glands in the skin, which produce natural oils. The excess oil blocks the skin pores, forming blackheads and whiteheads. The oils in the resulting swellings are broken down by the normal BACTERIA on the skin, forming irritant acids that may lead to painful inflamed red sores that eventually become pimples and burst, or dry up without doing so.

■ SAFETY FOR THE SEMI-MOBILE CHILD A crawling baby should not be left alone. Many potential dangers, from glass ornaments to poisonous plants, are obvious but you cannot predict every eventuality.

Steps will be crawled down; corners bumped into; furniture pulled over. Rearrange the room, if necessary, so that he does not bump into sharp corners. Ensure that anything he might pull himself up on to will not topple over.

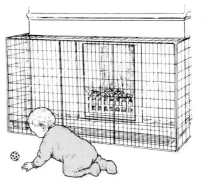

■ Keep a gate on the stairs, and across the doorway of any room which has not been baby-proofed. Beware of baby walkers, infants can scoot through doors and topple down stairs so easily.

■ All open fireplaces, wood stoves and hot radiators should have barriers around them to prevent eager hands from being burned.

■ Take him to the door or telephone when you have to answer it, or put him in a play-pen at such moments. Do *not* leave him where he can move about unobserved.

■ Pick up everything small enough to swallow, and put it out of reach.

■ Cover electric wallsockets with safety plugs. Electrical burns to the mouth are serious.

■ Allow nothing breakable within 3 ft (one m) of the floor.

■ Don't leave wires trailing, especially wires to electric irons and other appliances.

■ Keep poisons in high locked cupboards.

■ Move all the dangerous chemicals from the cabinet under the sink or fit a lock or child-proof latch.

■ Check that none of the plants he can reach are dangerous. Your poison control center can advise you on this.

■ Check that he cannot crawl through the banisters on the landing or balcony.

■ Keep hot cups of tea and coffee up out of reach.

■ Put away table-cloths for a year or so. He can easily pull everything on top of him if he tries to use the cloth to pull himself up.

■ Keep drawers closed. If a child pulls up and leans forwards, the drawer can close on his fingers.

■ Watch for children's fingers on the hinged side of the door.

■ Swinging doors are dangerous for babies.

■ Wedge doors open.

■ Wedge books into bookcases with folded newspapers.

■ SAFETY FOR THE MOBILE CHILD Once he starts moving about the house you will need to extend your child-proofing further.

■ Once he can walk, he will also climb. Keep all windows locked.

■ Never leave him alone near water. A child can drown in 2-3 in (5-7½ cm) of water left in a bathtub or wading pool.

■ Keep all medicines in a locked cabinet.

■ Keep all cleaning materials out of reach.

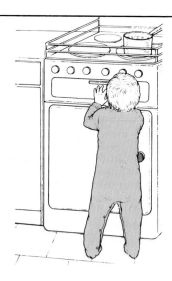

■ Don't leave a toddler in the backyard unsupervised, a fenced play area is safer.

■ Make sure swimming-pool gates are always locked such that a young child cannot jiggle them open. Never ever leave a young child alone in the pool area even for a minute.

■ Make sure garden sheds and garages are locked.

■ Make sure weed-killer and other garden poisons are out of reach, in case he does get into the garage.

■ Don't leave lighted barbecues or fires unguarded.

■ Make sure his clothes are flame resistant.

■ Use the back burners on the stove, and turn all pots and pans so that the handles cannot be knocked or pulled off the stove.

■ Be sure he cannot reach the iron or knock over the ironing board.

■ Don't polish your floors so well that he will slip.

■ Make sure rugs don't slip.

■ Make sure he cannot lock himself in the bathroom or any other room.

■ Make sure he cannot open the front or back doors by himself.

■ Never leave old refrigerators or freezers where he could climb inside – always remove the door from the hinges if it is waiting for trash removal.

■ Never let a child tie string or straps around his neck. These may get caught, twist and choke him.

■ Never let him play with plastic bags – he may smother.

■ Check your hot water tank, make sure it is set at the lower range. At the mid- and high-range setting, the tap water may be hot enough to scald and cause serious burns if accidentally turned on by your toddler or young child.

▓ ACTION Go round your house now and note all the hazards. Deal with them now, before the worst happens. Much can be achieved simply by moving all the most dangerous objects up and away from a child's normal reach. Do you need some extra high shelves, a cabinet that locks?

SAFE TO PUT IN HIS MOUTH?

How safe it is for him to put objects into his mouth depends on the objects:

■ Too small and it could be swallowed.

■ Mouth-width objects may get stuck.

■ Loose and furry, and he may choke on little bits.

■ Long and thin, such as a wooden spoon, and he may choke on it.

■ *Anything* sharp can cut.

■ If you are worried about the germs and dirt on toys, wash them with soap and water but remember all children put things in their mouths. It is impossible to avoid all germs.

ACNE

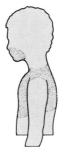

Acne commonly occurs on the face and upper trunk.

Development of spots

1   2   3

1 *Excess grease blocks the pores; blackheads or whiteheads form.*
2 *Normal bacteria breaks down the grease, producing irritant acids.*
3 *Painful red spots appear.*

▓ ACTION Don't dismiss acne as an untreatable hazard of growing up. It can be distressing for many teenagers, and mild acne can often be effectively treated by simple measures such as washing regularly and applying benzoyl peroxide creams.

▓ GET MEDICAL ADVICE if the acne persists, and you are concerned about it.

▓ TREATMENT Creams containing benzoyl peroxide may reduce the blockage of the pores by peeling off the top layer of skin. They also have an antibacterial effect. They can be bought at the drugstore without prescription. Your doctor may prescribe a vitamin A cream to be used in conjunction with the benzoyl peroxide cream. ANTIBIOTICS such as tetracycline, taken for long periods (weeks or months on occasion) reduce the bacteria on the skin and prevent the breakdown of oils to irritant acids. Occasionally, topical antibiotics are used. Older adolescent girls with severe acne may be prescribed a pill similar to the contraceptive pill. This contains female hormones and neutralizes the effect of the male hormones. This is only used in girls who have stopped growing. It is never used in boys.

If the acne is severe, and these treatments do not clear it, the doctor may refer your child to a dermatologist.

■ LONG-TERM MANAGEMENT
Antibiotics can be taken for several years if necessary. Not all teenagers outgrow acne, so long-term treatment may be required.

ADDICTION
See *ALCOHOL ABUSE, SOLVENT ABUSE, SMOKING, DRUG ABUSE.*

ADDITIVES IN FOOD
Substances used in the processing of food and drinks, typically as preservatives or coloring.

Pectin, used to gel jams, is a natural additive, as is lecithin, made from soya beans, and used to stop foods from separating. Some factory-produced additives are identical to natural substances; others are entirely artificial.

Additives are shown in the ingredients list on food packaging. The first ingredient listed is present in the largest amount, the last one in the smallest.

Additives fall into four groups:
1 Those that enhance the flavor and appearance of food. There are more than 50 permitted colors, the commonest being caramel, made by overcooking sugar. Another common one, beta-carotene, is a coloring extract of carrot converted to vitamin A in the body. There are no colorings in baby foods.

Flavor enhancers include monosodium glutamate and artificial sweeteners such as aspartame. Flavorings make up the largest group of additives, but are used in very much smaller quantities than the preservatives.

2 Those that act as preservatives: Potassium nitrate is a typical preservative: it kills micro-organisms, BACTERIA, yeasts and FUNGI, preventing food from rotting, allowing it to last longer and improving its safety.

3 Those that prevent food spoiling and maintain freshness: Antioxidant additives prevent or delay deterioration in fats by limiting the effect of oxygen, which causes fat to go rancid. VITAMINS are also preserved by antioxidant additives. They also prevent the discoloration of fruit and vegetables. Vitamin C is a commonly used antioxidant. The use of preservatives widens the range of available foods and can reduce the cost. of food.

4 Those that aid food processing: These include acids, which help release carbon dioxide gas necessary for raising bread; bleaching agents to whiten flour; bulking agents, emulsifiers, firming agents, freezing agents, glazing agents, humectants (to increase moisture), propellants, anti-caking agents, releasing agents (to prevent food from sticking to packaging) and thickening agents.

■ PROBLEMS WITH ADDITIVES
A tiny minority of people are affected by food additives. Those principally under suspicion are the yellow color tartrazine; the red color erythrosin; several antioxidants; and some preservatives.

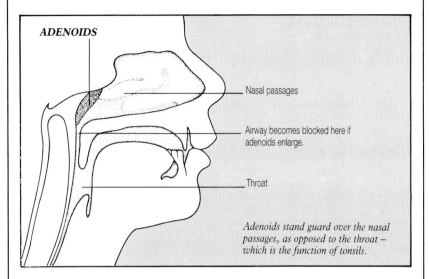

ADENOIDS

Nasal passages

Airway becomes blocked here if adenoids enlarge.

Throat

Adenoids stand guard over the nasal passages, as opposed to the throat – which is the function of tonsils.

Reactions include skin RASHES (URTICARIA), ASTHMA, HEADACHES and joint pains. Some asthmatics are sensitive to sulfites.

Although some authors claim a link between additives and HYPERACTIVITY, a number of placebo-controlled trials have failed to prove the association. Furthermore, the additive-free diets are quite difficult to follow and if too restrictive they may be detrimental to the child's health. Fashionable as the additive issue may be, research has shown that it is unlikely to be the cause of hyperactivity in most children.

ADENOIDS – ENLARGED

Adenoids consist of fleshy lymphoid tissue lying at the back of the nose. They have a structure and function similar to the tonsils, and guard against INFECTION. The adenoids are at their largest in the four- to seven-year age group; in individual children they may grow to be too big for the relatively small space they occupy, thus causing blockage of that space at the back of nose.

■ SYMPTOMS Persistent breathing through the mouth (the nose seems permanently blocked) and nasal speech.

■ ACTION If you suspect adenoid trouble, discuss the symptoms with your doctor.

■ TREATMENT Symptoms may remit spontaneously or be relieved by nasal decongestants. Severe obstruction may justify an operation to remove the adenoids but such a decision should take into account the views of your doctor and an ear, nose and throat specialist. In the past, the operation was performed more often than is now thought necessary. It was also common to remove the tonsils at the same time, but this is no longer done unless there are specific additional indications to remove the tonsils.

■ OUTLOOK As the child moves into adolescence, the facial bones enlarge, along with the space in which the adenoids lie. The child then literally grows out of the problem.

ADRENAL DISORDERS

The adrenal glands are situated on top of the kidneys, and their function is to produce various hormones. These secretions are vital for normal health. Over- or under-production causes a range of problems, which, for simplicity, are listed below under the names of the hormones involved.

The steroid hormones (cortisol and aldesterone) Too much cortisol causes Cushing's disease. This is a very rare disease in childhood. Over-secretion by the adrenal glands often indicates that an adrenal tumor is present. The effects of excess cortisol are much more commonly the result of high dosage treatment with cortisol-like agents such as prednisone. Clinically excess cortisol makes a child short, overweight and sometimes hairy.

Some children are born with a lack of both cortisol and aldosterone (the body's main salt-balancing hormone). This most commonly is the result of an abnormality in their production, which results in an overgrowth of the adrenal glands, termed congenital adrenal hyperplasia. The absence of the normal adrenal hormones causes serious problems in the first few days of life, which are life-threatening if not recognized. With treatment, however, the child can grow and develop normally.

Sex hormones In congenital adrenal hyperplasia the abnormal production of cortisol leads to formation of masculinizing hormones. These may result in an enlargement of the clitoris in a baby girl to the size of the male's penis so that sex identity may be difficult at birth.

In some children, over-production of sex hormones by an adrenal tumor can cause early or precocious PUBERTY.

Adrenal disorders are rare; their clinical presentation is not usually obvious nor of sudden onset. However, once considered they are generally easily recognized and treated by a specialist (endocrinologist). In most instances a complete cure can be effected, although this may require taking medications throughout life.

AGGRESSION

See also *BEHAVIORAL TREATMENTS, BULLYING AND TEASING, SIBLING RIVALRY, TANTRUMS.*

All children are aggressive at times, both within and outside the family. Problems can arise from the way aggression is expressed, such as by hitting, kicking, swearing, biting or spitting. The feeling of aggression is universal; its mode of expression is learned. Children punished physically are more likely to express aggression physically – imitation is a powerful expression of learning, and children copy adults as well as other children. Aggression that succeeds in being rewarded is likely to be repeated. It can be an effective way of gaining adult attention. With age, children normally learn greater self-control and how to channel aggression in socially acceptable ways. Boys are naturally more aggressive than girls.

▧ MANAGEMENT Don't retaliate aggressively. Don't allow aggression to achieve results. Ponder on situations in which your child has been aggressive, and ask yourself what may be causing it. When he fights, remove him from the 'arena' and leave him on his own for a few minutes to cool off. Explain briefly why it is wrong, and suggest an alternative method of dealing with the situation. In general, praise your child when he has shown self-control. Parents have different philosophies on the virtues of hitting back when children are hit by others. All children have to learn to stand up for themselves, but physical retaliation is not the only way.

Seek advice if your child is frequently aggressive, is difficult in a range of situations, and is constantly in trouble. All these can affect his relationships inside and outside the home. Your family doctor may suggest discussing the problem with a child psychiatrist or psychologist.

AIDS (ACQUIRED IMMUNE DEFICIENCY SYNDROME)

A condition of depressed immunity caused by INFECTION with the Human Immunodeficiency VIRUS (HIV).

Children are most commonly infected during pregnancy because the mother has been infected (as a result of intravenous drug abuse or through sexual intercourse with an infected partner). Another smaller group of children (including hemophiliacs) are infected through contaminated blood products given to them before the risk of AIDS was known and blood products screened for HIV before they were given.

▣ SYMPTOMS Many children remain symptom free for the first year after infection. Most then develop non-specific symptoms which may include fever, diarrhea, FAILURE TO THRIVE, enlargement of lymph glands and a tendency to repeated infections such as PNEUMONIA and oral CANDIDIASIS (thrush). Serious BACTERIAL infections and infections with unusual organisms may occur. Progressive neurological problems with DEVELOPMENTAL DELAY are common. More rarely, seizures, symptoms of ENCEPHALITIS such as drowsiness, blurring of vision, neck

stiffness and eventually COMA may occur.

Some children have BRUISING, ANEMIA, HEPATITIS or unusual skin conditions. In contrast to adults with HIV infection, cancer is uncommon.

▣ ACTION A correct diagnosis is essential, and this is difficult because no group of symptoms is diagnostic. Some children born to infected mothers will not develop the disease even though blood tests in the first few months of life may suggest infection. There are a variety of blood tests available but results can be difficult to interpret, especially in the first year of life. Expert advice should be sought in the interpretation of any test performed.

If a mother knows she is infected with HIV, she must consider whether breast feeding is advisable. Recent studies suggest that the risk of transmission through breast milk is small compared to the risk of transmitting HIV to the baby during the pregnancy and delivery.

If a child is proven to be infected, it seems likely, judging from current evidence, that he will eventually develop AIDS, although information is still limited because of the small numbers known to be infected. Early diagnosis and prompt treatment of the infections may prolong survival. Close follow-up is important. Get medical advice at the first sign of any symptoms that suggest infection.

▣ TREATMENT There is no drug known for AIDS. Clinical trials of antiviral agents such as AZT (zidovudine) are under way, but their long-term effectiveness is still not known. Some centers give intravenous gamma globulin regularly;

others do not. Regular therapy with cotrimoxazole can decrease episodes of lung infection with *Pneumocystis carinu*, a common problem in these children. All children infected with HIV should receive routine immunizations against diphtheria-tetanus-pertussis (DTP), the killed or inactivated polio vaccine and the *Hemophilus influenzae* b conjugate vaccine. Since measles may be very severe in HIV-infected children, measles, mumps and *Rubella* vaccine should also be given. Influenza virus vaccine and pneumococcal vaccine are also recommended.

There is no evidence that infected children can pass AIDS on to their playmates, and they should not be segregated.

Counselling and social support for families is crucially important, especially as the condition progresses.

▓ OUTLOOK is worst if symptoms develop early after infection.

▓ PREVENTION HIV infection is primarily a sexually transmitted disease. Adolexcents should be educated about the risk factors, including unprotected sexual intercourse, and intravenous drug abuse with shared needles or syringes. Sexual contact with multiple partners or a partner who has had multiple partners increases the risk of infection. Regular and proper use of condoms can decrease the risk of sexual transmission.

ALBINISM
A group of rare inherited conditions in which there is absence of the pigment melanin in the skin.

▓ SYMPTOMS Affected children have white hair, pale skin, blue-grey irises in the eyes, and abnormal vision, also due to lack of pigment.

▓ CAUSE The inheritance of generalized albinism is recessive, which means that in a family, one in four children will be affected when both parents are carriers (see *INHERITED DISORDERS*). A separate form of albinism affecting only the eyes is inherited as an X-linked recessive, where some boys are affected and girls are carriers.

▓ ACTION Children with this relatively rare condition should be under the care of a specialist. There is no effective treatment, but sunblocking creams will help protect the skin from burning.

ALCOHOL ABUSE
Alcohol is the socially acceptable drug. Studies indicate that 35-40 percent of adolescents in school in the United States are 'moderate drinkers' and more than 25 percent have a drinking problem. Regular and even occasional drinking carries health risks for children and adolescents. Adolescents often abuse more than one drug, further complicating the problem.

▓ SYMPTOMS of acute intoxication are the same as for adults, only more pronounced and often quicker to take effect. The smaller the body size, the smaller the volume of alcohol taken that causes acute intoxification. You will probably notice uninhibited behavior, excitement and a loss of judgement; poor coordination, slurred speech, unsteadiness and a proneness to sustain accidents; and finally drowsiness, that eventually leads to coma, with the danger of death by inhalation of vomitus. Regular alcohol abuse may be associated with falling school grades, a change in friends and activities, withdrawal from the family, truancy and blackouts. If an alcohol-dependent stops drinking, withdrawal symptoms may include tremors and hallucinations.

■ PREVENTION Alcohol is a powerful drug with the potential to disrupt life and permanently damage health, especially in the young. Many schools have programs aimed at preventing drinking and driving, a lethal combination for many adolescents. Adolescents need to learn having a good time socially does *not* require alcohol.

Effective education, from as early as primary school age, is the key to developing a responsible attitude towards alcohol, but it is often negated by parents and other adults setting a poor example.

■ ACTION for acute intoxication: Make sure the child does not harm himself accidentally. If you think he has drunk a great deal get medical advice. Alcohol in large amounts can be poisonous.

■ ACTION for suspected alcohol abuse:The treatment of DRUG ABUSE, alcohol or other has three phases: acute (withdrawal), short-term (motivation to change) and long-term (rehabilitation). Adolescent alcoholism is best dealt with by an experienced team. Ask your doctor and school guidance councillor for advice and help if you suspect alcohol abuse. Do *not* delay or ignore the problem. It rarely cures itself.

■ TREATMENT If the child (or teenager) is unconscious, place him in the RECOVERY POSITION. It is safe to let the youngster sleep off mild intoxication at home; hospitals occasionally admit children and adolescents recovering from exceptionally heavy bouts of drinking.

ALCOHOL IN PREGNANCY

Alcohol is best avoided, especially in early pregnancy. The occasional alcoholic drink, in the later stages of pregnancy, is probably harmless. Increasing amounts, for example the equivalent of two to three ounces of hard liquor each day, may cause LOW BIRTH WEIGHT, PREMATURITY and CONGENITAL ABNORMALITIES. A higher intake, that is, over five ounces each day, may lead to fetal alcohol syndrome: severely stunted growth, mental retardation and abnormal facial features.

ALLERGY

An abnormal reaction by the body to certain molecules, most commonly proteins (ANTIGENS or allergens), that are foreign or extraneous to the body. The reaction results in the production of ANTIBODIES. Subsequent exposure to the same antigen results in an antibody-antigen interaction that stimulates a cascade or chain of biochemical steps resulting in the allergic reaction.

■ INCIDENCE Allergy in one form or another affects 15-20 per cent of the population, and is an important cause of chronic illness in childhood. It tends to run in families, but not every member of the family will have the same type of allergy, or be allergic to the same things. Many experts believe that prolonged breastfeeding offers some protection against the development of some allergies.

■ CAUSES Common antigens include the house dust mite, pollens, animal hair, feathers, drugs, food and insect stings. A child may be allergic to one or many allergens.

■ SYMPTOMS depend on the type of allergy, and include ECZEMA, HAY FEVER, ASTHMA, CONJUNCTIVITIS, URTICARIA and FOOD ALLERGY.

Anaphylaxis is a severe allergic reaction consisting of difficulty with breathing, a drop in BLOOD PRESSURE and a rapid heart rate. It is a rare but life-threatening condition.

■ ACTION 1 Try to determine what causes the allergy by careful questioning and detailed observation of the child:

– Determine the places where allergy is worst; indoors, out in the cold air, in a grassy meadow.
– Decide whether contact with animals has any effect.
– If allergy is seasonal, a pollen could be the cause.
– Skin and BLOOD TESTS may help establish the likely causes of allergy (see below). 2 As far as possible avoid situations that you recognize may provoke an allergic reaction in your child:
– Exposure to house dust mite may be reduced by keeping the area where your child sleeps and plays as dust-free as possible. For example, plush toys and bedroom wall to wall carpeting are difficult to keep dust-free, and should be avoided.
– Pollen is difficult to avoid completely, but it is usually possible to take some avoiding action and thereby keep exposure to a minimum.
– Pets' hair can only be avoided by not having pets in the house and avoiding homes of friends who do have pets. Finding new homes for pets is, of course, easier said than done. You should seek your doctor's advice as to the likelihood of helping

the allergic symptoms by removing the pet.
– Foods can be excluded from the diet: reintroduction may clarify whether or not they cause symptoms. This should only be done with medical supervision: long-term dietary manipulation can in extreme situations lead to serious nutritional deficiencies.

■ TESTS Blood tests may show whether allergy is likely to be present. If the allergies are serious, your family doctor may refer your child to an allergist for skin testing. Minute amounts of common allergens are introduced superficially into the skin. Redness and itching develop if the child is allergic to an allergen. Otherwise these tests are without discomfort. While skin testing can be helpful, it cannot always identify every allergen. Food allergies are not easily identified by any current laboratory or clinical test.

■ TREATMENT
– Antihistamines may relieve the symptoms but may cause drowsiness, which in turn may affect school performance. Some recently developed antihistamines have a less sedative effect.
– Anti-allergic drugs such as sodium cromoglycate block the release of histamine. They are used to prevent allergic reactions, but are not useful in treating symptoms once they have developed.
– Steroids are often effective against allergies, and when used locally (for example as a nasal spray or inhaler), have very few side-effects. When taken by mouth, particularly in high doses and for a prolonged course, the side-effects can be severe.
More details of treatment are given under specific allergies.
– Desensitization (termed hyposen-

sitization by some physicians) involves giving frequent repeated injections into the skin of small doses of the allergen. The dose is gradually increased until the child no longer reacts to the allergen.

Unfortunately desensitization is not a particularly successful form of treatment because a child is often allergic to more than one substance; any protective effect wears off in time; desensitization can only be performed for certain specific allergies, such as house dust mite, pollen, animal hair and insect venom.

There is also a small risk of a severe allergic reaction to a desensitizing injection.

▓ LONG-TERM MANAGEMENT Allergies cannot be cured. Avoidance remains the best treatment, but when this is impossible, use the smallest dose of medication possible to relieve symptoms. If the allergy is seasonal, it may not be necessary to continue treatment all year round.

▓ OUTLOOK Allergic reactions tend to become less frequent and less troublesome as a child grows up. About a third of allergic children are free of their symptoms by the time they reach adulthood.

ALOPECIA
Hair loss or baldness from any cause.

▓ CAUSES Many babies are of course born bald, or become bald soon after birth, before their proper hair grows. This is normal. The hair growth cycle follows a pattern of 80-90 percent of the scalp hair actively growing, 5 percent in transition phase and 10-15 percent in a resting phase. Fifty to 100 hairs are normally shed per day. This normal

pattern may be disrupted by severe illness, fever, emotional stress, and so on. Increased shedding and thinning of the hair is noted two to three months after the stress, followed by regrowth of the hair.

Abnormal hair loss can also be caused by: friction – babies who habitually lie on their backs often develop a bald patch; pulling – either as a habit (known in older children as trichotillomania), or as a result of over-vigorous use of curlers or tight braiding; drugs – used for treating CANCERS; and INFECTION of the scalp by RINGWORM (a fungus). Additionally, hair loss may occur locally (*alopecia areata*) or more generally (*alopecia universalis*) for no identifiable reason.

▓ SYMPTOMS Ringworm infection of the scalp is likely to cause itching and irregular or oval patches with broken-off hairs; otherwise a completely bald patch is the only sign of alopecia.

▓ ACTION Unless the cause is obvious, such as the baby's bald patch, or using curlers that are too tight, a doctor's opinion should be sought.

▓ TREATMENT Infections of the scalp are treated by oral antifungal agents prescribed by your doctor. *Alopecia areata* may resolve without therapy. Steroid creams and/or injections and other medications are occasionally recommended. Trichotillomania may be a sign of underlying emotional problems, for which psychological treatment may be necessary. It may, however, simply be a habit that will stop after suitable explanation and reassurance to both child and parents.

▓ OUTLOOK Hair lost during anticancer drug treatment always grows again as does hair loss associated with severe stress. *Alopecia areata* usually resolves in time; *alopecia universalis* is generally permanent.

AMNIOCENTESIS
See *PRENATAL DIAGNOSIS*.

ANAL FISSURE
Straining to pass a hard stool can sometimes result in a small, superficial skin tear at the outer edge of the anus. If the child continues to be CONSTIPATED, the skin may stretch uncomfortably again and again and healing may be delayed. There may be slight bleeding at the site, and the child may become distressed before, during or after having a bowel movement.

◼ **ACTION** Avoid constipation. Inspect the skin around the anus if your child cries when passing a stool, or if there is blood on the toilet paper when his bottom is wiped. If there is a tear, make sure the area is kept clean and apply a soothing antiseptic cream two or three times daily. It will probably heal within three or four days. If it does not heal rapidly, get medical advice.

ANAPHYLACTIC SHOCK
The most severe form of ALLERGY, which occurs within a few minutes of contact with a drug or other substance (see *BITES AND STINGS*) to which the child is allergic. An itchy URTICARIAL rash appears suddenly; there is rapid severe swelling of the face and neck with severe breathing difficulty, a hoarse voice, rapid pulse and SHOCK. This is a medical emergency. Call an ambulance immediately. If you have an adrenalin kit, use it. An adrenalin injection can be life-saving. If you have none, start resuscitation if the child has stopped breathing. Prevention is best:

avoid drugs and substances to which your child is allergic.

ANEMIA
Deficiency of hemoglobin, the blood's oxygen carrier. This can occur because there are too few red blood cells; or because they don't contain enough hemoglobin, even though they are present in adequate numbers. There are several different types of anemia, described below.

◼ CAUSES Deficiency of the substances necessary to make hemoglobin gives rise to IRON-DEFICIENCY ANEMIA.

Excessive destruction of red blood cells produces the HEMOLYTIC ANEMIAS, which include THALASSEMIA, SICKLE-CELL ANEMIA and GLUCOSE 6-PHOSPHATE DEHYDROGENASE (G6PD) DEFICIENCY. A further form of the disease, APLASTIC ANEMIA, is caused by under-production of red blood cells in the bone marrow. Finally, many chronic illnesses, kidney disease, INFECTION, and LEUKEMIA can all cause anemia.

◼ SYMPTOMS are similar, regardless of the cause. If the problem develops gradually, the symptoms may go unnoticed until the anemia is severe.
– Tiredness, listlessness, loss of APPETITE and irritability are typical. The child may seem pale: his lips and the membranes of the lower eyelids are the best places to look. Don't suspect anemia just because a child's cheeks are pale: this often happens, regardless of whether or not a child is anemic.
– The child may be breathless when he runs about, and generally disinclined to exert himself.
– Other symptoms occur, specific to the different types of anemia: see the

separate entries.
– Severe anemia can cause HEART FAILURE.

■ ACTION If you suspect anemia, get medical advice. A BLOOD TEST is necessary to confirm the diagnosis, and the doctor may suggest treatment with iron since iron deficiency is the most common cause of anemia in childhood. See *IRON-DE-FICIENCY ANEMIA.*

Further action will depend on the type of anemia.

■ TREATMENT depends on the cause. BLOOD TRANSFUSION may be necessary if the anemia is severe. Heart failure is treated in the usual way.

■ OUTLOOK depends on the cause of the anemia; see the separate entries.

ANESTHETICS
Drugs used to make surgical operations painless. General anesthetics act on the brain to make the patient unconscious. Local anesthetics block the action of the nerve supply to a specific part of the body with no effect on consciousness.

General anesthetics may be given singly or in combination by inhalation, injection into a vein or, occasionally, as an enema. Prior to a general anesthetic for major surgery, it is common to give premedication with a tranquillizer. A drug is also given to dry secretions and protect the heart from excessive slowing of reflexes in response to procedures such as passing an airway (endotracheal tube) through the larynx. Today's general anesthetic typically causes light unconsciousness but, combined with an analgesic, is also a powerful painkiller. The child wakes up quickly afterwards, and although

ANAESTHETICS

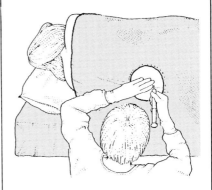

Inserting an epidural anesthetic.

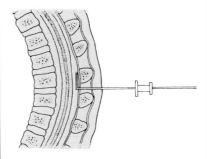

some children feel 'hung over', most do not. This type of anesthetic is also suitable for procedures such as CESARIAN SECTION, in which case sedative effects on the baby are to be avoided.

Some general anesthetics, however, cause deep unconsciousness and are used for major or prolonged operations.

It is common to give a paralyzing drug as part of the anesthetic in order to relax muscles. This allows, for example, a tube to be passed through the larynx, and it generally makes the surgery easier to do. Meanwhile breathing is controlled by artificial ventilation.

Local anesthetics are solutions given by injection. This may be given into the tissue under the skin where a local operation is to be carried out, or it may be given into the tissue round the nerve supply (nerve block), for example at the base of a toe for ingrowing toe-nail surgery, to the nerve going to a tooth or to nerves in the neck that supply the arm and hand.

Anesthetizing the lower half of the body to perform some abdominal, pelvic and leg operations (including CESARIAN SECTION) is done by spinal anesthesia whereby an anesthetic solution is injected into the spinal canal of the lower back. This form of anesthesia is used only in older children and adolescents.

Prepare your child for a general anesthetic by explaining that it will simply put him to sleep for a while. See also *HOSPITALIZATION.* Many hospitals have outpatient visiting programs to acquaint children with the anesthetic and surgical equipment prior to a scheduled operation. Parents should always be encouraged to stay with their child while an anesthetic is taking effect and while it wears off. The child may not be allowed to drink any fluids after waking, but if he is, give him only a few sips. If he does not feel sick, let him drink more.

The range of modern anesthetics means that there is a safe one for almost everybody, although there remains a remote but real risk of a child reacting adversely – and gravely. However, children are at no greater risk than adults. So *before* your child goes into the hospital, make a note of everything you can about former illnesses, previous anesthetics, any drugs the child is taking, especially steroids; any allergies, especially to adhesive tape or bandages; and any problems with anesthetics experienced by a member of the family. See *HEATSTROKE.* Ensure that the doctor in charge of your child at the hospital has all this information.

ANOREXIA NERVOSA

Self-induced weight loss by voluntary starvation, which usually occurs in teenage girls, and is sometimes associated with BULIMIA. Younger girls and some boys may also be affected. Once the child or adolescent is 10 to 15 percent below the average weight for height, there is cause for concern.

■ CAUSES There is no single definite cause, but the illness often occurs in intelligent, hard-working and intense young people. An interest in health foods, diet and fitness may antedate the weight loss. A VIRAL illness with loss of appetite is sometimes seem at the start. Uncertainty about growing up and independence may also be present, though perhaps not admitted to by the individual.

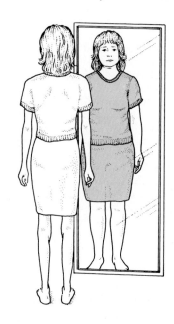

How these diverse features come together to cause this potentially serious illness is not understood.

■ SYMPTOMS Dieting that does not stop when a reasonable weight is reached; dieting that is disguised; increased interest in food (sometimes with eating binges), sometimes with the preparation of elaborate meals for others; a sudden increase in exercise, even after dramatic weight loss. Menstrual periods stop, but the girl does not seem concerned. After serious weight loss, fingers and toes may become cold and redened with cracked skin, and downy hair grows on the trunk; the girl prefers to wear bulky clothing even in summer. Sometimes self-induced vomiting or the use of laxatives are added to promote or sustain weight loss (this last is characteristic of bulimia). An important sign is the girl's denial that dieting or weight loss is a problem; often she is reluctant to seek help and is convinced that she is overweight despite her thinness.

■ ACTION If your daughter is looking thinner than usual (especially if not overweight before) check her weight yourself. Take her to the doctor to be examined, and to establish what her weight should be. Discuss her diet with her; make sure it is a balanced one; and find out what is happening with her periods. The best chance of controlling or containing the disease probably lies in early recognition, with sympathetic attention to the girl's diet, weight and underlying worries.

If your daughter continues to diet, don't ignore it even if she makes excuses. Check her weight weekly and go back to the doctor; defiance of parental authority is part of the illness, which is harder to treat

the longer it goes on.

If weight loss continues, you will probably be referred to a specialist in adolescent medicine, clinical psychologist or psychiatrist. You may be seen by the consultant with your child (see *FAMILY THERAPY*) or separately, and hospital admission may be necessary.

■ OUTLOOK Most recover, but some have lasting difficulties in maintaining normal weight. Extreme cases are rare, but include a risk to life. Early detection and treatment improve outlook.

ANTIBIOTICS

These are drugs used to treat bacterial INFECTIONS. Most antibiotics work by killing the BACTERIA; others prevent the bacteria from multiplying and rely on the body's defenses to eliminate them. Many infections suffered by children (COMMON COLD, throat infections and DIARRHEA) are mainly caused by VIRUSES that are not destroyed by antibiotics. Occasionally, a bacterial infection may follow a viral infection, extending the illness; it may then be appropriate to treat the child with antibiotics.

It is sometimes difficult to be certain whether an illness is the result of a viral or a bacterial infection. It is then reasonable for your doctor to prescribe antibiotics, particularly when an infection fails to improve over several days. Certain illnesses are particularly likely to be caused by bacteria, as in the case of URINARY TRACT INFECTION.

■ ADMINISTRATION Antibiotics may be given by mouth in liquid, capsule or tablet form. The daily dose depends on the age and weight of the child, the type of antibiotic and the focus of the infection, and needs to be given at the intervals specified on the medication bottle's label. The duration of treatment will depend on the nature of the infection and the pattern of the child's recovery. Antibiotics are most often prescribed for courses of treatment between five and ten days duration. It is important to complete the prescribed course. If an antibiotic is not given regularly, or stopped too soon, the remaining bacteria may reestablish the infection.

The particular antibiotic prescribed will be determined by the type of bacteria likely or known to be causing the infection. If the child has received an antibiotic recently, the bacteria may have become resistant to its action; the doctor may then take account of this probability and choose to prescribe an alternative antibiotic. Other factors affecting the choice of antibiotic are the type and severity of the illness and the presence of other disorders, notably liver or kidney disease. Antibiotics may be changed during an illness if the child does not show signs of responding to therapy, or if laboratory tests show that the bacteria causing the illness are not destroyed or inhibited in their multiplication by the antibiotic.

If a child is very ill, antibiotics may be given intravenously or by intramuscular injection, and more than one antibiotic may be given.

■ SIDE-EFFECTS of antibiotics vary with the type of drug used, but are usually mild and may include nausea, diarrhea and loss of appetite. Uncommonly an ALLERGIC REACTION may occur, usually in the form of a skin rash. Your doctor should be notified at once and is may or may not advise stopping the drug. Abrupt onset of wheezing and difficulty breathing may on very rare occasions follow the injection or in-

gestion of an antibiotic; this is an emergency, and you should take your child at once to the nearest hospital emergency room.

■ OVER-USE OF ANTIBIOTICS Parents have reason to be anxious about the excessive use of antibiotics. Side-effects may occur, and bacteria resistant to the commonly used antibiotics may proliferate.

If it is not clear whether an infection is due to a virus or a bacterium, and if your child is not very ill, it is better to wait and see. If there is no improvement within a few days, it is more likely to be a bacterial infection and the use of antibiotics may be necessary. If your doctor uses antibiotics frequently, discuss with him or her the possibility of reviewing the situation after a few days, rather than using antibiotics immediately.

ANTIBODY
A protein produced by white blood cells when they come into contact with an ANTIGEN. The antibody's function is to help protect against INFECTION and other foreign agents. Antibodies react with the antigens and help to destroy them.

A BLOOD TEST can detect antibodies that often remain in the blood. This can help in the diagnosis of some current or previous infection, and also helps in the diagnosis of ALLERGY. However, antibody tests are not available for all viruses.

Antibodies that remain in the blood are a marker for IMMUNITY to that particular infection in most cases.

ANTIGEN
A chemical, usually a protein, that the body perceives as foreign. Proteins on VIRUSES, BACTERIA, FUNGI and PARA-

SITES may constitute antigens, as may components of environmental particles such as pollen, animal hair and the house dust mite. An antigen may stimulate the body's IMMUNE system to produce an ANTIBODY and/or sensitized cells, specifically matched to the antigen's chemical make-up. This is part of the body's defense responses serving to eliminate foreign substances.

An organ that is transplanted into an individual also contains proteins that the body recognizes as foreign (see *TRANSPLANTED ORGAN*). Proteins that are eaten are digested into smaller particles called amino-acids before they are absorbed into the body. As the amino-acids are normally present in the circulation, they do not of themselves result in an allergic reaction.

ANTISOCIAL BEHAVIOR
See *AGGRESSION, STEALING, SCHOOL ATTENDANCE PROBLEMS, TANTRUMS, LIES AND FIBS*.

ANTIVIRAL DRUGS
These are drugs used to treat some viral infections. Most antiviral agents prevent the multiplication and/or uptake and release of virus particles by cells. The body's own defenses are an important component of successful antiviral therapy.

The available antiviral agents are active against only a few viruses. For most viral infections, such as the common cold, there are no useful antiviral agents.

■ ADMINISTRATION Each antiviral agent has its optimal route of administration depending on the drug, the site and the severity of the infection and the age of the patient.

Oral, intravenous and inhaled routes are used. The length of treatment depends upon the virus and the severity of illness. Many of these drugs are only used in hospitalized patients.

■ SIDE-EFFECTS of antiviral agents vary from minimal to very serious depending upon the drug, the dose and the patient. Ask your doctor.

ANUS, IMPERFORATE
This is a CONGENITAL ABNORMALITY that is detectable at birth – part of the routine examination of a new-born baby is to carefully examine the anus.

■ TREATMENT If the anus is obstructed, MECONIUM and subsequent bowel contents cannot be evacuated. The obstruction varies from a relatively thin diaphragm of tissue to complete lack of development of the anus. The complexity of the operation to open up the passage depends upon the abnormality.

ANXIETY
A normal experience of all children (and adults), both useful and necessary for keeping children safe (see *SEPARATION ANXIETY*) and making them think ahead, plan and prepare carefully, especially for new, strange or risky situations.

It is highly unusual for a child to be able to describe feelings of anxiety before adolescence. It is much more common to show behavior that results from anxiety: being clinging or whining; having a tummy ache or headache, which keeps the child at home and close to his parents; finding reasons not to stay quietly in his own bed at night time; being nervous or tearful before a test at school. From an early age some children are by nature more cautious and fearful than others, and will show this type of behavior more readily.

Anxiety only becomes a problem if it seems to be extreme and prevents the child from developing new skills and acquiring independence, or if the symptoms, or coping with them, occupy a major portion of your or your child's attention.

▇ IN PRE-SCHOOL CHILDREN

Separation anxiety is an important way for a child to show anxiety at this age. He may also show excessive SHYNESS about speaking in front of strangers. Routines and rituals are often developed as a way of coping with anxiety: many bedtime routines are an example of coping with anxiety about being left alone in the dark and your child may insist on your following these routines precisely; see *SLEEP PROB-LEMS*. Such routines are only a problem if there are too many of them, if the time they take is excessive or increasing (see *PHO-BIAS*). Sometimes a timid or anxious child may have tremendous temper tantrums or outbursts either unpredictably, or if the routines are not followed. These should be handled in the same way as any other TANTRUM.

▇ IN SCHOOL AGE CHILDREN

Many of the symptoms of anxiety in younger children may persist into the school years, in particular routines, rituals and phobias. They may also reappear at times of stress or upheaval for the child, or for the family generally. At this age, anxiety is often shown by the child through physical symptoms such as head-aches and stomach-aches. You will be able to observe how these symp-toms arise in relation to stressful events, rather than as specific phys-ical illnesses.

▇ ACTION Explain to the child that you know of his worries, talk about them and plan how he is going to prepare for the test, outing, new class or night away from home. Your confidence that he can cope after some preparation will help him more than will avoiding the issue, which will raise his anxiety even more when the next challenging occasion comes along.

Most children can quickly learn to cope with new or anxiety-provoking situations. If your child is not doing this, think about whether you may be contributing to his anxiety. Is this an area in which you had problems as a child and could this be making you uncertain about how he will cope? Do you feel worried because, for any reason, your child has special difficulties? If so, remember that your child will be less anxious if you have confidence in him; and if you have talked to him about how he will handle each situation, how he will behave and who will help him if problems do arise.

With this type of preparation, he will gradually master his anxiety. Praise him for his achievements and remind him of what he will gain from overcoming his anxiety. Always break preparatory talks down into small, manageable steps. If your child continues to be exces-sively anxious despite such prepara-tion, look for help in the setting where the problem arises.

APGAR SCORE

A rating to assess a baby's condition immediately after birth. It is named after the famous American pediatri-cian, Dr Virginia Apgar, who devised the scoring system. The doctor present at the delivery grades the baby accord-ing to heart rate, breathing, color, re-sponse to stimulation and muscle tone.

Zero, one or two points are given for each component of the score, amounting to a maximum of ten for the whole observation. The results indicate whether the baby at one minute and at five minutes of age has adapted to birth adequately. Scores of less than five indicate severe central nervous system depression and the need for vigorous ressussitation.

APLASTIC ANEMIA

A rare form of ANEMIA, caused by faulty production of blood cells in the bone marrow.

■ CAUSES It can be present at birth, or caused by certain drugs and environmental toxins. Sometimes it occurs later in life for no apparent reason.

■ SYMPTOMS are the same as for any anemia. Sometimes only the production of red blood cells is affected, but if insufficient white cells and platelets are produced, INFECTION and bleeding may also result.

■ TESTS BLOOD TESTS will reveal a decreased number of red blood cells.

■ TREATMENT BLOOD TRANSFUSIONS will relieve the acute problem. White blood cell and platelet transfusions may also be needed, and infection must be treated as soon as it occurs. Steroids may stimulate the bone marrow to function better. Bone marrow transplantation may be a possibility for long-term treatment. When this is not possible, immune-suppressing drugs may be used.

■ OUTLOOK depends on the cause. Severe anemia, bleeding and infections are hazards.

APPENDICITIS

Inflammation of the appendix, a small finger-like outgrowth of the intestine situated at the junction of the small and large bowel. The cause(s) of appendicitis are unknown; there is no known way of preventing the condition.

■ SYMPTOMS Appendicitis usually begins with ABDOMINAL PAIN of fairly recent onset, often affecting the central area round the navel first, spreading to the right lower part of the abdomen within a few hours. The child is usually unable to sit up comfortably or walk upright. Children of any age may be affected; it is rare, however, in infants and toddlers. There may also be vomiting, fever, diarrhea or constipation. See

APPENDICITIS

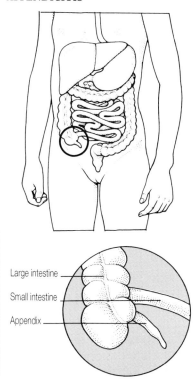

Large intestine

Small intestine

Appendix

PERITONITIS for details.

■ TREATMENT is surgical: an operation is performed to find and remove the inflamed appendix.

■ OUTLOOK Expect the child to be in the hospital for several days, after which recovery should be complete, with no complications. If the appendix has ruptured, a more prolonged hospital stay with intravenous ANTIBIOTICS may be required.

■ COMMENT Chronic or recurring appendicitis probably do not exist – see *ABDOMINAL PAIN*.

APPETITE

Children vary enormously in their eating habits. Parents are often gratified by a child who eats vigorously, and worried by a child who 'picks at his food' (see *FEEDING PROBLEMS*). If the child is growing normally (see *GROWTH PATTERNS*), loss of appetite is usually no cause for concern; but in a child who normally eats well, it may be an early sign of illness.

■ CAUSES (Apart from normal variation among children): hot weather; any feverish illness; sore throat or mouth (see *TONSILLITIS*); unhappiness or emotional upset (see *ANOREXIA NERVOSA*; excitement; as a concomitant of a variety of serious diseases.

Increased appetite may accompany or precede a growth spurt or recovery from illness.

■ ACTION and INVESTIGATIONS If you are worried by your child's sudden loss of appetite, especially if this is accompanied by weight loss, you should contact your doctor. BLOOD, stool or URINE TESTS may also be suggested, to check for a variety of possible causative conditions.

■ TREATMENT None is usually needed, unless investigations reveal a significant underlying cause.

■ SELF-MANAGEMENT Try to make sure your child drinks at least as much as usual, even if he refuses to eat. Dehydration causes more problems in the short term than lack of food.

■ OUTLOOK Changes in appetite usually accompany another disturbance. The eating pattern should settle as the underlying problem is resolved.

ARRHYTHMIAS

Abnormalities in the heartbeat, which may be too fast, too slow, or irregular. Rare in childhood.

■ CAUSES Slow heart rates (bradycardia) can be present at birth as in congenital complete heart block. In older children, it is found occasionally in association with heart-disease.

Rapid heart rates (tachycardia) can occur in infancy and childhood as a result of abnormalities of the conduction network of the heart muscles. Sudden 'attacks' of very rapid beating of the heart (as in supra-ventricular tachycardia) can present as pallor, fainting or panic episodes. Tachycardia can also occur in association with other HEART-DISEASE or generalized illnesses with fever or shock.

Some degree of irregularity of the heart rate is normal in childhood, as when the heart rate quickens and slows with breathing in and out (sinus arrhythmia). Greater irregularities occur in association with heart-disease.

▓ SYMPTOMS Slow heart rates may cause no symptoms, or there may be some tiredness or shortness of breath. Occasionally dizziness or fainting can occur.

Rapid heart rates can cause breathlessness, palpitations (sensation of the heart beating rapidly), dizziness and occasionally chest pain.

Irregular heart rate can give a sensation of a heart missing a beat, or palpitations.

▓ TESTS Principally, an ECG (ELECTROCARDIOGRAM). Sometimes a continuous tracing of the heart rhythm over 24 hours is recorded. Other tests may be done if heart-disease is suspected.

▓ TREATMENT Slow heart rates don't usually need treatment in childhood. If fainting is due to a slow heart rate (it is usually a manifestation of a complex irregularity of the heart rhythm), and requires the placement of a pacemaker. However, fainting is a rare problem in childhood and a pacemaker is rarely necessary.

Rapid heart rates are usually treated with drugs such as digoxin. Irregular heart rates may not need treatment unless they cause symptoms, in which case treatment is usually with drugs.

▓ OUTLOOK will depend on whether there is associated heart-disease. In isolation, the outlook is normally good.

ARTHRITIS

Pain and swelling of one or more of the joints. There are many causes including: certain BACTERIAL and VIRAL INFECTIONS; injury (in children with HEMOPHILIA, minor injury can cause severe bleeding into a joint); JUVENILE RHEUMATOID ARTHRITIS.

There are also many other rare causes of arthritis such as LEUKEMIA, LYMPHOMA, SICKLE-CELL ANEMIA, HENOCH-SCHONLEIN PURPURA, IDIOPATHIC THROMBOCYTOPENIC PURPURA and RHEUMATIC FEVER.

▓ SYMPTOMS Pain in the affected joint or joints, may become worse with movement; swelling of the joint, which also makes movement difficult; the joint often feels hot, and there may be redness of the skin over the joint.

These symptoms may develop slowly or rapidly, depending on the cause of the arthritis. Many children have vague pains in their joints, particularly if they have a viral infection. This is not arthritis and is usually not serious if it does not persist.

▓ ACTION Any painful, swollen joint should be examined by a doctor: infection in a joint can rapidly cause severe damage, so don't delay in seeking help.

▓ TESTS are often necessary to make the diagnosis. These include BLOOD TESTS and X-RAYS. Special types of SCANS are now also being used in some centers.

Occasionally it is necessary to insert a needle into the joint, to remove some fluid in order to test for infection. This is done under a local or general anesthetic – not in itself painful.

▓ TREATMENT Analgesics are usually necessary for the pain, acetamenophen being the usual first choice. With juvenile rheumatoid arthritis, aspirin or other anti-inflammatory drugs may be prescribed. These may have serious side-effects (see *REYE SYN-DROME*), especially in high doses. Never give more than the recommended dose without consulting your doctor.

Rest is usually necessary at the onset of a painful episode. Special splints can be used to rest joints in a position in which they do not become stiff, and can function well.

Bedclothes can press uncomfortably on painful knees and ankles: a 'cradle' to raise the bedclothes can help.

If there is a bacterial infection in a joint, aspiration of the joint or an operation may be necessary to remove the infected fluid. ANTIBIOTICS are also used to treat the infection; see also *OSTEOMYELITIS*.

Joint injury usually improves if the child gets some rest. If there has been bleeding into the joint, it may be necessary to remove the blood with a needle.

Once the inflammation has been treated, the child should exercise to prevent joints from becoming stiff and muscles from becoming weak. The first exercise sessions are best done under the supervision of a doctor or a physiotherapist. Exercises can be made into games so that they don't bore the child.

■ OUTLOOK depends on the cause.

ASPERGER SYNDROME

A rare condition in which children relate to others in an unusual way from early in life, thought to be similar to a mild form of AUTISM. The child's gestures and speech are odd, he has problems in making friends, behaves in an uninhibited way in social situations, is noticeably clumsy, and has peculiar and engrossing interests for a child of his age. Most grow up to lead normal, if eccentric, lives.

ASPHYXIA

See *EMERGENCY RESUSCITATION*.

ASPIRIN

See *REYE SYNDROME, POISONING*.

ASTHMA

The commonest cause of recurrent cough and wheezing in childhood. The disorder frequently runs in families. Its physiology is explained in detail below and in the illustration.

■ INCIDENCE One in ten individuals display features of asthma during childhood, but the majority grow out of it by adulthood.

■ CAUSES There is no one cause of asthma. Many factors predispose and interact, prominent among which are ALLERGIES to the ANTIGENS of the house dust mite and molds (found in all homes), animal fur and grass pollen. Allergy to specific foods such as milk may in rare instances precipitate asthmatic symptoms. Attacks of asthma may be provoked in susceptible children by the COMMON COLD or other VIRAL INFECTIONS, exercise, by changes in atmosphere and air temperature, and by exposure to air pollutants, such as tobacco smoke.

■ SYMPTOMS are intermittent: children with asthma rarely have symptoms all the time. Wheezing (a continuous or 'musical' sound heard when the child breathes) is caused by three changes in the airways of the lungs: spasm of the muscular walls (bronchospasm), swelling of the inner lining, and excess mucus (sticky fluid) production. These three reactions lead to a narrowing

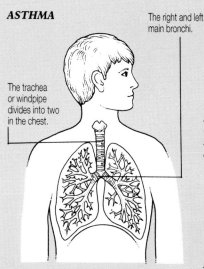

ASTHMA

The trachea or windpipe divides into two in the chest.

The right and left main bronchi.

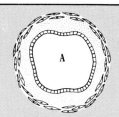

A shows a (much magnified) normal bronchiole. The muscle is the thin band of surrounding cells. (Actual width may be as little as one mm.)

Right and left bronchi divide into ever-smaller bronchi, and then into bronchioles.

In B the muscle has contracted, narrowing the air passage. In a really bad attack, the bronchiole may be blocked completely.

of the air passages, which prevents air getting into and out of the lung and causes breathlessness and wheezing. Most asthma is mild to moderate, interfering little with a child's normal life. Occasionally it can be severe, requiring emergency hospital attention.

Not all children have an audible wheeze: some only have a cough at night, or after exercise.

■ ACTION 1 If you suspect your child has asthma, get medical advice. It is not wise to use home remedies or other people's medicines for children who might have asthma. 2 If a child is known to have asthma, give the medicine or inhaler exactly as prescribed by your doctor for use in an attack. Do not give more medicine than prescribed, since this may cause problems. See *INHALERS, NEBULIZING MASKS.*

■ GET MEDICAL ADVICE if an attack of asthma gets progressively worse, or does not improve with the treatment.

■ RUSH THE CHILD TO HOSPITAL if he becomes cyanosed (blue) around the lips or unable to speak. Err on the side of caution: it is easy to underestimate the severity of an attack.

■ TESTS Lung function can be tested simply with a PEAK FLOW METER. In this way the effectiveness of treatment can be objectively assessed. Skin tests may occasionally be used to identify specific allergies.

■ TREATMENT Drugs are used either to prevent bronchospasm or to treat attacks when they have started. Salbutamol and other bronchodilators, given by mouth as sugar-free syrup or by inhalation in various forms, are the most commonly used drugs for treating attacks. Aminophylline and theophylline given as pills, capsules or syrups, may also be used as part of routine treatment. Inhaled sodium cromoglycate and steroids such as beclomethasone are used as preventive drugs. Steroids such as prednisone are given for severe attacks, and very occasionally on a long-term basis to prevent attacks if a child has severe asthma.

Desensitization to house dust mite, molds and pollen through a series of injections over long periods of time may be attempted – see *ALLERGY*.

■ LONG-TERM MANAGEMENT Avoid those things that you know will bring on an attack, such as playing with a friend's dog, or rolling in a hay field in the summer months, or going out in very cold weather in the winter months. If your doctor has advised long-term treatment, such as inhaled sodium cromoglycate or steroid twice daily, encourage your child to use it consistently as directed. Many children can master an inhaler by four years of age, with suitable training.

■ OUTLOOK Most children with asthma lead normal lives. For those who suffer from severe asthma, it should still be exceptional to miss time from school if a treatment plan is well devised and carried out. Occasionally severe attacks do occur which require expert and urgent hospital management.

ASTIGMATISM
A normal eyeball is more or less spherical, like a ball. If it is flattened – say into more the shape of an egg – astigmatism may result. The shape of the eye is important because it plays a part in the eye's ability, as a lens, to bend rays of light, focusing them on the retina at the back of the eye. Imperfect curvature of the eyeball means distortion of the image formed on the retina. The strain incurred in attempting to focus may cause HEADACHES and/or PAIN IN THE EYE.

If your child complains of difficulty seeing with or without headaches, an EYE TEST should be performed and EYE GLASSES prescribed if necessary.

ATHLETE'S FOOT (RINGWORM OF THE FEET)
The common name for a FUNGAL INFECTION of the skin on the feet. Uncommon in young children, but common in adolescents.

■ SYMPTOMS Common features include a fine blistery or scaly rash with itching and soreness, uncomfortable red fissures between the toes, and the unpleasant 'cheesy' smell of the feet. Slight redness extending over the surface of the feet may be noticed.

■ CAUSE Fungal infection: the fungus is quite contagious and may be transmitted simply by going barefoot at swimming pools or in shower rooms.

■ TREATMENT Topical application of an antifungal cream such as miconazole, tolnaftate, or a similar preparation. Such creams are available at the drugstore without a doctor's prescription. Proper foot hygiene is important and includes keeping the feet dry and cool; gentle cleaning; thorough drying between the toes; and use of a foot powder. Recurrence is common. Occasionally, for severe infections, your doctor may prescribe oral antifungal drugs.

ATRIAL SEPTAL DEFECT
See *CONGENITAL HEART-DISEASE.*

AUDIOMETRY
A test of hearing, performed either to detect DEAFNESS (partial or profound), or to measure the type and degree of hearing loss. There are several types of audiometers used, depending on the age of the child and the purpose of the test. Some require the child to respond to a particular sound, made through headphones (pure-tone audiometry), while others measure the elasticity of the child's eardrum by applying slight pressure through a tiny tube inserted into the ear canal (impedance audiometry). Younger children are tested in a special room, where specific sounds are made under controlled circumstances and the child's behavior is observed (free-field audiometry).

In every case, the results need to be interpreted by a specialist, and often to be repeated before the exact degree of deafness can be determined.
See also *DEAFNESS.*

AUTISTIC CHILD
A condition or group of conditions in which a child does not communicate normally in speech, gesture or eye contact.

■ CAUSES The 'cause' of autism is unknown. There is no evidence that parents cause autism through improper childrearing.

■ INCIDENCE One child in 3,000.

■ SYMPTOMS Some autistic children may appear normal for the first year of life. Others seem different from birth. Features of autism, which usually become evident before the child is five, are:

– He does not relate to others normally: he shows little interest in adults, in physical affection or eye contact; he is solitary and unresponsive; he seems to be in a world of his own, although sometimes enjoying rough and tumble play.
– He plays in an absorbed, repetitive and non-creative way. He may, for example, repeatedly spin the wheels of a toy car, but never use it as a car.
– His speech development is delayed and his speech is abnormal when he does learn to speak. He may repeat what is said to him (echolalia). Sometimes the child never learns to speak at all.
– His development is delayed in many areas: most autistic children have serious LEARNING DISORDERS.

■ ACTION Take your child to your doctor. The diagnosis is never clear at first. It may require months or years of observation and consultation with a pediatrician, developmental specialist and/or child psychiatrist to reach a firm conclusion.

■ TREATMENT There is no specific treatment for autism. Many children can be helped by special nursery or school programs, often with speech therapy. Psychologists may assist with therapy for behavior difficulties. Some authorities employ 'holding' as a technique, aiming to assist the autistic child with making physical contact. Other authorities feel this is of doubtful value. Discuss the treatment alternatives with your doctor.

■ OUTLOOK There is a range of disorders covered by the term autism. At its mildest, the outlook for an independent adult life is good; at its most severe, the prospect is currently one of substantial handicap.

B

BABY-BOTTLE CARIES
See *BOTTLE FEEDING*.

BACTERIA
Micro-organisms that occur ubiquitously in our environment. Most bacteria do not cause disease and some are beneficial, such as those found in the digestive tract. Recognition of the type of bacteria causing an INFECTION is important, since specific ANTIBIOTICS are only effective against certain bacteria but not others. Bacterial identification is achieved by taking a sample of material from the infected source (skin, urine, blood) and placing it in a culture medium to grow the bacteria.

■ TREATMENT of bacterial infection is usually with antibiotics. The choice of antibiotic can be assisted by testing the bacteria grown in the culture against a range of antibiotics to see which is best.

Certain types of bacteria are more likely than others to cause particular infections, such as TONSILLITIS or URINARY TRACT INFECTION. It is therefore sometimes possible to predict which antibiotic is likely to be effective before the test results are available.

BALANITIS
A BACTERIAL INFECTION of the foreskin and tip of the penis that may be seen in uncircumcised babies. It causes redness and swelling, and often a slight discharge. A baby may cry when passing urine. You should keep the penis clean by bathing with warm water, change his diapers regularly and get medical advice. Your doctor may take a sample of the exudate for laboratory examination, and he may prescribe ANTIBIOTICS.

Once treated, your baby should have no further problems. Boys with recurrent balanitis may develop PHIMOSIS and require CIRCUMCISION.

BALDNESS
See *ALOPECIA*.

BCG
See *TUBERCULOSIS*.

BEDWETTING (ENURESIS)
Control of the bladder is acquired through physiological maturation – until this stage is complete a child cannot be dry at night. The age at which children become dry varies: some are dry at two years; by the age of five about 15 percent still wet the bed; by the age of ten this drops to about 5 percent of boys and 2 or 3 percent of girls.

No consistent differences in depth of sleep, bladder capacity or other physical factors have been found between children of the same age who are wet or dry at night. Bedwetting tends to run in families. Some children suddenly stop bedwetting, while for others the process is more gradual. The first sign may be the occasional dry or drier bed. See also *TOILET TRAINING*.

If a child is worried about wetting the bed – and many are once they are in the early school years – or if wetting the bed elicits negative responses from parents, this can add a degree of anxiety to the problem. It is extremely rare for a child to wet his bed deliberately. Bedwetting can be a sign of emotional stress, particularly in children who have been completely dry in the past, and a small number of children wet the bed because of URINARY TRACT INFECTIONS or other medical conditions, such as DIABETES.

▨ ACTION Minimize the inconvenience as far as possible by using a plastic sheet that can be easily washed between the mattress and bed sheets. Minimize the effect of bedwetting on your child by a matter-of-fact reaction to the problem: wash or bathe your child and change his bed sheet each morning (if at all possible) to avoid unpleasant odor of urine. Handle the subject tactfully so that the child is not teased or embarrassed because of it.

▨ GET MEDICAL ADVICE if bedwetting becomes a real problem for either you or your child, or if your child starts bedwetting again after a long period of dryness for no obvious reason.

▨ TREATMENT is rarely suggested if a child is under six years of age. Your doctor will advise how best to deal with the problem. The most effective preventive measure, if used correctly, is the enuretic alarm – a

safe wire mesh placed between the bed and plastic sheets connected to a buzzer that should wake the child when the bed sheet first becomes damp. Other preventive measures include rewards for dry nights and exercises to improve bladder control. There is little evidence of the effectiveness of drugs such as imipramine.

BEHAVIORAL DISORDERS
See *AGGRESSION, STEALING, SCHOOL ATTENDANCE PROBLEMS, TANTRUMS, BEHAVIORAL TREATMENTS*.

BEHAVIORAL TREATMENTS
Commonly used to help parents of children with behavioral problems. Such treatments fall broadly into two categories.

▨ BEHAVIOR MODIFICATION aims to teach new skills and to increase sociable behavior. It is based on the theory that anyone is likely to repeat behavior if it is rewarding. This applies to good and to bad behavior: a child who has a temper tantrum in a supermarket and is given candy to keep quiet is likely to do so again. The psychologist would say that the child has learned that having a tantrum is a way of getting what he wants. Likewise, most parents praise children who oblige during toilet training. Genuine praise and attention are potent rewards and the toddler feels encouraged to try to do the same thing again.

In behavior modification, rewards are used to build up desirable behavior; bad behavior is ignored and not rewarded in any way. Rewards in this context are not the same as bribes. Bribing means telling the child that he will only get something if he does what is wanted. A true reward is given straight after the good behavior and not discussed beforehand.

Ignoring bad behavior, though effective, can be difficult to achieve in practise. 'Time out' is perhaps the main technique: it usually involves simply putting the child alone somewhere for a few minutes to defuse the situation. Another approach is to encourage good behavior which is incompatible with bad behavior. For instance, the child who helps his mother with the shopping will not need to lie screaming on the floor to get attention.

Consistency is essential to behavior modification. The parent should try to reward good behavior and deal with bad behavior in the same way every time so that it is clear what is expected of the child. Consistency between parents is crucial. If one parent responds with attention for bad behavior, this undermines the whole process.

Parents use these techniques in day-to-day dealings with their children without having to be guided by professionals. When problems get out of hand a psychologist may sometimes have a role to play. He or she will probably help to devise a systematic and practical way of applying behavior modification. *COGNITIVE BEHAVIOR THERAPY* is a treatment for ANXIETY, PHOBIAS and mood problems. The individual works with a therapist to define and understand the thoughts, feelings and behavior involved in difficult situations. Relaxation, gradual practice and confidence-building exercises are used to overcome problems. Because children understand comparatively little about their difficulties, these methods are generally not useful before adolescence unless parents are actively involved.

BEREAVEMENT

Losing a close relative or friend may be just as upsetting for a child as for an adult, and sometimes more so. The situation is complicated by the child's level of understanding of death, how close the child felt to the person (which is not the same as how much time they have spent together), and how the loss affects other people in the family. Many of the reactions children show after a death are similar to those shown when facing DIVORCE, which is a kind of bereavement for many children.

◼ BELOW SEVEN YEARS, children don't understand the finality of death. Often, they may not appear particularly upset if told a relative or friend has died. This does not mean they did not care about the person. They may ask practical questions about where the person is, what they are doing or eating. It is best to answer these questions in as straightforward a way as you can. They will often be asked several times as the child tries to make sense of what has happened, and of your being upset. If a child had felt angry or in some way upset with the person who died, he may feel responsible for the death. It is important to reassure the child that wishing that someone will die or be hurt does not make it happen. Some children may continue to behave normally; others will show SEPARATION ANXIETY, or have problems with eating, sleeping or behaving properly, especially if the child's routine has had to be disturbed. In this younger age group, children may take anything you say literally: if, for instance, you say "Grandad died because he was sick" your child may think that if you (or he) is sick, you (or he) will die too. So you will need to explain that death is a natural process. Reassure the child that his memories about the dead person will always remain and that you will be happy to talk about this any time. The exact form of explanation will depend on your child's age and level of development, and on your personal and religious beliefs. Your library is a good source of books that may help you and your child discuss these difficult issues.

▓ ABOVE SEVEN YEARS children understand better that death is final and irreversible. Still, they may, like younger children, feel in some way responsible for what has happened if they had angry or negative feelings about the person. They are likely to show that they are upset in more obvious ways, but this may fluctuate frequently in the period after the bereavement: children's moods don't always last as long as adult's, but this does not mean they do not care.

Older children may well show changes in their pattern of eating, sleeping, concentrating and behavior at home or at school; and such changes may last for several months. This will depend on the child's feelings and on how much the bereavement has affected everyone in the family, and its routines.

▓ ACTION If your child is still showing a marked change in any aspect of his life a few weeks after the event, check how he is functioning at school. If this confirms your worries, see your doctor and discuss the possibility of help from a clinical psychologist or child psychiatrist. Many reactions to bereavement can be quickly helped by a few sessions

in which to talk about the feelings involved. This can prevent long-term DEPRESSION, or problems at school.

BILIARY ATRESIA
A CONGENITAL obstruction of the bile duct system that leads from the liver to the intestine. It is a rare condition without an identified cause, although VIRAL INFECTION during pregnancy has been considered.

Obstruction may be partial or complete. Bile is prevented from draining from the liver, which becomes inflamed.

▓ SYMPTOMS Persistent JAUNDICE with pale BOWEL MOVEMENTS lacking the usual brown pigment. The abdomen may be distended by an enlarged liver, and there may be associated CONGENITAL ABNORMALITIES.

▓ ACTION Jaundice lasting longer than one week in a full-term baby, or two weeks in a premature baby (born at or before 37 weeks), should be investigated, although jaundice caused by biliary atresia tends to occur later than other types of jaundice that affect new-born babies.

▓ INVESTIGATIONS BLOOD TEST checks on liver functions and ULTRASOUND SCANS of the upper abdomen will help to make the diagnosis.

▓ TREATMENT The diagnosis must be made early (within two months) for surgery, which connects the liver directly to the small intestine, to be successful.

A diet of easily digestible fats will be necessary. The child will be given extra VITAMINS, particularly vitamins D and E and minerals, for example iron and zinc.

■ COMPLICATIONS BACTERIAL IN-FECTION may affect the liver, causing a high FEVER and a worsening of the jaundice. ANTIBIOTICS may be needed. Biliary cirrhosis may develop (see *CIRRHOSIS*). Failure to take vitamin supplements may lead to RICKETS or neurological disorders.

■ OUTLOOK The life span in untreated biliary atresia is less than two years. The results of surgery are variable and there are complications, but children with this problem can survive into adult life. While liver transplantation can cure the problem, this is an expensive procedure hampered by a very limited supply of organ donors, and requires lifelong immunosuppressive therapy after the transplant. Thus it is not an option for many children with biliary atresia.

BIRTH ASPHYXIA
Lack of oxygen at birth. Before birth, the baby receives oxygen via the placenta. If this supply falls below a certain level there will be signs of FETAL DISTRESS during labor and the baby may have to be delivered swiftly. After birth, he may have a low APGAR SCORE.

■ CAUSES are usually uncertain. Factors that increase the risk of birth asphyxia include prolonged pregnancy (more than 42 weeks), extreme PREMATURITY, MULTIPLE PREGNANCY, HYPERTENSION (as in toxemia of pregnancy), and the separation of the placenta from the uterus.

■ PREVENTION Prenatal care identifies problems in pregnancy. Monitoring during labor reveals whether a baby is showing signs of FETAL DISTRESS. If asphyxia is anticipated,

BIRTH ASPHYXIA

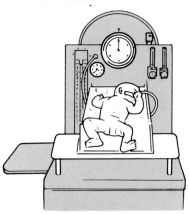

Oxygen provided by mechanical ventilator in hospital intensive care unit.

then qualified medical staff may expedite rapid delivery and should be present at the birth.

■ TREATMENT is resuscitation. Most babies are given oxygen from either a face mask or a breathing tube placed into the trachea (wind pipe). Babies with severe asphyxia may subsequently need INTENSIVE CARE.

■ OUTLOOK Three to four minutes after resuscitation, most babies are pink and active; such babies will not usually develop long-term problems. A very small minority are severely asphyxiated, and may develop some degree of handicap or CEREBRAL PALSY.

BIRTH INJURIES
Injuries to the baby during DELIVERY. They may result in damage to the bones, nerves or skin.

■ BONES Fractures are rare, affecting less than 1 percent of babies.

They are often associated with difficult births, breech deliveries and large birth weight. The majority are fractures of the clavicle (collar bone), often only noticed when a hard lump or callus develops on the bone after a few days. No treatment is necessary. Fractures of the bones of the legs and arms are usually recognized immediately. The baby usually does not move the fractured limb. Treatment is simple splinting; the fracture normally heals quickly and without deformity. Fractures of the skull bones usually follow difficult deliveries during which FORCEPS are used. Such fractures are usually minor, give no symptoms and need no treatment.

■ NERVES Injuries to the nerves are rare. However, during delivery the nerves in the neck known as the brachial plexus may be stretched and cause three types of injury. Erb's palsy is the most common and affects the nerves supplying the upper arm muscles. The arm hangs loosly at the baby's side and is turned inwards. Klumpke's paralysis is rare. It affects the nerves to the hand so that it looks like a claw. Very rarely there is a combination of both types of injury in which the whole arm is affected. Sometimes the nerve to the eye is damaged, resulting in a droopy eyelid and small pupil.

The nerve supplying the face may be damaged by FORCEPS, causing the side of the mouth to droop. Recovery is usually complete but takes a few days: until then, extra care may be needed with feeding.

■ SKIN After a forceps delivery, the baby's face may have minor scratches or bruises. After a breech delivery the baby's bottom and genitalia may be bruised for 24 to 48 hours. Birth pressure on the head during normal deliveries may result in CAPUT or CEPHALOHEMATOMA.

BIRTH, PROBLEMS OF
See *AGPAR SCORE, BIRTH ASPHYXIA, BIRTH INJURIES, BIRTHMARKS.*

BIRTHMARKS
A general term for various skin abnormalities apparent at or soon after birth.

■ SYMPTOMS Birthmarks are either red, due to abnormal blood vessels in the skin, or dark, due to skin pigment (melanin).

There are two main types of red birthmarks: the strawberry hemangioma, which is a raised swelling resembling a strawberry; and the port wine stain, which is flat. The strawberry hemangioma is not always visible at birth, but soon appears and enlarges for up to age 18 months. From the age of about three years, it begins to shrink and disappear; and most have disappeared (leaving a fine papery non-pigmented area of skin) by six years of age. They tend to develop on the face or upper trunk, and very occasionally become large and disfiguring.

Port wine stains do not disappear. They may be present on any part of the body, most notably the face or neck, and can be extensive and disfiguring. There is a risk with port wine stains on the face and scalp of associated abnormality of the blood vessels within the brain (Sturge-Weber syndrome). Such children should at some stage be assessed by a child neurologist.

Pigmented birthmarks are less common than ordinary MOLES, which develop in later childhood. They are usually small and light to dark brown in color; rarely a 'bathing trunk' nevus is present, which covers a large segment of the trunk.

Many babies born to parents of African, Asian and Mediterranean origin have blue areas of pigmentation in one or more areas over their backs and buttocks. These are known as 'Mongolian spots'. They become less evident with age. It is important not to confuse them with bruises resulting from trauma (see *CHILD ABUSE*).

■ ACTION Since by definition a birthmark will be noticed at or soon after birth, advice will usually be available from a doctor at that time. However, in the case of cosmetically worrisome marks, you may wish to discuss with your doctor whether a dermatologist's or plastic surgeon's opinion would be helpful.

■ TREATMENT Strawberry hemangioma: treatment is rarely needed and may lead to scarring. Port wine stains can be covered by cosmetic or masking creams. Laser beam treatment has proven effective is some cases. Pigmented birthmarks need no treatment if small, but extensive ones may be removed surgically.

■ LONG-TERM MANAGEMENT Children with permanent unsightly birthmarks of the face may be helped by cosmetic counsellors, whose services are available at most plastic surgery clinics. Ask your plastic surgeon for advice on where to buy such cosmetics. Occasionally additional psychological support is indicated.

■ SELF-HELP Treat the birthmark in a matter-of-fact way; don't discuss it casually with others within earshot of the child. A word to the school teaching staff may be helpful.

■ OUTLOOK Strawberry nevi disappear in four to six years. The port wine stains do not, but advances in plastic surgical techniques (including the use of lasers) offer reasonably good cosmetic results.

BITES AND STINGS

Animal bites can be especially dangerous to children – see RABIES.

■ SYMPTOMS The bites of mosquitoes and other blood-sucking insects are trivial, but to children often excessively irritating. The reaction is caused by ALLERGY to the saliva of the insect, injected before it starts sucking blood. This results in an itchy lump, similar to URTICARIA.

Bee and wasp venoms contain poison which damages blood vessels, causing swelling and pain. Individuals who have been stung by wasps or bees can develop an allergy to the venom, leading to far worse reactions on subsequent stinging, the most severe form being ANAPHYLACTIC SHOCK. When a bee stings, it leaves behind a tiny barbed rod (stinger) which should be gently removed with tweezers. A wasp's stinger is retractable, so can be used repeatedly; it is also likely to carry the germs of TETANUS.

Snake bites can be serious and even fatal if the venom is poisonous (see *SNAKE BITES AND VENOM DISEASES*).

Jelly fish stings See the separate entry.

■ ACTION *Mosquito and other bites*: common-sense precautions, such as protective clothing at dusk and insect-repellents can help. However, these measures are never 100 percent effective.

Bites themselves can be relieved by an antihistamine taken orally.

Bites can become infected through being scratched, and may then need an antiseptic cream.

Bee and wasp stings: acetamenophen reduces pain; reassurance that the sting will not cause serious damage may be just as important. If an allergic reaction develops, or if the child is known to be allergic to bee or wasp stings, immediate treatment with adrenalin should be given. Adrenalin kits are available as pre-prepared adrenalin in a syringe with an attached needle for injection. These should be carried by all individuals allergic to bee and wasp stings on advice from their doctor.

Desensitization with a series of injections is often prescribed for severely allergic individuals.

■ OUTLOOK Allergy to bee and wasp stings is potentially fatal: children who have reacted badly to stings should be seen by a specialist for advice on further treatment. Avoiding contact with bees or wasps is essential. Your doctor can advise you on how this can best be done.

BLACK EYE
BRUISING of the tissues around the eyeball usually resulting from the direct impact of a blow. A black eye, if spontaneous, may reflect an underlying disease such as a bleeding disorder, but this rarely occurs. Normally, after injury, despite the dramatic swelling and vivid color of the bruise, healing relatively quickly: the blue-black turns to yellow-green and the discoloration usually fades in two weeks. No treatment is called for, unless there is pain around the eye after the injury, in which case it can be relieved with acetamenophen and an ice-pack.

BLACK-OUT
See *FAINTING, EPILEPSY, CONVULSIONS, GRAND MAL SEIZURE.*

BLEPHARITIS
A generalized inflammation of the skin of the eyelid margins. The lid margins look red, swollen and feel sore and itchy. It may result from an infection of the eyelids (see also *CONJUNCTIVITIS*), allergy or both. It also occurs in children who have a tendency to greasy skin (seborrhoic dermatitis, CRADLE CAP).

■ TREATMENT is to keep the eyelids from becoming crusted (in infants this may require bathing the lids with clean cotton balls and warm water) and, as far as possible, dissuading the child from rubbing his eyes.
  If the lids become unusually inflamed an infection may have developed. You should then get medical advice. Your doctor may prescribe an ANTIBIOTIC ointment.

BLINDNESS
In developed countries, typically one in 2,500 children are registered as blind or partially blind.

■ CAUSES These include: CONGENITAL ABNORMALITY of the eye; CONGENITAL INFECTION; CATARACTS; damage to the optic nerve, which carries the impulse for sight to the brain; damage to the area of the brain that deals with vision (see HYDROCEPHALUS and CEREBRAL PALSY); retinoblastoma (see *TUMOR OF THE EYE*).

■ SYMPTOMS Suspect a problem if your baby takes no visual interest in objects when a few weeks old. He may have obvious STRABISMUS, or his eyes might wobble from side to side (nystagmus) when trying to look at something.

■ ACTION If you suspect any problem with a child's sight, you must of course contact your doctor. If a problem is noted the child will be referred to an eye specialist (opthalmologist) for assessment including EYE TESTS. The opthalmologist may well ask about any family history of blindness or eye problems.

■ TREATMENT The major goal of treatment is to maximize and preserve whatever vision is present and then to help the child and family adapt to this problem. Cataracts can be treated by surgery. Unfortunately, complete or partial blindness due to most other causes cannot be cured, or even improved upon.

■ SELF-HELP Babies with impaired vision need extra stimulation of the other senses to encourage learning. Plenty of holding and touching are also essential to convey love and reassurance. Speech, noise (but not so that it startles), different textures and smells can all be used to enhance the baby's awareness of his environment.

When he begins to crawl, parents have to provide an extra-safe environment. See *ACCIDENTS IN THE HOME*. Don't despair about his co-ordination; it will improve with practice. Toys he can operate to produce a noisy response will help.

Mixing with other children and encouraging independence will improve his confidence in his own abilities. Some visually handicapped children can distinguish light and dark or see bright colors. Large, bright toys can encourage learning in these children.

Since visual cues are absent, talking to these children is especially important in building up communication skills.

Many communities have special nursery school and pre-school programs for the visually handicapped.

■ EDUCATION The decision about which school suits your child needs to be made with the help of professionals. Special schools may cater to the needs of visually handicapped children along with those who have other handicaps. Alternatively, a regular school with special attention and extra help may be appropriate. The decision often depends upon the seriousness of the visual problem, the presence of other disabilities, the types of schools available and the desires of the parents and child.

The classroom will need to be well illuminated. Tape recorders and typewriters or word processors can help overcome the inherent problems of reading and writing. Braille will probably be taught in the specialist school.

Adolescence is a difficult time of change with exaggerated demands on the youngster for identity and independence. Skills acquired at school and the possibility of further education help the transition to independence.

BLISTERS

Thin-walled, dome-shaped 'bubbles' on the skin containing clear fluid.

■ CAUSES There is usually a local cause: friction, BURNS or an insect BITE; blisters are rarely due to a generalized skin disease. A blistering rash is common following skin contact with POISON IVY, poison sumac or poison oak. Particular types of blisters (called vesicles) are characteristic of CHICKEN POX.

Grouped vesicles at the edge of the lip (COLD SORES) are due to herpes virus.

▩ ACTION Ordinary blisters, as from ill-fitting shoes, should be protected by a simple dressing. Avoid bursting them; this invites INFECTION. See *BURNS* for the treatment of these. Insect bites may result in irritating blisters. No treatment is needed, but an antihistamine cream can ease the itching.

▩ GET MEDICAL ADVICE if the blisters have no obvious cause, especially in a young baby, where they may be due to a serious infection of the skin, IMPETIGO, or may very rarely be the first pointer to rare and serious diseases such as neonatal herpes virus infection. OUTLOOK Depends on the cause. If in doubt, your doctor may refer your child to a dermatologist.

BLOOD GROUP INCOMPATIBILITY

When mother and baby have different blood groups, the baby having inherited the father's. Why this occurs is not fully understood.

The incompatibility (which is relatively uncommon) can cause problems when the baby's red blood cells cross the placenta into the mother's blood during pregnancy. If these cells are of a different group than the mother's, she is likely to produce ANTIBODIES against them. If antibodies are produced in sufficient quantities, they too can cross the placenta into the baby's blood circulation, and destroy the baby's red blood cells.

The result is usually mild ANEMIA and JAUNDICE in the baby during his first few days of life; there are usually no long-term problems if mild.

Blood group incompatibility, also known as ABO incompatibility, may occur during a first pregnancy, or during a subsequent one. See also *RHESUS INCOMPATIBILITY.*

BLOOD IN STOOLS
See *ANAL FISSURE, CONSTIPATION, ULCERATIVE COLITIS.*

BLOOD IN URINE
See *HEMATURIA.*

BLOOD PRESSURE

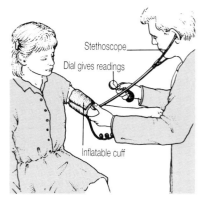

Stethoscope

Dial gives readings

Inflatable cuff

BLOOD PRESSURE

The pressure of the blood measured in the arteries. It is lower in a younger child and increases to adult levels during adolescence. Raised blood pressure is called hypertension.

To measure blood pressure, an inflatable cuff is placed around your child's upper arm and the pressure in the cuff increased until it is above the pressure in the artery. As the pressure in the cuff is released, the blood begins to flow in the artery and the resultant pulsation can be felt at the wrist or heard at the bend in the arm with a stethoscope. The procedure is not painful, but creates a sensation of pressure which a child may find alarming.

Blood pressure can be raised if a child is crying. It is necessary for the child to be lying or sitting quietly to obtain an accurate reading.

BLOOD SUGAR
See *DIABETES MELLITUS.*

BLOOD TESTS
There are many different types of blood tests: blood can be tested to:
– diagnose disease;
– determine the response to treatment;
– measure the function of organs such as the liver and kidneys;
– check the levels of certain drugs in the blood, to ensure that the correct doses are being given;
– assess blood loss after injury;
– match a patient's blood with that of a donor's if a transfusion is necessary.

Small amounts of blood can be taken by a finger prick, or heel prick in the case of young babies; larger amounts are taken from a vein with a needle. After the initial prick the procedure is not usually painful. You may prefer to hold your child yourself while this is done. Small children need to be held very still to complete the procedure as quickly as possible. Nurses are trained to do this, so either ask them to show you how best to hold your child, or let the nurse do it. If you become distressed this could further upset your child, so it is best if you can remain calm and reassuring. If you are anxious about it, discuss this with your doctor when the tests are suggested.

BLOOD TRANSFUSION
Giving blood taken from a healthy person to someone else who needs it. Likely reasons for blood transfusion include severe bleeding and ANEMIA.

New-born babies may require an EXCHANGE TRANFUSION.

Before blood can be given, a sample of blood must be taken from the child to identify his blood group. There are four main blood groups (A, B, AB and O). Only blood of a compatible group can be given. The child's blood must then be cross-matched with the blood which he will receive, to reduce the likelihood of an adverse reaction when the blood is given.

The amount of blood given depends on the weight of the child and the severity of the blood loss or anemia.

A blood transfusion is never given unless it is absolutely necessary: transfusions can result in complications including a rash or a feverish reaction. The HEPATITIS B VIRUS and AIDS virus have, in the past, been transmitted by blood transfusion. This is now unlikely in developed countries because all donated blood is screened to be sure these viruses are not present.

BLUE BABY
See *CONGENITAL HEART-DISEASE.*

BOILS
Superficial skin INFECTIONS caused by BACTERIA, commonly *Staphylococcus* or *Streptococcus* strains. Most children suffer the occasional boil, but if they recur frequently the doctor may suggest some tests to rule out an underlying problem. In older children and teenagers boils tend to occur in sweaty places – armpits, groins, buttocks.

■ TREATMENT Most small boils will clear up within a week – keep the area clean and dry if possible. If the area is very painful, red and angry, take the child to the doctor, who will decide whether it needs a small incision to let out the infected pus, or whether ANTIBIOTICS are necessary.

In babies and infants boils should not be neglected, especially if accompanied by indications of general illness.

BONDING

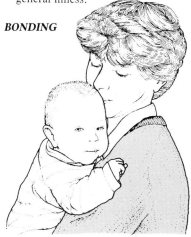

BONDING

Bonding describes the formation of the powerful emotional tie that develops between a parent and a new baby. The term refers generally to the mother-child relationship but a father also normally bonds with his baby.

Although parents are encouraged to hold their babies within moments of the birth to help develop feelings of attachment, those unable to do this (as, for example, following a CESARIAN SECTION or if the baby is sick at birth) can still bond successfully. Bonding is not necessarily an instant process and feelings of deep affection for and attachment to the baby develop over the first few weeks. How a parent reacts initially may depend on a number of factors such as the length of labor, previous experiences and personality.

Parents who are concerned about their feelings towards their new baby should consult their doctor. Mixed emotions are common and discussing your concerns will be helpful. Occasionally mothers who feel detached from their babies are in fact suffering from postpartum depression.

BONE TUMORS

Abnormal, undisciplined cell growth affecting the bone. Benign (noncancerous) bone tumors grow slowly, do not spread to other parts of the body and are not life threatening. Malignant tumors – bone cancers – can spread around the body, destroying normal body tissue and cause death.

■ SYMPTOMS usually start as a bone swelling. There may be pain and redness of the skin over the swelling. Occasionally there is weight loss or fever. Sometimes a FRACTURE can occur at the site of the tumor, because the tumor has weakened the bone.

■ ACTION Early diagnosis makes treatment more effective, especially of malignant (cancerous) tumors.

If your child has any unexplained swelling or pain over a bone, see your doctor.

■ TESTS are necessary to confirm the diagnosis. X-rays can show a tumor and whether it has spread. An X-ray of the chest is performed to see whether the cancer has spread to the lungs. A bone scan and sometimes a scan of the whole body will help in the diagnosis.

Biopsy is often necessary to find out what type of tumor is present, and what treatment is best. This may be done by aspirating a portion of the tumor through a needle or by cutting part of it out at a minor operation. BLOOD TESTS may also be done.

■ TREATMENT Surgical removal can cure most benign, and some malignant, tumors. The type and extent of the surgery varies. In some cases amputation may be necessary but this can sometimes be avoided by just removing the tumor and replacing the area with a bone graft or splint. The type and extent of the surgery depends upon the type of tumor and how far it has spread.

Radiotherapy (X-ray treatment) and anti-cancer (cytotoxic) drugs can halt the growth of malignant tumors. Treatments are steadily improving with the introduction of increasingly effective drugs.

The child will probably be looked after by an orthopedic surgeon, a pediatrician and a cancer specialist so that the different forms of treatment can be co-ordinated.

■ OUTLOOK with benign tumors is good and long-term problems are unlikely.

Survival rates of children suffering from malignant bone tumors are improving.

BOOSTER SHOT

This is a further dose of a vaccine after the initial IMMUNIZATION. It stimulates the body to produce more ANTIBODIES so that the child remains immune to that particular INFECTION.

BORNHOLM DISEASE

See CHEST PAIN.

BOTTLE FEEDING

Formula milks are made to have a nutritional content similar to breast milk. There are, however, important differences: formula milks do not contain the beneficial ANTIBODIES provided by breast milk. The protein used in formula milk is usually derived from cow's milk; soya bean protein is an alternative. Soya-based formulas are sometimes used for babies thought to have COW'S MILK ALLERGY.

There are many different types and brands of formula. However, for most babies a regular formula with added iron is satisfactory. Your doctor will advise you if you are in doubt as to which one to choose. There is normally no need to change the baby's formula until he progresses to baby and junior foods and regular cow's milk.

Bottle feeding offers a degree of convenience that may be necessary for some families, for example, mothers who must work fulltime. It also allows a father the opportunity to feed his baby. However, strict attention to hygiene in cleaning the bottle and nipple, and preparing the formula, is essential. This is especially true in tropical countries: if bottles cannot be properly cleaned, and if made-up formula milk stands around and becomes a breeding ground for BACTERIA, there is a serious risk of GASTROENTERITIS. Proper formula milk preparation is also essential since too dilute or too concentrated solutions can make your baby ill. Follow the package instructions carefully.

The recommended average intake for a 24-hour day is around 2, oz of formula for each pound of the baby's weight (150 ml per kilogram), this amount being spread over four to eight feedings. The amount taken and pattern of feeding is, of course, highly variable from baby to baby. Babies should not be left with the bottle propped in the crib: feeding should always be supervised because of the risk of vomiting and inhalation of the milk into the lungs. Older babies and toddlers should never be put to bed with a bottle of milk, formula or juice since this can lead to baby-bottle caries (decay of the front teeth). Advice on all these matters should be available from your doctor, who will also be able to weigh the baby to check for steady weight gain.

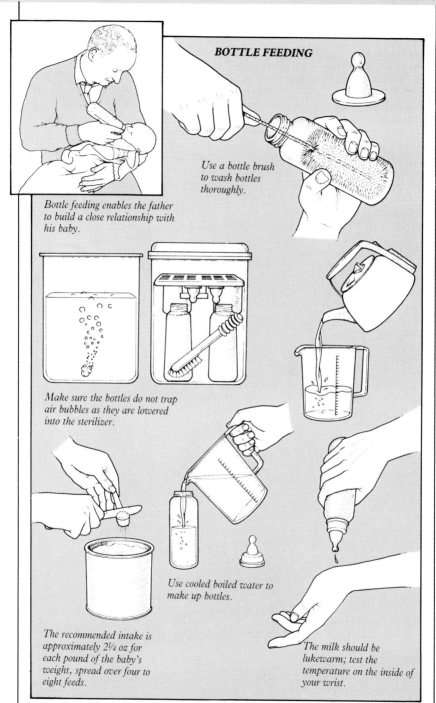

BOTTLE FEEDING

Bottle feeding enables the father to build a close relationship with his baby.

Use a bottle brush to wash bottles thoroughly.

Make sure the bottles do not trap air bubbles as they are lowered into the sterilizer.

Use cooled boiled water to make up bottles.

The recommended intake is approximately 2¼ oz for each pound of the baby's weight, spread over four to eight feeds.

The milk should be lukewarm; test the temperature on the inside of your wrist.

BOW LEGS

Normal in infants and young children. In older children, bow-leggedness can be due to RICKETS, OSTEOGENESIS IMPERFECTA or other very rare bone abnormalities.

■ SYMPTOMS are unlikely. You may notice that your child has bow legs, or this may be pointed out by a relative or friend.

■ ACTION If you are worried, get medical advice.

■ TREATMENT depends on the cause, but ordinarily no treatment is required.

BOW LEGS

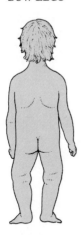

BOWEL MOVEMENTS

The sticky dark green substance passed by a new-born baby is known as MECONIUM. It is replaced within a few days by semi-solid bowel movement (stool) – golden-yellow in the breast-fed baby, and greenish-brown in the bottle-fed one. As the child begins to take baby foods, the stool changes again. The consistency and color vary with the diet and with the individual make-up of the baby's digestive system. Most babies have a bowel movement daily or every other day with no evidence of discomfort. Occasionally, particularly at a time of change from breast feeding to regular milk or formula, babies may become CONSTIPATED (strain and pass dry stools at irregular intervals). This can usually be managed by simply adding extra water or fruit juice to the diet. If this becomes a problem, get medical advice. See also *DIARRHEA, CONSTIPATION, BLEEDING* and *MALABSORPTION*.

BRAIN DAMAGE

Permanent harm to the brain as a result of illness or injury. Once nerve cells in the brain are destroyed, they can no longer grow or be replaced. Brain damage is a general term, and does not simply refer to problems arising at birth.

■ SYMPTOMS Effects of brain damage depend on the portion of the brain that is damaged. Damage to the front part of the brain (frontal lobe damage) causes disinhibition, lack of initiative and concentration, and loss of ability to plan or control movements. Damage to the back portions of the brain can lead to blindness; damage to the mid-portions may lead to loss of language; difficulties perceiving shapes and distance; loss of sensation and varying degrees of paralysis. EPILEPSY is a common consequence of brain damage.

■ CAUSES Trauma; infective illness (including viral ENCEPHALITIS, MENINGITIS); biochemical disturbance (lack of oxygen or glucose; inborn chemical disorders); POISONING (typically from lead or carbon monoxide); lack of blood supply (cardiac arrest); bleeding (SHOCK) or raised pressure within the brain itself (for example in HYDROCEPHALUS).

■ INVESTIGATIONS depend on the circumstances, but emergency medical help is required if brain damage is suspected following an accident or in an acute illness. See *HEAD INJURY, CEREBRAL PALSY, MENTAL HANDICAP.*

■ TREATMENT depends on the cause. If there is acute damage after injury, neurosurgery may reduce its effects. In acute illness, ANTIBIOTIC or biochemical treatment may help. In either case, life support in an INTENSIVE CARE unit is usually required, including respiratory support, intravenous fluid and control of pressure in the head. If damage is of long standing, treatment is with physiotherapy, occupational therapy and speech therapy whereby most bodily and everyday living functions are relearned.

■ OUTLOOK It does not necessarily follow that damage will lead to loss of function; although the damage is irreversible, related parts of the brain can sometimes compensate for these losses.

Most mentally handicapped children with symmetrical cerebral palsy have not suffered brain damage, but show the effects of abnormalities of brain development before birth.

BRAIN TUMORS

These result from abnormal growths of brain cells; they may be benign (slow growing and confined to one site), or malignant (rapid growing and capable of spreading to more than one site). They may be primary (derived from brain cells) or secondary (from another part of the body). After LEUKEMIA, brain tumours are the commonest of the childhood CANCERS.

Primary brain tumours may arise from the lining of the brain (meningioma), cranial nerves (neuromas), the pituitary gland (for example craniopharyngioma), choroid plexus (which secretes cerebro-spinal fluid), glial cells (glioma) or nerve cells. The commonest are gliomas.

■ SYMPTOMS include convulsions, and symptoms of raised pressure inside the head such as headache and vomiting (especially in the morning), deterioration in intellectual function, development of double vision STRABISMUS or loss of vision, loss of balance or change in behavior. Occasionally specific local effects of the tumor give rise to particular changes in body function, such as passing large amounts of very dilute urine, and developing enlarged breasts.

■ INVESTIGATION may include a brain scan, an electroencephalogram (EEG), and occasionally the injection of an X-ray opaque dye into the blood supply to the brain (angiogram).

■ TREATMENT depends on the site and nature of the tumor. Benign and malignant tumors can be removed surgically, either in part or totally. Surgical removal of malignant tumors is often combined with radiation (radiotherapy) and drugs (chemotherapy). If a tumor causes increased pressure inside the skull and cannot be removed, additional steps may be taken, such as the use of steroid drugs to reduce swelling of the surrounding brain, or the insertion of a shunt, a plastic tube that drains the high-pressure cerebro-spinal fluid into the abdomen.

■ OUTLOOK A few malignant brain tumors are cured; for the rest, treatment is aimed at securing quality rather than quantity of life. Survival rates are highly variable, from a few weeks to many years. A child with a brain tumor can usually lead a full and active life for a long time after appropriate treatment.

BREAST FEEDING

A natural way for a mother to feed her baby. The alternative is BOTTLE FEEDING, in which case the baby receives a substitute for the mother's breast milk of modified cow's milk or soya bean-based milk.

'Breast is best' is a slogan that symbolizes the return to fashion of breast feeding in many developed countries. There is evidence to suggest that breast-fed babies may suffer less from allergies. Breast feeding is also encouraged because of the intimate contact and BONDING it promotes between a mother and her baby. It is also, of course, much less expensive than bottle feeding.

■ ACTION 1 Put the baby to the breast as soon as possible after birth, and allow him to feed for as long and as frequently as he wishes in the first few days. In this way your milk production will be stimulated. The first milk is a clear fluid (colostrum), which is rich in protein and ANTI-BODIES and valuable for your baby; within three to four days milk flow will increase and the milk itself becomes more creamy. 2 Be patient. A healthy baby needs no other sustenance than colostrum and milk in the amounts naturally available, increasing over the first week after birth.

The majority of mothers comfortably establish breast feeding to their great satisfaction, and that of their baby.

Some mothers, especially with their first babies, need some expert assistance, particularly in ensuring that the baby is correctly positioned at the breast. This is especially so in the first week when the breasts become full and swollen.

Difficulties may arise from confused and conflicting advice. Discuss problems with your doctor. Avoid giving your baby bottled water or formula (unless specifically prescribed by a doctor): such supplements will reduce your baby's appetite, and hence the feeding stimulus to your milk production.

3 Breast care: A feeling of fullness of the breasts is normal in the first few days, as blood flow to the breast and milk production increase. If this becomes uncomfortable, or if your nipples feel sore when your baby is feeding, then ask for help from your doctor or a breast feeding league. Most of the discomfort associated with breast feeding is avoidable if the baby is correctly positioned at the breast and feeding on demand. 4 Good positioning is essential. The nipple and most of the pigmented area around it (areola) should go into the baby's mouth. This is best achieved by ensuring that your baby's mouth is wide open as he attaches to the breast. Allowing the baby to attach to the nipple alone will make you sore, and will not promote milk production and flow. 5 Don't let anyone worry you about the quantity of your milk supply. Your supply will naturally adjust to meet your baby's needs and demands. Let a 'hungry' baby feed often. Both breast-fed and bottle-fed babies need to have their weights checked routinely at the doctor's office or clinic to verify that growth is adequate.

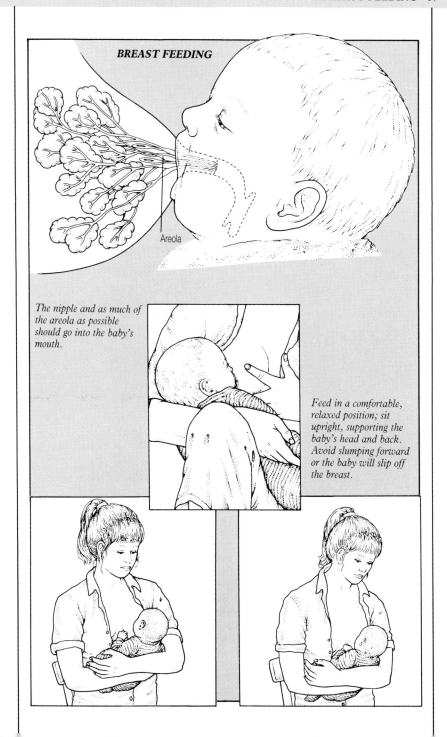

BREAST FEEDING

Areola

The nipple and as much of the areola as possible should go into the baby's mouth.

Feed in a comfortable, relaxed position; sit upright, supporting the baby's head and back. Avoid slumping forward or the baby will slip off the breast.

■ <u>OUTLOOK</u> The great majority of mothers succeed in smoothly establishing and maintaining breast feeding. If you are having difficulties, get expert advice. This may be availabe from your doctor or one of the voluntary expert groups that exist to support breast-feeding mothers.

BREATH-HOLDING ATTACKS
A child holds his breath or refuses to breathe: after a minute or so, his face turns blue and he may lose consciousness. Breathing then resumes normally. Breath-holding attacks may occur during TANTRUMS and are a common expression of anger in toddlers. They are alarming for parents to witness, but the child is not at risk: the body's natural response to shortage of oxygen is fainting, which allows normal breathing to return automatically. If your child has an attack, stay calm; there is no need to intervene, but make sure he is in a safe position. Don't try to stop the attack by startling, slapping or splashing him with water. This is not effective, does not discourage future attacks and only increases tension in your child and yourself.

BREATHLESSNESS (SHORTNESS OF BREATH)
Difficulty in breathing usually associated with *rapid*breathing.

■ <u>CAUSES</u> Breathlessness while exercising is of course normal; but if it occurs on minimal exertion, such as climbing a single flight of stairs, there could be something wrong.

ANXIETY can cause rapid or irregular breathing: see the entry on *OVER-BREATHING*.

ANEMIA, with its associated lack of oxygen in the blood, tends to make the lungs work extra hard to increase the amount of oxygen in the blood, and so causes breathlessness.

HEART-DISEASE, another cause, causes extra blood to accumulate in the lungs. This in turn makes them stiff, and breathing becomes difficult.

Several lung diseases, particularly ASTHMA, CYSTIC FIBROSIS and PNEUMONIA may result in rapid, labored breathing, as can obstruction to the upper airways, as in CROUP or when an object is inhaled (see *FOREIGN BODY ASPIRATION*). Onset with foreign body aspiration is usually sudden.

SHOCK is a rare cause of breathlessness. It may be due to bleeding, anaphylaxis or any other cause of a drop in BLOOD PRESSURE.

■ <u>ACTION</u> Try to determine whether your child is unusually breathless by comparing how he behaves when exercising moderately with a child of similar age. More than 50 breaths per minute is never normal, except just after strenuous exercise.

If a baby becomes breathless when feeding, get medical advice. Also get medical advice immediately if a child has a sudden onset of rapid breathing, particularly if it is noisy.

■ <u>TESTS</u> will depend on the suspected cause. They could include chest X-ray, BLOOD TESTS to look for anemia, and an ECG (ELECTROCARDIOGRAM). Sometimes lung-function tests are done by blowing into a special machine.

■ <u>TREATMENT</u> will depend on the cause. See the separate entries listed above.

■ <u>LONG-TERM MANAGEMENT</u> If your child has a CHRONIC ILLNESS causing breathlessness, find out from your doctor whether he needs to limit his activities. In almost all cases, a child can be allowed to determine his own limits. As long as he is allowed to rest when he becomes breathless, there is no danger.

BRONCHIECTASIS
A rare condition in which parts of the air passages (bronchi) in the lung become abnormally enlarged and infected.

■ CAUSES Bronchiectasis is occasionally inherited; more commonly, it is a complication of PNEUMONIA, severe attacks of MEASLES OR WHOOPING COUGH, or a result of CYSTIC FIBROSIS.

■ SYMPTOMS The child has a persistent cough, producing colored sputum with an offensive odor. If large portions of the lungs are affected, he will be breathless after exertion. With infection, the child is tired and often feverish.

■ ACTION Children with this condition require specialist treatment, and prescribed routines should be carefully followed.

■ INVESTIGATIONS A chest X-ray will usually be performed, but more specialized X-rays of the lungs and/or bronchoscopy (looking directly at the bronchi through a lighted tube) may also be needed to show exactly where and how widespread the trouble is. Pulmonary function (breathing) tests may be used to follow the course of the disease.

■ TREATMENT Physiotherapy is the key: a physiotherapist teaches parents how to help clear lung secretions from the chest. This may be re-

quired once to three times daily. ANTIBIOTICS are usually prescribed, in higher doses and for longer periods than for simple infections.

Occasionally, if the disease is not controlled by the other methods, the damaged portion of the lung is removed by surgery.

■ OUTLOOK One third of affected children recover completely, and more improve as they reach adolescence provided the disease is not due to cystic fibrosis.

BRONCHIOLITIS
A serious chest INFECTION of young children occurring in epidemics, mainly in winter months.

■ CAUSE The respiratory syncytial VIRUS (RSV) is the major cause.

■ PREVENTION Attempts to produce a vaccine against RSV are still in progress.

■ SYMPTOMS The baby, typically under 12 months, develops a cold, which rapidly progresses to involve the chest. Breathing becomes difficult and rapid, with a dry COUGH. Often, an older child in the family will recently have had a cold. There may be a FEVER, but it is not usually very high – say 100°F to 101°F. Some infants are at risk from more severe disease. These include those infants with CONGENITAL HEART-DISEASE and those with certain lung problems such as CYSTIC FIBROSIS.

■ ACTION Whenever a baby or young child develops rapid breathing and is in obvious distress, get urgent medical advice. Most children with bronchiolitis are treated in a hospital, but mild attacks can be managed at home.

■ TREATMENT Treatment is aimed at assisting the breathing with oxygen, and providing adequate fluids and nutrition, sometimes by tube feeding or intravenous fluids. For many infants hospitalized with bronchiolitis, this is sufficient. If severe respiratory difficulty occurs, however, assisted mechanical ventilation may be needed. Ribavirin, a drug active against RSV, can also be used in more serious cases. It is given by small particle aerosol in a tent or oxygen hood and appears to be helpful in some cases.

■ OUTLOOK Most cases recover after about one week. Some infants are left with a tendency to wheeze, which appears to be a form of ASTHMA.

■ LONG-TERM MANAGEMENT Most will recover completely. For those left with a persistent wheeze, treatment is the same as for asthma.

BRONCHITIS

An INFECTION of the bronchi, or air passages. In childhood, infection usually involves other parts of the respiratory tract as well.

■ CAUSES VIRUSES are normally responsible for bronchitis. Less commonly, BACTERIA may infect the bronchi, but this is more likely if the child already has a disease such as CYSTIC FIBROSIS or BRONCHIECTASIS.

■ SYMPTOMS The child has a COUGH and wheezes, and may have a FEVER. In severe cases, wheezing (see also ASTHMA), breathlessness and breathing difficulties may occur, which may interfere with drinking or feeding. ACTION. If your child is known to have asthma and you recognize his symptoms as a

BRONCHITIS

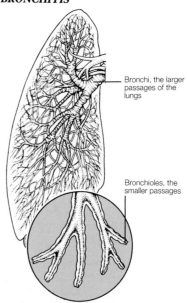

Bronchi, the larger passages of the lungs

Bronchioles, the smaller passages

Inflamed bronchioles: repeated infection damages their linings and makes them vulnerable to further infection.

mild asthma attack, then treat him accordingly; otherwise he should see the doctor. You should give acetamenophen to lower the child's temperature, and plenty of fluids to prevent dehydration.

■ TREATMENT ANTIBIOTICS may be prescribed, but are not required by most children. A drug such as salbutamol that dilates the bronchi often helps the child who is wheezing.
Recurrent 'bronchitis' usually turns out to be asthma, which may flare up with a cold. Your child may need treatment over a prolonged period of time (see ASTHMA). If there is no other problem, an attack of bronchitis usually clears up quickly and completely.

BRUISING

Bruising is caused by blood oozing from broken blood vessels into the tissues under the skin. During the week following the injury, the blood is denatured and reabsorbed by the tissues. This causes color changes in the skin. Bruised areas are not necessarily painful; the pain arises from injured nerve endings and from the inflammatory process that causes swelling of an injured area, which often disappears before the color changes do.

Toddlers and young children often get bruises on face, shins, forearms and back in the course of ordinary rough-and-tumble play. The patterns of bruising are characteristic, and the 'age' of the bruises corresponds with the timing of the injuries that have caused them.

Bruising that does not conform to these patterns may need investigation and tests. There are two main categories of 'abnormal' bruising which call for special tests. **1** Disorders of bleeding and clotting. Hemophilia is an example: an hereditary bleeding disorder, causing bruising without injury, swelling of joints due to internal bleeding, and other unusual symptoms. Another example is vitamin K deficiency, which disrupts the clotting mechanism in premature babies. There are many other disorders of bleeding and clotting, all of them rare. They can be distinguished only with blood tests. **2** Non-accidental injury – see *CHILD ABUSE*. If this is suspected from abnormal patterns of injury seen on the child, X-rays and BLOOD TESTS may be needed to rule out other possible causes such as CONGENITAL ABNORMALITIES of bones and blood.

■ ACTION Bruising is not itself painful; but pain arising from injury can be greatly relieved by acetaminophen or by an ice-pack. A bag of frozen peas from the freezer makes an excellent instant ice-pack.

BULIMIA

Secretive eating of large amounts of food, followed by self-induced vomiting or the use of laxatives. It is associated with ANOREXIA NERVOSA and is a psychological condition almost always affecting girls, from the teens onwards.

BULLYING and TEASING

A sad – if toughening – fact of life both at school and at home for most children at some time or another. If the child is obviously different from others (being short or overweight, wearing glasses), the problem may be long-term.

If your child is frequently upset by teasing, try to help him think up some techniques for constructively dealing with the teasing. This is far more helpful than if you overprotect him. Try to discover from his teacher whether this is a widespread problem in school and ask for the teacher's help. Children who bully others are often insecure and unhappy themselves, and in need of help. Explaining this to your child may help him to be hurt less by the teasing. Feeling the pain of teasing may also make him more sensitive to the needs of others.

BURNS AND SCALDS

Burns are to blame for some 10 percent of accidental deaths of children under five years of age.

■ IMMEDIATE ACTION *Minor burns and scalds*: Immerse the affected area in cold running water – from the tap, shower, or in a bowl or bucket. Continue immersion for ten minutes or so, or until the pain subsides. Remove any constricting clothing, including shoes and

BURNS AND SCALDS

Three essential steps in treating a burn: thorough irrigation under cold running water; cutting away clothing, but only if not sticking to the burn; dressing the area with sterile gauze.

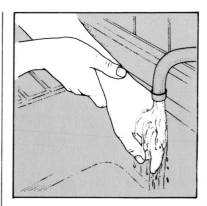

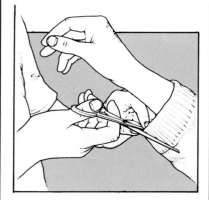

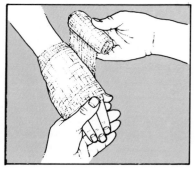

watches, from the burnt area before it starts to swell. At this stage get medical advice. If not readily available, then dress the area with sterile gauze. Don't burst blisters, or put on any lotions (butter, oil or grease) or use adhesive dressings.

Severe burns and scalds: Put out the flames. Smother flaming hair or clothes with a blanket, towel, coat or whatever is handy. Remove the child from source of the heat. If the child's clothing has been on fire, prevent him from running outside (breezes can fan the flames). Lie the child down, burnt side up, and put water (preferably cold) on the burnt area until the pain has stopped. Quickly remove the child's clothing but do *not* remove clothing, or anything else, that is sticking to the burn. Call for an ambulance, or take

the child to your nearest hospital. If you have called an ambulance, keep the child warm with blankets, lying down, and stay with him until the paramedics arrive. If you are taking him to the nearest hospital yourself, keep him wrapped in a blanket to keep him warm on the way.

Serious burns can bring on SHOCK. See that section for treatment.

A child with any but the mildest burn should be taken to the hospital for a check.

■ OUTLOOK With modern skin-grafting techniques, much of the horrifying damage can be repaired; but severe burns can still result in death, or permanent disfigurement and attendant psychological problems.

C

CANCER IN CHILDHOOD

Except for LEUKEMIA, cancers are very uncommon in childhood. See *NEPHROBLASTOMA, TUMOR OF THE EYE, BRAIN TUMORS.* See also *CHRONIC ILLNESS, THE DYING CHILD.*

CANDIDIASIS

An INFECTION caused by the *Candida* species of FUNGUS, also known as moniliasis and, in infants who only have involvement of their mouths, as 'thrush'. It thrives throughout the environment, and in the mouth, gastrointestinal tract and vagina of healthy persons. A baby is often infected while passing through his mother's vagina during birth, but the fungus can be present in baby-bottle nipples, pacifiers and anything else that is sucked by the baby. In older children the infection is usually associated with prolonged ANTIBIOTIC treatment that kills normal BACTERIA present in the bowel and allows the *Candida* to flourish. Children with depressed IMMUNITY are also at risk, and certain diseases such as DIABETES, LEUKEMIA and HODGKIN DISEASE can predispose to thrush.

■ SYMPTOMS White patches or plaques are seen inside the mouth, on the sides of the cheeks, on the tongue and on the roof of the mouth. If scraped off, the underlying mucosal surface may bleed. The areas around the thrush patches may be inflamed and sore, which occasionally can hinder feeding.

In the diaper area, the *Candida* infection causes reddened skin, extending right into the skin creases, unlike the usual DIAPER RASH. There are also small red spots that may extend from the diaper area. The rash can occasionally occur in other skinfold areas such as those around the neck and under the arms.

Candida infection can occur in a girl's vagina. This usually causes redness, white plaques and intense itching.

■ ACTION Thrush is common in babies. Check his mouth from time to time before feedings, particularly if he is reluctant to feed. Because *Candida* are excreted in stools, *Candida* diaper rash accompany oral thrush or another form of candidiasis. If you suspect thrush, get medical advice.

If your child has thrush or another form of candidiasis, mention this to a doctor if he or she intends to prescribe an antibiotic. Most antibiotics have a tendency to make thrush worse.

If you suspect, during pregnancy, that you have a vaginal *Candida* infection, make sure that it is properly treated before the baby is born.

■ TREATMENT is simple and effective but it must be continued for long enough to clear the infection completely. Although response to treatment is usually rapid, the infection tends to recur if not fully eliminated.

Oral thrush is treated with nystatin drops in the mouth given after each feeding. Treatment should be continued for seven to ten days. Baby-bottle nipples can cause reinfection, so these should be boiled after every feeding: ordinary chemical sterilizing agents do not kill *Candida*. If you are breast feeding, the infection can get into your nipples and so pass back to your baby. Nystatin cream will help to prevent this.

Candida diaper rash is treated with antifungal cream. As the infection comes from the bowel, it is usual to give nystatin drops by mouth as well. Since *Candida* thrives in a warm moist environment, frequent diaper changes with thorough cleansing and drying of the skin will also help treat and prevent recurrence of the rash.

Vaginal *Candida* infections can be treated with a special vaginal nystatin cream. Treatment should be continued until one week after the symptoms have disappeared.

If *Candida* infections occur whenever your child is given an antibiotic, it may be best to treat for candidiasis at the same time.

■ OUTLOOK Resistance to infection increases with age, so this is a diminishing problem as the child gets older.

CAPUT
The soft swelling that gives some newborn babies' heads a distorted shape. It is caused by normal pressure on the scalp as the baby passes through the mother's pelvis. Caput disappears in a day or two. A swelling that remains may be a CEPHALOHEMATOMA.

CARBUNCLE
See *BOILS*.

CARDIAC MASSAGE
See *EMERGENCY RESUSCITATION*.

CARDIOMYOPATHY
Permanent damage to the heart muscle. The cause is usually unknown. See *HEART-DISEASE*.

CATARACTS
The lens of the eye becomes clouded. This can affect the whole lens, or only a small area in an otherwise clear lens. Rare in children.

■ CAUSES Can be inherited: the child may be born with a cataract, or the problem may develop within the first few years. Cataracts can occur in children whose mothers contracted RUBELLA during the pregnancy. But in many cases the cause is uncertain.

■ SIGNS AND SYMPTOMS Parents may notice a white, clouded area within the pupil. If your child is old enough, he may complain of difficulty seeing.

■ TREATMENT There is no way to reverse the clouding which is like a scar. However, the cataract can be removed by a simple operation performed at any age.

■ OUTLOOK After the removal of the cataract, EYE GLASSES and/or contact lenses are needed to replace the affected lens. This is essential to bring a focused image (what is seen) to the retina at the back of the eye.

It is important to treat cataracts early, so sometimes the operation is performed on babies only a few weeks or months old. In these cases, soft contact lenses are prescribed.

Regular follow-up eye examinations are necessary to change the strength of the lenses.

How successful the treatment will be depends on a number of factors, including how old the child was when the cataract developed, and the presence of any other eye disease.

CATARRH
See *POSTNASAL DRIP, COMMON COLD.*

CELIAC DISEASE
A chronic illness caused by intolerance of wheat and rye protein (GLUTEN). It is characterized by MALABSORPTION; an abnormal small bowel inner lining; and improvement when wheat and rye cereals are excluded from the diet.

Celiac disease may be detected at any age in childhood, or in adult life.

▓ FEATURES Poor APPETITE and FAILURE TO THRIVE in infancy soon after the introduction of cereals to the diet, usually at three to four months of age. Abnormal BOWEL MOVEMENTS (pale, large, foul-smelling, greasy, with a tendency to float in the toilet bowl and difficult to flush down the toilet), ABDOMINAL SWELLING, thin muscles (usually buttocks and thighs) and floppiness may be noticed. The child is usually miserable. RICKETS may be associated.

A celiac crisis is unusual, but consists of ANOREXIA, VOMITING, DIARRHEA and generally feeling very sick with marked swelling of the abdomen.

Some patients are diagnosed in adult life with ANEMIA, bloating of the abdomen and recurrent diarrhoea.

Celiac disease must be differentiated from other causes of malabsorption such as prolonged GASTROENTERITIS or bowel INFECTIONS, SUGAR INTOLERANCE, COW'S MILK ALLERGY, and CYSTIC FIBROSIS.

▓ TESTS The diagnosis of celiac disease is based upon demonstration of a flattened, abnormal small intestine inner lining on biopsy, which reverts to normal after removal of gluten from the diet. Thus, an intestinal biopsy is necessary before and after treatment (to confirm that healing has occurred): this is safe and involves passing a fine tube through the stomach into the small bowel, under sedation. A cutting device painlessly collects a tiny piece of tissue, which is examined under a microscope. In celiac disease, the fine projections of the normal lining of the bowel are flattened by inflammation. When the biopsy is repeated after treatment, the inner intestinal lining should have returned to normal, healthy state.

Other tests to determine the severity of the malabsorption, such as blood tests for anemia and oral sugar (xylose) absorption, may be done. Some centers also measure antibodies to gluten.

▓ TREATMENT All foods containing flour or cereal from wheat or rye grain should be removed from the diet. A dietician will advise on a gluten-free diet and where to buy such food. Eliminating gluten takes effort but should be continued indefinitely to avoid recurrence of the symptoms.

▓ OUTLOOK This is usually a permanent problem. However, a repeat biopsy after reintroducing gluten into the diet may confirm in later childhood that the initial illness was due to a temporary intolerance.

A child with true celiac disease who stays on the appropriate diet will feel well and gain weight satisfactorily, although it may take some time to catch up on his delayed growth.

CELLULITIS

A spreading BACTERIAL INFECTION of the skin and soft tissues.

■ SYMPTOMS The site of infection is irritated and red, often with a raised edge. The skin feels hard, hot and tender. The child is generally sick, and has a FEVER.

■ ACTION This condition needs urgent medical treatment: the child should see a doctor as soon as possible.

■ TREATMENT An ANTIBIOTIC, chosen for its action on the bacteria that usually cause cellulitis, given by mouth or, if necessary, by intramuscular injection or intravenously.

■ OUTLOOK If not treated, cellulitis may progress to form an abscess, and from this the infection can spread to involve the lymph glands. Blood stream infection (septicemia) may occur. Correct antibiotic treatment is normally rapidly effective, and the condition heals with no long-term effects.

CELLULITIS OF THE EYE

See ORBITAL CELLULITIS.

CEPHALOHEMATOMA

A collection of blood under the skin covering the skull bones of a new-born baby. It is caused by bruising during the BIRTH (see also BIRTH INJURIES). It can be felt as a soft bump, on one or both sides of the back of the head. It is harmless and generally subsides over four to six weeks.

CEREBRAL PALSY

Cerebral palsy as a term covers an enormous range of problems. The most minor may be no more than an infant who is a late walker and grows up to be a somewhat clumsy child. The most severe represents a major lifelong challenge for the child and his family.

Disorders of posture, movement and co-ordination usually become apparent in late infancy or toddlerhood. Although the effects of cerebral palsy change as the child grows, the disease does not get worse.

Cerebral palsy (CP) may be classified into several types, according to how the different parts of the body are affected. Spastic cerebral palsy is the commonest (two-thirds of the cases). The child's muscles show increased resistance to passive movement and tightness on exertion.

Athetoid cerebral palsy involves writhing movements of the arms, legs and mouth muscles, which are outside the control of the child. Ataxic cerebral palsy is characterized by a lack of balance of the trunk and general unsteadiness of co-ordination. Cerebral palsy severely affecting all four limbs accounts for about 5 percent of CP patients.

If all four limbs are affected, this is called quadriplegia; diplegia means the legs are most affected. When one half of the body is affected, it is described as hemiplegia. Ataxic diplegia means a lack of trunk balance, plus spasticity in the legs.

Associated conditions include EPILEPSY; MENTAL HANDICAP or retardation; visual or hearing defects (up to a tenth of cases); language and communication problems; and in the more severely affected, drooling of saliva and FEEDING PROBLEMS.

About two in every 1,000 children suffer from cerebral palsy.

▨ CAUSES Damage to the developing brain during pregnancy, birth or the early postnatal period. Causes include: CONGENITAL ABNORMALITIES, INFECTION in pregnancy (including RUBELLA, cytomegalovirus), BIRTH ASPHYXIA, complications of PREMATURITY (despite INTENSIVE CARE), MENINGITIS or ENCEPHALITIS, or physical injury in early infancy.

▨ TREATMENT Since CP is a complex manifestation of structural BRAIN DAMAGE, there is no cure or simple treatment. Management includes a wide-ranging and long-lasting programme of special education with particular attention to physiotherapy, speech therapy and occupational therapy. Aids, appliances, adapted footwear or orthopedic surgery may be required. Psychological and social support for the child and whole family may be indicated.

Drugs may have a place for such associated problems as epilepsy or CONSTIPATION.

With a well-planned, co-ordinated and concerted effort, the child may achieve more than may seem possible as judged in infancy. Occasionally athetoid children, thought to be mentally retarded in infancy, turn out to be of average or above average intelligence, but require special communication systems before they can express their abilities.

▨ OUTLOOK Facilities for children with cerebral palsy tend to be based in child development centers or in special schools; adolescent and young adult rehabilitation services are also available. Many countries, including the United States, have organizations and societies established that are very effective in supporting individuals and families with CP.

Most children with CP can be expected to live a normal length of life.

CESARIAN SECTION

The DELIVERY of the baby through an incision in the abdominal wall and uterus. The use of Cesarian section varies from country to country. In the United States, for example, it accounts for 17 percent of births. It is generally done to facilitate the safe delivery of the baby.

Some Cesarian sections are anticipated, for example: if the mother has needed one at a previous delivery; if the baby's head is too large for the mother's pelvis; if the baby is in an unsuitable position – breech (bottom-first') or transverse (crosswise); or if the placenta is lower than the baby's head (*Placenta previa*).

Some Cesarians may become necessary for various reasons during labor: if, for instance, there is FETAL DISTRESS or the umbilical cord becomes trapped between the mother's cervix and the baby's head, hindering the flow of blood to the baby; or if there is failure of the labor to progress normally.

Cesarian section is performed either under an EPIDURAL or a general ANESTHETIC. Both will usually be offered if the DELIVERY is not an emergency. In an emergency, a general anesthetic is given. With an epidural anesthetic, the mother remains awake during and after the delivery. The pubic hair may be shaved and a catheter (a small tube) inserted into the bladder to keep it empty (some maternity units avoid these procedures). Fluids and medication are given intravenously as necessary. When the anesthetic has taken effect, a 'bikini line' incision is usually made through the abdominal wall and then into the uterus. The baby is eased out either by hand or, less often, by using FORCEPS. The umbilical cord is cut and the baby is handed to his mother, or to his father if the mother is under general anesthetic.

■ COMPLICATIONS After delivery the scar is sore and medications to relieve the pain may be needed. The mother may not be able to move around easily, and will need help at first to care for her baby. Most mothers are up and about by 24-48 hours, albeit with some pain. Abdominal discomfort and constipation are more likely following a Cesarian section. It is helpful to be up and about as soon as possible after birth in order to minimize the risk of thromboses (blood clots) forming in the legs.

A mother who has had a Cesarian section will usually stay in the hospital for about seven to ten days after the delivery. She can, however, still get out of bed and play her full role in the care of her baby.

CHALASIA
See *GASTROESOPHAGEAL REFLUX.*

CHEST PAIN
An unusual symptom in childhood.

■ SYMPTOMS The nature of the pain and other symptoms present may well indicate the cause.

If the child has a sharp pain in his chest which is made worse when breathing, suspect an injury such as a bruised or torn muscle or a FRAC-TURED rib. The commonest cause of chest pain is in fact a minor muscle injury.

A similar type of pain can be due to inflammation of the lungs (as in PNEUMONIA and PLEURISY) or a VIRAL INFECTION. There is usually a cough (which can make the pain worse), fever and sometimes general muscle aches and pain.

Pain caused by HEART-DISEASE is always related to exercise, lasts for a few minutes, and is relieved by rest. It is best described as a tight feeling in the center of the chest and, in childhood, is very rare. The common 'stitch' in the side of the chest or sharp chest pain with vigorous exercise is usually due to local muscle spasm and not heart attack. An older child may be concerned that such a pain could be due to a heart problem and explaining these facts to the child may be reassuring.

Young children may complain of pain in the chest when its cause is due to a disease in the abdomen.

■ ACTION Look for signs of injury, typically BRUISING. Determine whether the pain is associated with coughing or breathing, or is related to exercising. Take your child's temperature to establish whether an infection is likely.

Get medical advice if the pain occurs with breathing or when exercising, or if it persists for more than a few days.

■ TREATMENT Muscular pain needs no specific treatment, but a painkiller such as acetamenophen may help. Chest-wall injury is normally also treated with a simple painkiller.

Pain from pneumonia, pleurisy or a viral infection is also treated with a painkiller, but the child must see a doctor in case treatment with an

ANTIBIOTIC is needed.

Chest pain that could be due to heart-disease must be evaluated by a heart specialist (pediatric cardiologist).

▣ TESTS A chest X-ray helps to diagnose a fractured rib, pleurisy, pneumonia or heart-disease.

An ECG (ELECTROCARDIOGRAM) will be necessary if heart-disease is suspected.

CHICKEN POX (VARICELLA)

A highly INFECTIOUS disease, mainly but not exclusively confined to childhood, caused by one of the herpes group of VIRUSES called varicella-zoster virus. It is transmitted by direct contact or airborne spread from an infected person. It is most infectious one to two days before the RASH appears, so it is very difficult to prevent your child from coming into contact with a child or person who has it. The disease tends to be mild in children (but may be more severe in adults). The INCUBATION PERIOD is 14-21 days.

▣ SYMPTOMS **1** There is often a mild FEVER, HEADACHE and a feeling of being ill, particularly in older children. **2** The rash occurs mainly on the body, but in severe cases it develops on the face, scalp, arms and legs. It consists of raised red spots which rapidly turn into itchy blisters. These gradually dry to form crusts that can last for a few weeks. They do not leave a scar unless they are scratched too much, or get infected. New spots occur in batches, so while some are forming crusts, others may be appearing for the first time.

There are few serious complications but PNEUMONIA or ENCEPHALITIS do occasionally occur. In children with reduced IMMUNITY, including those on steroids and those who have leukemia, chicken pox can be severe and life-threatening.

▣ ACTION The fever can be treated with an analgesic such as acetamenophen; give cool baths if necessary.

Keep your child's nails short and clean to prevent him from scratching, and infecting the spots. Calamine lotion will help to reduce the itchiness.

Bed rest is unnecessary, unless your child is more comfortable there.

If you suspect PNEUMONIA or ENCEPHALITIS (see separate entries), get urgent medical advice.

Your child is infectious until new blisters have stopped appearing – usually about a week after the rash started. The crusts are not infectious.

▣ TREATMENT If the itchiness is really causing problems, your doctor may prescribe an antihistamine, usually as a syrup. Creams containing antihistamines can cause ALLERGIC reactions and are not generally used.

Minor skin infection can be treated with an antiseptic soap or cream, but more severe infection may require ANTIBIOTICS. Don't ignore spots that are much more red or painful than the rest of the rash: infection can spread rapidly.

For very severe cases, an intravenous antiviral drug called acyclovir helps to control the infection.

▣ OUTLOOK There are few long-term problems, but a child who has had chicken pox may develop shingles or zoster many years later. The virus lies dormant in the nerves of the spine. The shingles rash contains the virus, and this can cause chicken pox in someone who has not had the disease. However, a child with chicken pox will not pass on shingles to an adult; but he may, of course, pass on chicken pox to anyone who has not developed immunity by having had the disease.

CHILD ABUSE

The main forms of child abuse are non-accidental injury, neglect, psychological or emotional abuse and SEXUAL ABUSE.

▓ INCIDENCE Accurate information on the frequency with which child abuse occurs is impossible to obtain because there is no single standard of parental care and children who are abused rarely report it to persons outside the family. However, one child in every 300 or 400 is at risk for abuse at one time or another.

▓ SIGNS include bruises, welts or burns for which no satisfactory explanation can be given. Neglect and emotional abuse result in DEVELOPMENTAL DELAY, FAILURE TO THRIVE, apathy or BEHAVIORAL PROBLEMS, including DEPRESSION, stealing or AGGRESSION.

▓ ACTION If you suspect that a child is being abused, contact your local social service department. A child abuse team including a doctor will assess the case. If there are reasonable grounds for suspicion, and the child is thought to be in immediate danger of further serious abuse, he may be moved from the family home to a safe place. This is not a step that is taken lightly. Social workers are trained to balance the need to protect a child against a concern for individual liberty, and the possible harmful effects of removing a child from home.

▓ INVESTIGATIONS The child is carefully examined and then may have tests for bleeding tendencies and X-rays for evidence of recent or old bone fractures. The family and other persons who care for the child will be interviewed – usually by a doctor and/or a social worker. Within days, a case conference of all professionals who know the family and representatives of relevant social agencies will be called. It may be that further information revealed at this time will dispel suspicion.

▓ TREATMENT The aim is a long-term plan of action for protecting the child. This typically includes everyday support for the family from an experienced social worker. Ways of reducing pressure on the child, and on the abuser, will be sought: the problem will be looked at in the light of everything that affects the family. Prosecution of the abuser will be considered. If there is no alternative, the child may be placed for care in a foster home. The aim, not always the reality, is that this should be a temporary measure. Only if continued abuse is considered inevitable or extremely likely is long-term care away from the family contemplated.

▓ PREVENTION Better education in school about standards of behavior could make a difference. Housing, employment, recreation, child care, benefits and support services – indeed anything that affects the quality of family life – has a bearing on this social problem.

▓ SELF-HELP Parents or other persons who have abused children and have learned to cope, with support, can sometimes help families experiencing this kind of trouble for the first time.

■ OUTLOOK Abuse of any type has grave long-term consequences for abnormal physical, mental and emotional development of a child. Abused children often abuse their own children.

CHILD PSYCHOTHERAPY
A psychological treatment for children with emotional problems based on the theories of psychoanalysts such as Anna Freud or Melanie Klein. It involves the child and often his family in regular discussion sessions with a therapist, usually over a matter of months or years. PLAY THERAPY may be used to help the child in hospital deal with anxieties or fears; it may also serve to distract the child and combat boredom.

CHLAMYDIA
Chlamydia is a SEXUALLY TRANSMITTED DISEASE (STD) due to a BACTERIA. If a mother is infected when giving birth, her baby may develop CONJUNCTIVITIS and later PNEUMONIA. Both can be treated with ANTIBIOTICS. Older children can catch the infection from an adult carrier through SEXUAL ABUSE. Chlamydia is a more common STD in sexually active adolescents and adults than GONORRHEA but infection with both can occur.

Vaginal infection with chlamydia may be asymptomatic or it may cause a vaginal discharge. In boys, asymptomatic infection is common but discharge from the penis and burning with urination may occur.

Swab tests can confirm the diagnosis. Treatment with antibiotics is effective.

CHOANAL ATRESIA
A rare congenital obstruction of one or both nostrils. If both sides are blocked a breathing tube must be passed from the mouth down the throat into the windpipe (trachea). If this is not done, the baby will be unable to breathe. Surgery is then required to open the obstructed nasal passages.

CHOKING
Whole or partial blockage of the airway, interfering with the child's breathing. It occurs typically when a child inhales an object such as a peanut or button. Though rare, a baby may choke if left unattended with a propped-up bottle.

■ IMMEDIATE ACTION If possible, ask someone to call for an ambulance. Then remove anything tight from around the child's neck. If your child is at risk of dying from airway obstruction, then start EMERGENCY RESUSCITATION. If the chest fails to rise, take the following steps: *In babies and children under two years*: Hold the child on his stomach dropped over your knee, with his head lower than his feet. Bang four times on his back between the shoulder-blades with your fist. This should dislodge the object and allow the child to spit it out. Turn him over and give four compressions to the chest as in cardiac massage (EMERGENCY RESUSCITATION, step C). Repeat this back-pounding action if not successful first time. If this fails, start artificial ventilation (EMERGENCY RESUSCITATION, steps A and B) in the hope of forcing air past the obstruction.

In children above two years: If blows to the back (as for younger children, above) fail to work, try the Heimlich maneuver. (Since this is a potentially dangerous procedure, it should only be used with severe choking not responding to blows on the back.)

CHOKING

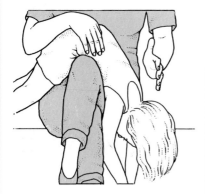

Action for children under two years.

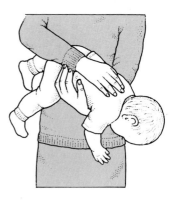

Action for babies.

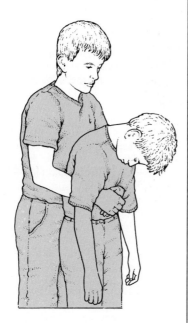

The Heimlich manoeuvre, for children over two years.

First, make sure that someone has called for an ambulance. Stand behind the child. Wrap both your arms firmly around the child just below the rib cage. Pull sharply and quickly inwards. This is meant to force the object upwards and out of the airway. Repeat if not successful at first.

If the object is obviously within reach at the back of the mouth, hook it out with your finger(s).

If all these efforts fail, start artificial ventilation (EMERGENCY RESUS-CITATION, steps A and B) in the hope of forcing air past the obstruction. *If the child is unconscious:* Turn him on his back and immediately start artificial ventilation (EMERGENCY RESUSCITATION, step B). If this is unsuccessful, try to dislodge the obstruction as described above. Check whether the object has moved by looking in the mouth. If the choking continues, repeat artificial ventilation and once more check whether the obstruction has been dislodged. Again, make sure that an ambulance has been summoned. Keep repeating until the obstruction is dislodged, and the child is breathing. Put him in the RECOVERY POSITION and arrange transportation to the hospital.

CHOREA

Sudden, jerky, non-repetitive involuntary movements. These may be associated with athetoid CEREBRAL PALSY or may occur after streptococcal throat infection (Sydenham's chorea). Chorea due to Huntington's disease occurs in adulthood. The childhood concern with Huntington's chorea relates to matters of genetics and counselling.

CHROMOSOMES

Parts of a cell which contain the GENES. They transmit the inherited characteristics from parent to child. Each gene has a particular place on a chromosome. Every nucleated cell in the body contains 23 matching pairs of chromosomes. An ovum and a sperm each have one of every pair, so the new cell produced at fertilization contains 46 chromosomes. The two chromosomes from each pair are identical in size and shape, except for those in the 23rd pair. These determine sex. Females have two identical sex chromosomes – the X chromosomes – while males have one X chromosome and a smaller Y chromosome. The sex of a child depends on whether an X or a Y chromosome is inherited from the father. An X chromosome from the father together with one of the X chromosomes from the mother will result in a female. A Y chromosome from the father together with one of the X chromosomes from the mother will result in a male.

Chromosomal abnormalities may cause an abnormality of development so that the baby dies before birth (and is miscarried), or is variously malformed; this is evident at birth as a CONGENITAL ABNORMALITY.

CHRONIC EPSTEIN-BARR VIRUS INFECTION

See *CHRONIC FATIGUE SYNDROME*.

CHRONIC FATIGUE SYNDROME

Following an apparently minor viral infection, a few people, including children, may complain of debilitating fatigue that persists or relapses for at least six months. Other symptoms of this syndrome may include HEADACHE, muscle aches, joint complaints, FEVER, SORE THROAT, painful lymph nodes, muscle weakness, SLEEP PROBLEMS, depression and concentration disturbances. In the mid-1980s this symptom complex was attributed to chronic Epstein Barr virus (infectious mononucleosis virus) infection. Recent studies cast doubt on this. The symptom complex was renamed chronic fatigue syndrome.

There are no specific laboratory tests to confirm the diagnosis. Treatment requires a combination of medical and psychological support, with incentives for recovery.

CHRONIC HEPATITIS

Inflammation of the liver continuing without improvement for longer than six months. It is uncommon. The problem can be caused by a variety of conditions including chronic infection of the liver by certain VIRUSES, some drugs and certain INHERITED DISORDERS. In some cases no cause is identified. See also *HEPATITIS*. Some patients respond to immunosuppressive therapy with steroids such as prednisone. Stopping the offending drug may help drug-related cases. Some cases progress to CIRRHOSIS and some may develop liver cancer as adults.

CHRONIC ILLNESS, CHILD WITH

The principles of care of children with chronic medical conditions and those with mental or physical handicaps are similar in many respects. Whether your child has, for example, ASTHMA or DIABETES, or a physical or mental handicap, certain restrictions on activity may make him different from others. Parents, too, have their own problems in coping. A child with a chronic disease has specific needs, but these are in addition to, and not instead of, those of other children. He requires a loving, stable, stimulating environment. Contact with other children is also important.

■ ADJUSTMENT WITHIN THE FAMILY It takes time to accept that a child has a problem. Discuss your worries with your doctor. Your whole family is involved. An ill child takes up time that would otherwise be shared with the rest of the family. If your partner and the other children take part in the decision making and the day-to-day activities of your ill or handicapped child, they are likely to feel more involved and understanding. Frank discussion with your other children will help them to accept the situation better.

■ GENERAL ADVICE
– Make sure that any medical, social service, educational or other professionals who see your child in consultation or at school or community agencies inform your doctor of their opinions regarding diagnosis and management. Your doctor is often the person your child sees for general medical care and in emergent situations, and can only advise you properly if he or she is fully informed of these matters.
– Don't be ashamed to ask for help if you need it. Stress can affect your judgment and ability to handle difficult situations.
– Look carefully at all educational possibilities and obtain the best advice about school placements and individual educational plans for your child.

– Get an accurate idea of what your child's potential is so that you will not expect too much or too little of him.
– Don't over-protect your child.

■ PRE-SCHOOL Your child will be largely in your care. Support from friends is invaluable and local self-help groups can offer practical advice. Such support is important: if you are having difficulty coping, the family will suffer. It is especially important to help the child build his self-confidence by praising his achievements.

■ SCHOOL Once your child is approaching school age, you should seek advice regarding the future. Your doctor will usually co-ordinate special services and facilities for the child with particular needs. A pediatrician or educational psychologist may help define the capabilities of your child and help you to make decisions on the appropriate goals for his education.

If your child is attending a regular school, inform teachers and the school nurse about his illness or disability. Many schools have programs that support placing disabled children in regular classrooms ('mainstreaming') and may be able to adjust their program to suit your child's needs. They should know: what treatment he is receiving; what symptoms to look for; and what to do in an emergency; if there are any restrictions on his physical activity; and what learning problems he may have. If your child is not doing well (or is unlikely to do well) at the local school, discuss the problem with all the health and educational professionals involved, before deciding to send him to a special school.

Special schools have advantages and disadvantages. They may have better facilities for specific handicaps, such as ramps for wheel chairs and special educational equipment; also they assign fewer children to each teacher so that each child receives more individual attention. The disadvantages of special schools are that the child is in a protected environment and may later find it difficult to adjust to the real world. Also your child may have to live away from home in order to attend a special school, and most of these schools charge high fees. However, federal laws require that all public schools provide special educational programs and facilities for handicapped children (children with special needs).

■ ADOLESCENCE presents specific problems. The striving for independence can result in the rejection of authority, and long-term treatment is less likely to be adhered to regularly (as in DIABETES and ASTHMA). A young person with a severe handicap will have to rely on others for help with washing and dressing. The lack of independence and privacy may make him very resentful. He may also have problems meeting other young people and may experience problems with SEXUALITY. Sex education is essential and specific sexual problems should be discussed with your doctor.

CIRCUMCISION
The surgical removal of the foreskin, which covers the glans of the penis. The new-born baby's foreskin is attached to the glans and cannot be pulled back. It becomes progressively easy to retract it from one year of age onwards.

Circumcision is performed worldwide for religious and cultural reasons. Occasionally circumcision is necessary

on medical grounds; for example, following recurrent BALANITIS, for PHIMOSIS and paraphimosis (when the foreskin has been forcibly pulled back and is trapped in the retracted position). In the United States the operation is normally performed without using an ANESTHETIC.

CIRRHOSIS OF THE LIVER
Chronic (long-term) damage to the liver. It is an uncommon complication of HEPATITIS, or may be associated with other rare diseases; or the cause may be unknown.

■ SYMPTOMS Early signs of liver disease include skin changes and JAUNDICE. The child will be ill and poorly nourished. There may be generalized itching; also swelling – due to excess fluid – of the abdomen and limbs (EDEMA) caused by low protein levels in the blood and slowing of the blood circulation in the lower half of the body. The spleen may be enlarged. There may be internal bleeding. Eventually there may be liver failure, which can reduce brain function. There will be personality changes, tremor (fine shaking of the limbs), speech disorder and lethargy progressing to deep COMA and death.

■ INVESTIGATIONS Liver-function tests on blood samples; ultrasound, X-ray, CAT SCAN or radioisotope scan of the liver; liver biopsy.

■ TREATMENT In early cirrhosis, a high protein diet and fat-soluble VITAMINS will be necessary. Control of esophageal bleeding, BLOOD TRANSFUSION and correction of clotting disorders may be required. Surgery may be needed to control bleeding. Complications will be treated as required.

OUTLOOK There is no cure once cirrhosis is fully developed, but a liver transplant, if possible, may be life-saving.

CLEFT LIP
See *CLEFT PALATE*.

CLEFT PALATE
An abnormality of development in which the two sides of the roof of the mouth fail to join together, either totally or partially. Cleft palate is commonly accompanied by a cleft of the upper lip.

INCIDENCE Cleft palate, cleft lip, or both together, occur about once in 700 births.

CAUSES Unknown, but once it has occurred in a family, there is a slight risk of recurrence.

TREATMENT Feeding: is usually possible in the normal fashion by breast or bottle. Extra care and some expert advice may be needed. However, with the most extensive bilateral clefts, feeding by cup and spoon may be necessary.
Surgery: one operation to correct the cleft lip, another to repair the cleft palate. Usually a series of planned operations is required to improve the function and appearance of palate and lips. Opinion varies as to the best timing of the operations. Frequently correction of the lip is performed at about three months, while repair of the palate is initiated between three and six months.

LONG-TERM MANAGEMENT Cleft lip alone seldom leads to problems with speech, and the cosmetic result from modern surgery is ex-cellent. Cleft palate can result in 'nasal' speech, which may be improved by further surgery and by speech therapy.

OUTLOOK With a cleft palate there is an increased risk of MIDDLE EAR INFECTIONS and DEAFNESS. Regular hearing tests are advised. Teeth may not grow straight, so planned orthodontic care is necessary. However, children with a cleft lip or palate can expect to lead normal lives.

CLUB FOOT
The commonest CONGENITAL ABNORMALITY of the foot. One or both feet may be affected. The cause is not fully understood: an imbalance of the muscles of the foot may be implicated, with the muscles of the inner side of the foot pulling it inwards.

SYMPTOMS All new-born babies are examined routinely for evidence of club foot. Most have feet that turn in, but this can usually be corrected by gently moving the foot into the normal position.
In babies with a true club foot, this turned-in position is quite marked and the foot cannot be straightened. The range of movement of the ankle joint is restricted and the calf muscles are under-developed.

TREATMENT should be started soon after birth. The foot is manipulated into the correct position and then fixed by a plaster cast. This is usually done by a bone specialist (orthopedic surgeon).

If the foot is not back to normal after about three months, both on examination and on X-RAY, an operation is recommended. The tight ligaments and tendons on the inside of the foot are lengthened. After the operation, a plaster cast is worn for a few months to allow healing in the correct position.

Children who have not had early treatment usually need surgery. The same applies when the problem recurs after early treatment with casting.

■ OUTLOOK depends on the age at which treatment is started, and its effectiveness. Early treatment is usually successful; but even with prompt treatment, some children can have a relapse when treatment is discontinued. This is most likely in children who have especially underdeveloped calf muscles.

CLUMSINESS
The term covers a range of severity, from the normal child lacking in dexterity, to the child who has a clear specific MOTOR DEVELOPMENT difficulty. Clumsiness may affect balance, co-ordination, hand function or speech. Overall, about 2 percent of children might be termed 'clumsy'; as a group, they demonstrate the whole range of intelligence. In its more severe forms, however, it is commonly associated with learning problems.

■ MANAGEMENT Accept the problem and find activities in which the child can experience success, particularly those that can be shared with you, or hobbies that can be shared with other children. Occasionally speech therapy, physiotherapy or occupational therapy may be useful, as well as special help with handwriting.

■ OUTLOOK The majority of clumsy children grow into normal adults, who perhaps lack co-ordination skills in such things as handwriting, sports and dancing.

COARCTATION OF THE AORTA
A narrowing of the artery that carries blood from the heart (aorta). It is a CONGENITAL HEART-DISEASE AND IF SEVERE WILL CAUSE HEART FAILURE in infancy. If it is not severe, it may be noticed because the pulses in the legs are weak, a HEART MURMUR is heard, or hypertension is discovered. Tests will be necessary to show the severity of the narrowing. Surgery is usually necessary.

COLD SORES
Caused by the herpes VIRUS, which lies dormant in the body after an initial INFECTION, which may or may not cause symptoms. The sores tend to occur in older children and adults, and can be activated by an infectious illness, overexposure to sunlight or emotional upsets; but often no cause is found.

■ SYMPTOMS Initial infection can cause mouth and lip ulcers that are extremely painful and associated with a high FEVER. The lymph glands in the neck may be swollen and the illness can last for a week or so. There may be loss of APPETITE. Recurrent cold sores develop on the lips and around the nose and mouth when the dormant virus is reactivated. They begin as a tiny but painful crop of blisters. There is usually no fever, but the pain may be severe enough to make the child miserable. It lasts a few days and the sore then forms a scab.

■ ACTION 1 Initial infection: painkillers such as acetamenophen can be used against the fever and pain, particularly if a baby is not feeding well. A dose given about half an hour before a feeding may be useful. Occasionally, the pain and fever are so severe as to prevent feeding and cause DEHYDRATION, so keep a written record of how much your baby is taking and, if you are in any doubt, get medical advice. **2** Recurrent cold sores: Analgesics may be necessary if the pain is severe. Avoid excessive exposure to sunlight if this seems to be a cause. Prevent secondary BACTERIAL infection by discouraging scratching of the sore. Cold sores are infectious and can be spread by kissing. They can be especially severe in children who have ECZEMA.

■ TREATMENT Viral infections are generally difficult to treat because the virus is within the body's cells. However, there are several antiviral drugs, such as acyclovir, that can be given for herpes infections as a tablet or as a suspension, or for local application on the skin. If used early, they can clear the sore up quickly. They do not, however, usually prevent recurrences of cold sores.

■ COMPLICATIONS are rare, but herpes infection of the eye can be serious if not recognized and treated. In children with reduced IMMUNITY, such as those on high doses of steroids or those with LEUKEMIA, the herpes virus may spread through the body and cause severe illness. In these cases, high-dose intravenous acyclovir is used.

■ OUTLOOK Herpes mouth ulcers do not usually recur. Cold sores tend to recur less frequently with time.

COLIC

The term 'colic' in a baby essentially means spasms of abdominal pain (presumably of intestinal origin) and of severe crying. It usually occurs in babies less than three months old (three-month colic').

No single cause consistently accounts for infant colic. Alleged causes are excessive gas, a poor burping technique, or over- or under-feeding. There may be an unsatisfactory relationship between the baby and the mother, but this is often secondary to the mother's tension and stress caused by the colic. Allergy to COW'S MILK and possibly soya milk protein has also been claimed but colic can occur in breast-fed babies. Older infants and children may experience colicky abdominal pain with bowel obstruction or INTUSSUSCEPTION.

■ SYMPTOMS Bouts of infant colic are most common in the evening or at night. The attack usually begins suddenly, the cry is loud and continuous. The baby stops crying briefly when offered a feeding, but then starts to cry again during the feeding. The legs are often drawn up on to the abdomen. The face may be flushed, the feet cold. The attack may stop when the baby is exhausted but often relief comes with passage of gas or stool. Colicky abdominal pain with bowel obstruction is severe, spasmodic and griping. It is relieved only by release of the obstruction.

■ INVESTIGATIONS Diagnosis of infant colic is usually made from the history and, where possible, observation of the child. Other causes need to be excluded by the doctor.

■ TREATMENT For baby colic, holding the infant upright, permitting him to lie prone across the lap or on a warm (not hot) water bottle or heating pad may help. Some babies are soothed by rides in a car seat in the car or gentle rocking. Occasionally antispasmodic drugs may help. A stable environment, adequate burping and avoiding over- or under-feeding may help prevent attacks. Severe cases may need to go to the hospital for a few days for advice on feeding and handling. Most infants, however, lose their colic by three months of age and don't need such specific therapy. Severe colicky abdominal pain in any infant or in the older child may indicate an INTESTINAL OBSTRUCTION which needs investigation and treatment. Get medical advice if you are unsure of the basis of the abdominal pain.

COLOR BLINDNESS
Inability to distinguish between certain colors, typically red and green. It usually causes few problems.

It is much more common in boys than in girls: about 5 percent of males have some degree of color blindness. Some children may have difficulties at school if things are color coded. If parents and teachers are aware of the problem, appropriate allowances can be made.

COMA
A state of UNCONSCIOUSNESS that may last for hours, days or longer. It is not a disease as such, but a manifestation of disease in which brain function is disturbed.

Degrees of coma range from light unconsciousness with reactive pupils, restlessness and response to being touched, to deep unconsciousness with fixed dilated pupils, no response to stimuli and the need for artificial ventilation.

The outcome really depends on the underlying cause of the coma. In general, however, the lighter the degree of coma and the shorter it lasts,

the better the outcome. Full recovery from deep coma can occur, for example after barbiturate poisoning. Slow and progressive recovery from deep coma of other origins can continue over weeks or months.

▧ CAUSES include HEAD INJURY, ENCEPHALITIS, very low or persistently high blood sugar in DIABETES, drug poisoning, post-convulsive states, and brain swelling in a wide range of medical conditions, most notably liver failure.

▧ OUTLOOK If coma proves irreversible, it is taken to represent very severe brain damage. A point may then arise when a difficult decision has to be made on whether or not to continue life support treatment. The doctors will be looking for an agreed set of physical signs that indicate with a fair degree of certainty that the brain is damaged beyond any chance of recovery, so-called 'brain death'. The signs include no spontaneous breathing, no response to painful stimulation, no reaction of the pupils of the eye to light or no eye movements when the ears are syringed with ice-cold water. The tests are usually repeated after 12 to 24 hours; it is usual to involve at least two experienced doctors in making the decision that brain death has occurred. An EEG RECORDING (ELECTROENCEPHALOGRAM) may also be performed to confirm the absence of electrical activity of the brain. At this stage, it may be appropriate to discuss the prospects of the child being a donor of one or more organs for TRANSPLANTATION surgery. In that case, life support will continue until the organ or organs can be properly removed.

COMFORT HABITS
Automatic repetitive actions such as

thumb sucking, rocking and HEAD BANGING that appear to be reassuring because of their familiarity. They may be irritating to the parents, but are not directly harmful to the child. Punishment is both ineffective and inappropriate; distracting the child's attention or encouraging alternative actions may help. The habits frequently reflect anxieties and worries, which the child may be too young, or be otherwise unable to express.

COMMON COLD

A viral INFECTION of the nose and throat, that can be caused by many different VIRUSES. The exact way that cold viruses are spread is unknown, but direct contact with infectious secretions on skin or objects and contact with aerosolized (sneezed or coughed) droplets are the likely routes. Overcrowding favors the spread of colds. Cold weather does not cause colds. Infection by one of the cold viruses does not give IMMUNITY to others. The average child has about five to seven colds a year. Those in day care may have many more due to increased exposure.

■ SYMPTOMS The INCUBATION PERIOD is two to three days. The illness begins with sneezing, a sore throat, followed by a watery discharge from the nose which may block the nostrils. There may also be a low-grade FEVER and general feeling of illness. The symptoms usually last for a week. Colds may last nearly twice as long if there is smoke in the environment. Secondary BACTERIAL infection is rare: in such cases, swelling and inflammation caused by the virus block the air passages in the nose, ear, throat and lungs and allow bacteria to multiply, giving rise to such problems as SINUSITIS, OTITIS, PHARYNGITIS and PNEUMONIA.

■ ACTION 1 An older child (three years of age or more) often has mild symptoms, and it is not usually necessary to get medical advice. Rest in bed or at home is not necessary. 2 If a child under six has a fever and has previously suffered from a FEBRILE CONVULSION, be on your guard against a repetition. 3 Colds in small babies can be distressing for the infant and the parents. A blocked nose may interfere with feeding. In extreme cases you may need to feed your baby with a spoon. However, if you are BREAST FEEDING you should certainly continue if at all possible. 4 Encourage your child to drink plenty of clear fluids: both fever and breathing through the mouth can lead to DEHYDRATION.

■ GET MEDICAL ADVICE if the child:
– is under six and has a high fever;
– is not feeding properly;
– has not improved within a few days;
– has other symptoms such as EARACHE, VOMITING or a persistent COUGH.

■ TREATMENT There is no specific treatment. You can give medicines that you find helpful to relieve significant symptoms. Aspirin should *not* be given to children because of the risk of REYE SYNDROME.
– Acetamenophen is an analgesic that may help the sore throat and malaise, in addition to reducing fever.
– Decongestants, although designed to treat colds, are not very effective against them. They act by drying up nasal secretions and reducing the swelling of the nasal passages. Many contain antihistamines, which may cause drowsiness. They should not be given to children under one year of age.

– Decongestant nose drops act in the same way as decongestants taken by mouth. However, they can irritate the nasal membranes, causing further congestion, so do not overuse them. Saline nose drops (salt water) have fewer side-effects and usually work just as well.

– When buying cold remedies, choose single-ingredient medicines rather than those with an analgesic and decongestant combined, which reduce control over dose.

– ANTIBIOTICS are not indicated for the common cold, since they have no effect on viruses.

■ ALTERNATIVE TREATMENT There is a view that VITAMIN C reduces the severity and frequency of colds. Medical trials do not support this theory. It is inadvisable to give large doses of vitamin C to babies.

■ LONG-TERM MANAGEMENT Colds usually get better without treatment. Antibiotics are only indicated for secondary bacterial complications such as otitis and sinusitis. A child who has cold symptoms lasting for months probably has a nasal ALLERGY not a cold. A high number of colds suggests a high contact rate, for example a child in day care, while prolonged symptoms may indicate contaminated environment, for example smoking.

■ OUTLOOK The illness rarely causes serious complications.

CONCUSSION
A state of altered awareness following HEAD INJURY. The child is disoriented, confused, drowsy and may vomit. It is usually brief, with full recovery.

In younger children, if you judge that the blow to the head was other than trivial, or that the concussion lasts longer or is more severe than you think reasonable, get medical advice.

If the doctor is in doubt, he or she may advise an X-ray of the head (to look for a skull fracture), and perhaps overnight observation in hospital to ensure complete recovery.

CONGENITAL ABNORMALITIES
Any abnormality present at birth. Approximately one baby in 100 is born with a significant congenital abnormality.

During the nine months of pregnancy, vast changes take place. The results of conception progress from the fertilized egg to the embryo, to the fetus to the new-born baby. Any deviation from the normal process of this development can result in a congenital abnormality.

Congenital abnormalities may arise as a result of inherited factors or environmental factors, or the interplay of the two. In most instances, no simple or single cause or explanation for the occurrence of a congenital abnormality can be found. The frequency of such abnormalities may also be affected by the age of the mother: for example, a mother over the age of 35 is more likely to have a child with DOWN SYNDROME.

Most organs are formed in the first 12 weeks after conception, so any noxious influence acting during this time may result in a congenital abnormality. Such environmental factors include:
– certain specific infections such as RUBELLA and TOXOPLASMOSIS;
– disorders of the mother's biochemistry, particularly around the time of conception, as may occur, for example, in poorly controlled DIABETES;
– rarely drugs or medicines taken by the mother (note that any drug known to affect the developing baby will be either banned completely or carry a clear warning not to be taken in preg-

nancy). See *DRUGS IN PREG-NANCY.*

– Alcohol has been shown to cause congenital abnormalities (FETAL ALCOHOL SYNDROME). The precise quantity that will have an effect is unknown, but it is likely to be a combination of the frequency and amount taken during pregnancy. Recent U.S. reports indicate even very small amounts are harmful.

– X-rays of the mother's abdomen or directly of the developing embryo may slightly but significantly enhance the chances of the child developing cancer in later life. Thus while the result is not a visible malformation, it is a congenitally abnormal predisposition. This justifies the general advice to avoid exposure to X-rays throughout pregnancy.

Damage can be done in the first few weeks of pregnancy, even before you can be sure that you are pregnant. You should avoid all risks such as alcohol, smoking, drugs and X-rays if there is any chance of your being pregnant.

If there is a history of inherited disease or congenital abnormality in your family, it is advisable to seek GENETIC COUNSELLING before you become pregnant.

Some congenital abnormalities can be diagnosed during pregnancy (PRENATAL DIAGNOSIS).

The management of a baby born with a congenital abnormality will, of course, depend on its type and severity. In some cases no treatment is needed, or a simple operation can correct the problem: as, for example, with an extra little finger. If the condition is more severe, it may be necessary to embark upon a long-term plan of stage-by-stage reconstructive surgery, as in a severe CLEFT PALATE.

CONGENITAL DISLOCATION OF THE HIP

The hip is a ball and socket joint, the socket formed by the pelvis, the ball by

CONGENITAL DISLOCATION OF THE HIP

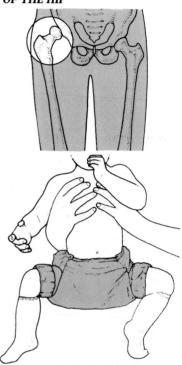

the top end of the thigh bone (the femur). If the socket is not properly formed, the femur tends to slip out – in other words to dislocate. The problem is often inherited. Girls are more commonly affected than boys, and if one girl in a family suffers from the abnormality, there is a high risk that her sisters will too.

■ SYMPTOMS All babies are checked at birth for the abnormality. In many there is a slight click as the hip is moved and the top (head) of the femur slips into the socket of the pelvis, but if the hip otherwise moves normally, it is unlikely to be dislocated.

If a child has a dislocation which was not discovered at birth or soon thereafter, this will show up when he begins to walk. He will probably walk late and may have a LIMP or an unsteady, waddling as he walks.

■ ACTION If there is a family history, tell your doctor so that particular care can be taken with the examination at birth and thereafter. Examination becomes increasingly difficult as the baby grows bigger and stronger, but he should be examined for the problem again at his monthly or bimonthly well-baby visits, so don't miss these routine checks.

If there is a click felt on examination of the hip, your doctor may suggest that the baby wear a double diaper. This holds the legs further apart than usual, keeping the head of the femur in the pelvic socket.

■ TESTS If examination suggests that there is dislocation, an X-ray of the hip is usually done to confirm this suspicion. An ULTRASOUND SCAN of the hip joint can also be used for early detection of dislocation.

■ TREATMENT If there is definite evidence of a dislocated hip, the child may have to be put in a harness or splint that keeps the head of the femur in the pelvic socket at all times. How long this will be required is determined by the natural growth of the hip joint. Eventually, the joint develops of its own accord so that it functions properly.

If dislocation is not discovered until the child is walking, traction on the leg is necessary to set the ball back into the socket, followed by a plaster cast to prevent it from coming out again. Sometimes an operation is the only option.

■ OUTLOOK If diagnosed before the child starts to walk, the problem is usually easy to manage. If dis-

covered late, ARTHRITIS may develop in the hip.

CONGENITAL HEART BLOCK
See *ARRHYTHMIAS.*

CONGENITAL HEART-DISEASE
Heart-disease that is present at birth. The heart is formed in the first 12 weeks of embryonic development. Any abnormality in this process can result in a heart that is not structurally perfect.

(Read this entry in conjunction with the general entry, HEART-DISEASE.)

■ CAUSES Usually no cause can be identified. Certain babies have a higher than average chance of having a congenital heart defect. These include: the infant of a mother with DIABETES (though the risk is higher than normal, it is still less than one case in 20); infants with CONGENITAL RUBELLA SYNDROME and with DOWN SYNDROME. Up to half of these will have a heart defect.

If you have had one child with congenital heart-disease, the chance of having another child so affected is about one in 50. If one child in a family has congenital heart-disease, it is advisable to seek GENETIC COUNSELLING to determine the risks to future children.

■ TYPES OF CONGENITAL HEART-DISEASE
Holes in the heart The common types are: ventricular septal defect, in which the hole is between the two ventricles (pumping chambers); atrial septal defect, where the defect is between the two atria (filling chambers); patent ductus arteriosus, where the blood vessel that communicates between the aorta and pulmonary artery fails to close after birth.

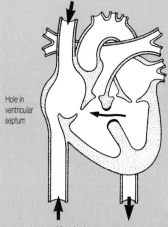

Hole in ventricular septum

Ventricular septal defect

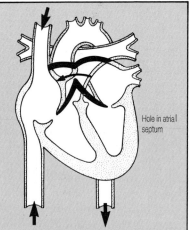

Hole in atrial septum

Atrial septal defect

CONGENITAL HEART-DISEASE

Types of congenital heart-disease: The three most common holes in the heart and (bottom) the two most basic valve abnormalities.

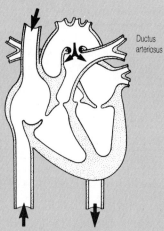

Ductus arteriosus

Patent ductus arteriosus

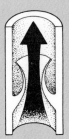

Valve opening is normal

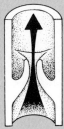

Valve opening is inadequate – stenosis

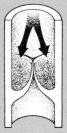

Valve closes normally

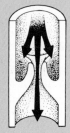

Valve closes inadequately – incompetence

Any communication between the right and left sides of the heart will result in blood passing from the high-pressure left side to the low-pressure right. If the hole is small, the amount of blood passing across will cause no problem, although a HEART MURMUR will almost always be present.

But if the hole is large, excess blood that accumulates in the right side of the heart is pumped into the lungs, resulting in increased blood flow and pressure within the arteries of the lungs. In time this causes damage to the tissues of the lung, which in turn causes pressure on the heart.

Valve abnormalities There are two basic varieties: narrowed (stenotic) valves, most commonly affecting the pulmonary and aortic valves, and leaking (incompetent valves). In this case any of the four valves in the heart may be affected (mitral, tricuspid, pulmonary or aortic).

If the valve abnormality is slight, there will be little effect on the heart, although a murmur may be heard. If the valve is severely affected, whether stenotic or incompetent, the heart has to pump harder to sustain the circulation. The extra work leads to enlargement of the heart and eventually to HEART FAILURE.

Coarctation of the aorta This is a special variant of stenosis in which the main great artery that leaves the left ventricle, the aorta, is itself narrowed beyond the site of the aortic valve. Clinical features include a heart murmur, absence or weakness of pulses to the lower half of the body coupled with high blood pressure in the upper half of the body. If severe, coarcation can lead to heart failure and will require surgical treatment.

Combinations of abnormalities, such as a hole and an abnormal valve, can occur. The effect is variable depending on the particular combination and severity. In some cases, blood containing low concentrations of oxygen passes directly from the right to the left side of the heart, and is pumped into the general circulation of the body without first going through the lungs to take up sufficient oxygen. This can result in the child appearing blue or cyanosed. Among the most common causes of this variety of cyanotic congenital heart-disease are Fallot's tetralogy and transposition of the great arteries.

▧ SYMPTOMS depend on the type and severity of the abnormality. Symptoms are not always present at birth, and if the abnormality is mild, symptoms may never develop and the only evidence of the defect may be a heart murmur (and in many instances the defect and murmur will disappear with age, especially in the case of small ventricular septal defects).

▧ ACTION If you suspect any of the symptoms above, get medical advice.

▧ TESTS See HEART-DISEASE.

▧ TREATMENT *Hole in the heart.* If the hole is small, no treatment may be required, although your child will usually be seen by a pediatric cardiologist at least once a year to ensure that there is no heart strain and to determine whether the hole is closing. If your child has a patent ductus arteriosus, he may need surgery, sometimes even in the newborn period (especially if the baby is very small or premature).

If a hole is large, medical treatment for heart failure may be required. Large holes seldom close on their own, and surgery is often necessary. A patch is usually sewn over the hole. The operation may be done during infancy, particularly if the child has symptoms of heart failure or signs that the pressure in the blood vessels of the lungs is high. *Valve abnormality*. Narrowing of the valve can be treated by stretching the valve with a flexible tube passed through a vein into the heart (cardiac catheterization); or by opening the valve surgically. This is only necessary if the narrowing is severe; milder degrees of narrowing may not require treatment.

Leaking valves can only be treated surgically. Repair, or replacement with an artificial valve, is a complicated procedure, only undertaken if the leak is severe. Drug treatment can help to improve heart function if the leak is not severe enough to require surgery.

Your child will need to see a cardiologist at intervals so that any change in the condition of the valve can be assessed.

The treatment of *combined and complex abnormalities* depends on the type and severity of the defect, and on the health and progress of your child. Heart failure is treated with drugs. If surgery is necessary, the age at which the operation takes place – and it may require a series of operations – will depend on many individual factors.

Many heart defects carry a risk of becoming infected: for example, if bacteria are released into the blood when a tooth is extracted, they can accumulate on the damaged valve and grow into a bacterial colony. For this reason most cardiologists recommend that antibiotics be given to children with certain congenital heart defects before certain procedures, especially dental treatments, are performed.

■ HEART AND HEART AND LUNG TRANSPLANTATION
There was a time when treatment of severe kidney disease in children by kidney transplantation seemed cavalier and experimental. Not so today. It seems likely that over the next decade some types of serious complex congenital heart-disease may also be treated by transplantation.

■ LONG-TERM MANAGEMENT and OUTLOOK
See HEART-DISEASE.

CONGENITAL INFECTION
See *RUBELLA, TOXOPLASMOSIS, CYTOMEGALOVIRUS.*

CONJUNCTIVITIS
An inflammation of the conjunctiva, the thin lining of the inside of the eyelid and over the front of the eyeball.

■ CAUSES Usually an INFECTION either by BACTERIA or VIRUSES, but it can also result from irritation of the eye by a foreign body, chemicals, trauma or an ALLERGY.

■ SYMPTOMS The eye is red and watery, and feels sore and itchy. There may be a discharge. Sometimes the eyelids are stuck together with yellow pus. The eyelids may look puffy.

■ TREATMENT Bathe the eye area frequently with water-soaked cotton balls to remove the pus and keep it clean. Search for any irritant particle. If found, it should be removed carefully – see EYE, FOREIGN BODY IN. In mild cases this may be the cure. If the symptoms continue, the eye is swollen or the child has a FEVER, get medical advice. If your doctor thinks the conjunctivitis is

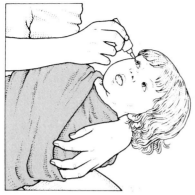

CONJUNCTIVITIS
Wrapping child tightly in towel helps keep him still when applying eye ointment or drops.

due to a bacterial infection, ANTI-BIOTIC eye drops or ointment may be prescribed. Putting drops or ointment into a child's eye can be difficult – see the illustration. There is no specific treatment for a viral infection of the eye.

The redness and itching may be caused by an allergy. This is likely to be a recurrent problem; in which case the allergen may be recognizable and should be avoided. Antihistamines taken orally may help.

Note: Do not confuse conjunctivitis with CELLULITIS OF THE EYE, a much more serious medical problem. If in doubt about the diagnosis, see your doctor.

■ OUTLOOK A seven-day course of antibiotics usually clears a bacterial conjunctivitis. Viral conjunctivitis usually clears spontaneously in a few days.

CONSTIPATION
True constipation is defined as excessively infrequent and dry BOWEL MOVEMENTS leading to pain on defecation or SOILING. Control of bowel movements is achieved by most children by three years of age.

Bowel movements may be in-fluenced by a number of factors. Inadequate fiber in the diet may be associated with hard bowel movements. A previous ANAL FISSURE may have resulted in pain on passing stools and subsequent constipation. Uncommonly, a simple external congenital narrowing (anal stenosis) may prevent the passage of stools. Constipation tends to be self-perpetuating since large, hard stools are often painful to pass leading to accumulation of large stools and injury to the anus (anal fissure) when they are passed.

The constipated child may suffer rectal bleeding and pass exceptionally large stools. Severe degrees of constipation may indicate HIRSCHPRUNG DISEASE. Inappropriate TOILET TRAINING (undertaken too early or with undue emphasis) and negative behavior can be factors in a pattern in which constipation also plays a part. A further factor may be the child who is too busy at school or play to take the time to go to the bathroom.

■ SYMPTOMS Withholding of stools and continuous distension of the rectum leading to a reduction in the normal urge to defecate: stools may be retained for several days. Liquid feces may escape past the hard stool to stain the underwear and there may be ABDOMINAL SWELLING.

■ ACTION If a child has hard, infrequent stools and difficulty having a bowel movement, get medical advice. Your doctor will ask questions about the child's diet, and try to establish whether there is an underlying bowel disorder, BEHAVIORAL DISORDER or other contributing cause.

Occasionally, referral to a pediatric gastroenterologist may be necessary.

■ INVESTIGATIONS General

examination may show abdominal swelling, with hard stools felt in the bowel. Often, however, these signs are not so obvious. The anus may be normal or appear to be pushed out. Examination of the rectum by the doctor may identify firm motions or, very occasionally, a tightness suggesting Hirschprung disease.

Abdominal X-ray will determine the extent of the constipation. A barium ENEMA may show a distended bowel above a narrowed segment in Hirschprung disease.

■ TREATMENT In most cases of constipation no underlying cause (such as Hirschprung disease) is found. Thus treatment is based upon bowel habit training. Helping the parents and child understand the process of digestion and bowel action can give results. Laxative agents to soften and clear the hard stools may be necessary in the early stages, although often added dietary fiber is enough.

A regular pattern of toilet training, particularly after meals, is important. A child-size toilet seat may make the young child feel more secure. Rewarding success by means of using a chart that indicates success by placing a gold star on it for every bowel movement made can provide positive reinforcement.

A child with marked problems may require oral mineral oil given two hours after meals to help soften the stool. It may take several days or weeks for this to work and may need to be continued for a long period of time until normal bowel habits are acquired. An anal fissure will need regular applications of anesthetic creams to stop the pain and allow the bowels to move normally.

Laxative agents may have to be continued for some weeks, and the distended bowel will need to return to its normal size before adequate bowel movements occur. Even after stopping laxatives, they may need to be used intermittently until regular bowel habits are established. Prolonged laxative use should only be continued under the supervision of your doctor. Surgery is necessary for anal stenosis and Hirschprung disease.

A psychiatrist's opinion or family therapy may be considered when the child is using constipation and soiling as a means of upsetting the family or drawing attention to his problems.

■ OUTLOOK depends on the cause. Surgical problems can usually be corrected. Dietary changes, laxatives and toilet training will help many children. When constipation is part of a behavioral problem, improvement may take a long time.

CONVULSIONS

Also described as fits, seizures or EPI-LEPTIC attacks, these are states of altered consciousness or behavior associated with involuntary stiffening/jerking (tonic/clonic) movements. They can affect the whole body (generalized) or only part of the body (focal) and are caused by transient, disorderly electrical activity in the brain. They are relatively common: one child in 20 suffers at least one seizure during childhood.

The essence of a convulsion is involuntary movement; but not all epileptic attacks are convulsive.

■ SYMPTOMS Twitching or jerking with associated states of mental confusion, stomach pains; dizziness or visual disturbances such as flashing lights. In some children, an aura (a warning sign such as strange tastes in the mouth or unusual smells) or focal seizures may precede a generalized convulsion.

Convulsions need to be distinguished from FAINTING, when the heart slows or stops; from OVER-BREATHING associated with ANXIETY; from BREATH HOLDING; from vertigo (a spinning sensation); from NIGHT TERRORS, shaking chills that occur with high FEVER, TANTRUMS and psychological attacks.

■ ACTION A child having a generalized convulsion should be placed in the RECOVERY POSITION until he awakens. With a focal convulsion, he should be kept safe and quiet until it passes. Rush the child to hospital if the convulsion continues for more than five minutes. The child should be transported in the recovery position. In any case, call a doctor once the child has recovered, unless he is a known epileptic.

■ CAUSES Between the ages of five and 15 years, convulsions can be provoked by flashing lights, looking at television or moving patterns, or light on the surface of the water. They can also be started by sudden high fever in infants aged six months to five years – FEBRILE CONVULSIONS. All of these may cease by themselves in later years. See also EPILEPSY. Convulsions can also be caused by genetic or biochemical disorders, brain malformation or BRAIN DAMAGE.

■ TREATMENT If convulsions are recurrent, prolonged or severe, they can be treated with anti-epileptic drugs. See *EPILEPSY*.

■ OUTLOOK Despite their disturbing aspects, convulsions are usually not harmful unless prolonged or frequent. There may be an epilepsy association in your area; give them a call – these organizations often have valuable information to help you cope with problems such as this.

CORONARY ARTERY DISEASE
Damage to heart muscle caused by blockage of the coronary arteries. Rare during childhood.

■ CAUSES are not always clear, but there are a number of risk factors that are thought to be important.

A diet consistently high in animal fats may raise the fat level of the blood (HYPERLIPIDEMIA), but probably only in those with a genetic predisposition. Hyperlipidemia is associated with an increased risk of coronary artery disease.

Cigarette smoking is known to be associated with damage to the coronary arteries.

OBESITY is an additional risk factor for coronary artery disease.

Coronary artery disease can be inherited. Certain types of hyperlipidemia are passed on as a dominant GENE, and appear in half the children of an affected parent. In these cases, coronary artery disease may appear early in adult life.

DIABETES and HYPERTENSION predispose to coronary artery disease.

■ ACTION Prevention is best. Although much remains to be learned about the precise risks and mechanisms involved, it is prudent to advise parents and children to avoid too much animal fat in their diet, not to smoke cigarettes, to avoid obesity and to exercise regularly, especially if there is a family history of coronary artery disease in young adults.

■ TESTS If there is a history of coronary artery disease occurring in young adults in the family, discuss with your doctor the possibility of BLOOD TESTS to check for the presence of familial hyperlipidemia.

■ TREATMENT If fat levels in the

blood are high, a low-fat diet plus certain medications are recommended that may succeed in lowering the level of fat in the blood.

■ OUTLOOK This is one of the most common causes of premature death in the developed world. International statistics suggest that lifestyle can influence the disease.

COUGH
The mechanism by which mucus or other foreign material is expelled from the passages of the lungs.

■ CAUSES Mucus may be produced in the nose and throat, as in COMMON COLD or HAY FEVER; or in the chest, as in ASTHMA, PNEUMONIA, CYSTIC FIBROSIS, or in TUBERCULOSIS.

■ SYMPTOMS depend on whether the mucus is produced in the nose or in the chest. If in the nose, it drains down the throat into the airways and the cough will be associated with a runny or blocked nose or sneezing, and is often worse at night. If produced in the chest, the cough may be associated with wheezing, rapid breathing, or other sounds in the chest.

■ ACTION A cough, in itself, can be treated by two entirely different types of medication:
– If the cough is caused by excess mucus production in the nose, it can be reduced by a decongestant or, in the case of hay fever, a specific anti-allergic preparation. It is important for the child to blow his nose regularly to minimize the amount of mucus draining into the throat.
– If the cough is caused by excess mucus production in the chest, medications may help to loosen the mucus and make it easier to cough up in some diseases. For example,

drugs such as bronchodilators not only ease breathing in asthma but allow mucus to be more easily coughed up. Chest physiotherapy and postural drainage with a directed cough may facilitate mucus clearance in cystic fibrosis.

A dry, unproductive cough may be caused by thick mucus in the chest. DEHYDRATION can make the secretions thicker, so encourage your child to drink plenty of clear fluids.
– If a dry cough is being caused simply by irritation in the throat, it can be suppressed, but cough suppressants are rarely necessary in children, and should only be used when there is no mucus in the chest and if the cough is exhausting the child and preventing him from sleeping. Cough suppressants are not appropriate for children with cystic fibrosis or asthma.

■ GET MEDICAL ADVICE if:
– a cough is accompanied by FEVER that lasts for more than a few days.
– the cough is associated with rapid breathing or shortness of breath.
– the mucus coughed up is green, yellow or contains blood.
– there is pain in the chest on coughing. See CHEST PAIN.
– the cough continues for more than ten days.
– your child has recently choked on something which could have been inhaled into the chest. See FOREIGN BODY ASPIRATION.

■ TREATMENT 1 Decongestants and anti-allergic medications usually contain antihistamines, and may cause drowsiness or irritability as side-effects. They should not be used for more than one week at a time. See HAY FEVER and ASTHMA. They also dry up secretions and should *not* be used in cystic fibrosis. **2** Expectorants and mucolytics are supposed to 'loosen' mucus, but there is little evidence to support their use. **3** Bronchodilators dilate the airways, making it easier to cough up mucus. They are used for asthma. **4** Cough suppressants such as codeine act on the cough center in the brain and suppress the cough. They should not be given to young children, or those with asthma or cystic fibrosis. **5** ANTIBIOTICS are seldom necessary as the most common causes of cough are VIRAL infection and allergy. **6** If foreign body aspiration is suspected, a bronchoscopy may be necessary. See *FOREIGN BODY ASPIRATION*.

■ TESTS If a cough persists, or if there are signs of chest infection, lung function tests (see *ASTHMA*) or an X-ray of the chest may be necessary. It is difficult to obtain a sputum specimen in a child, but if this is possible it can be tested.

■ LONG-TERM MANAGEMENT Chronic cough caused by hay fever, asthma and cystic fibrosis are discussed under the separate entries.

■ OUTLOOK Most coughs get better without treatment.

COW'S MILK ALLERGY

Intolerance of cow's milk protein affects primarily the gastro-intestinal tract, but also involves other organs of the body, some of which produce severe symptoms. It is not uncommon, but usually resolves by two years of age. Easily confused with LACTOSE INTOLERANCE.

■ SYMPTOMS There is a wide range, related to different organ systems in the body. Acute symptoms can be severe enough to cause SHOCK, general swelling as a result of excess fluid (angioneurotic EDEMA), URTICARIA, or VOMITING and acute DIARRHEA associated with DEHYDRATION – although these symptoms are more likely to be due to infective GASTROENTERITIS.

Babies who have early acute symptoms are likely to have a family history of ALLERGY – as may other members of their family, and will often later develop ASTHMA and ECZEMA.

Usually the effects of cow's milk allergy are gradual and consist of MALABSORPTION, persistent diarrhea, COLIC, ABDOMINAL SWELLING, FAILURE TO THRIVE, gastrointestinal bleeding and low protein levels in the blood. Diarrhea is of variable severity and is due to an immune reaction in the lining (the mucosa) of the small intestine, which may be a primary effect, or may occur after gastroenteritis, which leads to mucosa damage and intolerance to cow's milk.

The loose bowel movements contain blood, seen directly, or under a microscope. In the primary type, a milk-induced colitis (see ULCERATIVE COLITIS) can develop, with frequent stools containing mucus and fresh blood. Sometimes the baby vomits blood (hematemesis), or has iron deficiency ANEMIA. Excessive gastro-intestinal protein loss can occur with subsequent edema and MALNUTRITION, but this is rare. Symptoms can occur in breast-fed babies because of the presence of cow's milk protein in the mother's diet passing to the baby through her breast milk.

■ ACTION If symptoms suggest cow's milk allergy, discuss the baby's diet with your doctor; a change of milk may be considered.

■ INVESTIGATIONS The doctor who investigates the problem will want to know about any links between symptoms and feeding changes; gastroenteritis; and any family history of allergy. The baby will need a thorough examination to exclude INFECTION and to look for allergic manifestations such as asthma or eczema. The diagnosis is based on clinical criteria: there is no reliable laboratory test.

Internal examination of the colon is sometimes necessary and may reveal inflammation and ulceration. The main investigation, however, is a trial period with no cow's milk in the diet, giving instead alternative types of milk. Subsequent careful challenge with feeding a small amount of cow's milk, usually under supervision in a hospital, will be necessary.

■ TREATMENT Avoiding cow's milk in any form is, of course, the mainstay of the treatment. A dietician will help devise a workable new diet, often incorporating soya milk.

■ OUTLOOK Cautious reintroduction of cow's milk protein, starting with small amounts, and building up over a few days, can be considered, usually after the first birthday. A few children remain intolerant well after their first year. In some children, sensitivity to soya protein may also occur, in which case other milk formulae will have to be found. Babies whose families have a strong history of allergy and who are breast-fed may benefit from the mother excluding cow's milk and other dairy products from her diet.

CRADLE CAP
A common scalp problem in early infancy, consisting of thick scales that mesh with the hair to form a mat that covers all or part of the scalp.

■ SYMPTOMS None – the appearance is the only problem.

■ ACTION Frequent (at least daily) careful but firm washing of the hair, using a baby shampoo, will prevent cradle cap from forming, and can clear a mild cradle cap. When the build-up of scales is excessive, olive oil applied to the affected areas of the scalp and allowed to remain for eight or more hours (usually overnight) will gradually loosen the scales. There is no need to be afraid of injuring the soft part of a baby's head (fontanelle) while washing the scalp.

■ GET MEDICAL ADVICE if the cradle cap does not clear with these simple measures. Occasionally it can be a sign of another skin disease, such as ECZEMA or PSORIASIS.

■ TREATMENT Occasionally a simple cream to soften the scales is needed if the olive oil has not worked.

■ OUTLOOK Provided the baby's head is washed properly, cradle cap should not recur. Occasionally it is the first sign of seborrhea, a chronic skin condition characterized by a dry, scaling, red skin RASH.

CRAMP
Involuntary muscle spasm. It can be caused by exercise, particularly if warm-up exercises have not been done; if muscles are tensed to an exceptional degree; or if there is a deficiency of salt or other minerals in the blood. Often enough there is no apparent cause. Cramps often occur at night.

Gentle massage of the muscle will gradually ease the spasm . Children don't usually have severe cramp, but if they recur frequently, get medical advice.

CRETINISM
See *HYPOTHYROIDISM.*

CROHN DISEASE
An uncommon chronic inflammatory disease of the bowel that may affect any area of the intestinal tract, from the mouth to the anus, but most commonly concentrated in the lower end of the small bowel. The cause is unknown.

■ SYMPTOMS depend on how much bowel is involved and the degree of inflammation. They include:
ABDOMINAL PAIN, which may be acute and similar to APPENDICITIS; or intermittent and chronic. The pain is most often mainly in the right lower abdomen and can become worse on defecation. COLIC may occur from partial small INTESTINAL OBSTRUCTION.

DIARRHEA: mild and intermittent. Occasionally there is blood and mucus in the stools.

FEVER: frequent in Crohn disease in childhood; sometimes associated with ARTHRITIS or pain in the joints. Abdominal bloating, lethargy and fatigue may also occur.

ANOREXIA; poor APPETITE AND WEIGHT LOSS can occur, and over a long time this can be associated with growth retardation.

There may also be a lump (mass) in the lower right-hand side of the abdomen that a doctor can feel during his examination. There may be ulcers, abscesses, fissures or skin tags around the anus. Communicating channels (fistulas) may develop between the bowel and the skin near the anus. MOUTH ULCERS may de-velop. Rarely, a skin rash may be present and associated eye inflammation (uveitis).

■ INVESTIGATIONS BLOOD TEST. Examination of the bowel often under sedation, with biopsy of the bowel lining and the peri-anal skin, helps confirm the diagnosis. A barium enema and small bowel barium examination may show the extent of the disease. Checks on blood VITAMIN and hemoglobin levels and stool culture may be done. The erythrocyte sedimentation rate (ESR) blood test measures the degree of inflammation.

■ TREATMENT A high-calorie diet. In more severe cases, feeding of easily digested liquid food through a tube passed into the stomach, or intravenous feeding, may be required initially along with mineral supplements. Anti-inflammatory drugs such as prednisone and salicylazo-sulfapyridine can help. There are some side-effects with this treatment, especially from steroids (prednisone).

Other immunosuppressive drugs such as azathioprine may be needed if the response to steroids is poor.

Surgery may be necessary to deal with a peri-anal abscess or fistula, intestinal obstruction and other associated problems. This may include removal of portions of the bowel.

■ OUTLOOK Crohn disease is an upsetting, chronic problem with frequent recurrences even with therapy. However, the long-term outlook for most children is usually good.

CROSSED EYE
See *STRABISMUS.*

CROUP

The noisy cough younger children have with an INFECTION of the larynx, or the tissues around it.

■ CAUSES are VIRUSES, such as para-influenza viruses. Rarely, a BACTERIUM, *Hemophilus influenzae* causes a very serious form of croup called EPIGLOTTITIS. In the U.S. children are given a protective injection against this bacterium around the second birthday.

■ INCIDENCE Viral croup is usually a noisy manifestation of widerspread infection called LARYNGO-TRACHEO-BRONCHITIS. This is common, usually occurring in spring and fall. Once a child has had an attack, he is a little more likely to have further bouts of croup. Epiglottitis, while relatively rare, is very serious and if neglected can become life threatening over a period of hours.

■ SYMPTOMS The cough sounds like the bark of a sea-lion. In simple (viral) croup there may be no other symptoms, but the child will often have a runny nose and hoarse voice, or cry. Some children also have a FEVER, and seem generally unwell. The cough is often worse at night. If the croup is more severe, there will be noisy breathing, or STRIDOR. In epiglottitis, in addition to croup, the child is generally ill, looks toxic, is feverish, has difficulty in swallowing saliva (hence drools), and has distressed breathing with a heaving chest and drawing in of the space under the ribs.

■ ACTION For simple croup, fluids and acetamenophen will generally comfort the child and reduce the temperature. Some children may benefit from inhaling steam. You

may be able to provide this in the bathroom by running the hot water. Other children respond well to cool air out of doors or through a window.

■ GET MEDICAL ADVICE if your child has difficulty in breathing or swallowing, or if he becomes drowsy or distressed.

■ TREATMENT Antibiotics are not usually indicated since simple croup is caused by a virus. Children with severe laryngo-tracheo-bronchitis normally require admission to hospital for observation and treatment. Any child suspected of having epiglottitis must go to hospital as an emergency. See *EPIGLOTTITIS*.

■ OUTLOOK Even after a severe attack of viral croup, children recover fully and quickly. Although the croupy cough tends to recur, this becomes less common as their throats grow larger, and is rare after about five years.

CRYING

The universal dilemma of parenthood: is the baby (or toddler) crying because of some definite problem that ought to be corrected, or just because babies will cry?

The possible causes are perhaps best divided into three categories: **1** When there is no illness or injury: If the child has no obvious signs of illness or injury, crying can be due to discomfort, hunger, boredom, fatigue, fear, sadness, loneliness or frustration. **2** With minor illness, crying can be due to COLIC, TEETHING, FEVER or a COMMON COLD. **3** With definite disease, crying can be due to EARACHE, HEADACHE, SORE THROAT, MENINGITIS, other INFECTION or severe pain, typically ABDOMINAL PAIN.

■ ACTION If the child has no obvious signs of illness or injury, and can be pacified by food or other attention, it is reasonable to assume that the crying is not due to a major disease.

Anxiety on your part can be sensed by your baby and this can make him more irritable, so try to remain calm. Young babies need human contact, so don't hesitate to pick him up and cuddle him.

If you think the baby has colic, is teething or feels generally ill because of a common cold, a painkiller such as acetamenophen may ease the discomfort. In babies under three months of age this should only be given on a doctor's advice. See also *FEVER*.

If your child continues to cry, some undetected illness or injury should be suspected. A young child cannot localize pain well, and earache and stomach-ache can give the same apparent symptoms. If you remain uncertain, get medical advice.

Your child cannot injure himself by crying, but prolonged, intensive crying can make him vomit.

CURVATURE OF THE SPINE
See *SCOLIOSIS*.

CUSHING DISEASE
See *ADRENAL DISORDERS*.

CUTS AND ABRASIONS
■ ACTION Clean cuts and abrasions as soon as they happen, simply by rinsing them with water. This is the key to treatment because it painlessly and efficiently removes dirt, and with it the likelihood of INFECTION. Clean the surrounding skin with water applied with a clean wash cloth, paper towel or cotton ball. If you have a suitable antiseptic liquid or spray-on antiseptic, this may be applied to the wound. Some of these agents sting and may cause your child to cry out. Comfort the child afterwards. Don't dislodge any blood clots that form. To dry, pat gently. If bleeding does not stop, apply firm pressure over the wound. This stops bleeding by flattening the blood vessels in the area of the wound. Blood flows more slowly and encourages clots to form. Be prepared to keep up the pressure for five to 15 minutes. If something is buried in the wound, apply pressure beside and around it. If the wound is in an arm or leg or a hand or foot, raising it may reduce bleeding by reducing local blood circulation. Cover the wound with a sterile dressing.

■ GO TO THE HOSPITAL if there is glass debris or a foreign body in the wound: removing such material is best performed by a trained person. Large, jagged or gaping wounds will also need the attention of a doctor, preferably at your local hospital emergency room.

■ OUTLOOK Is the child IMMUNE to TETANUS? If not, get medical advice, even if the wound appears 'clean'.

CYSTIC FIBROSIS
An uncommon, chronic INHERITED DISORDER consisting of repeated chest INFECTIONS and MALABSORPTION with FAILURE TO THRIVE. There is excess salt in the sweat and thick mucus in the lungs and pancreas.

Incidence: one in 2,500 births.

■ CAUSE An unidentified abnormality of the cells, possibly also a deficiency of certain proteins and abnormal cellular salt transfer. This leads to production of thick secretions that block the ducts of the pancreas, lungs liver and other organs. The problems occur from birth and eventually lead to degeneration with fibrosis of parts of these organs.

■ SYMPTOMS Bowel problems: Sticky MECONIUM stools in infancy may obstruct the bowel (meconium ileus). The baby may vomit bile and have ABDOMINAL SWELLING. Similar symptoms can occur in an older child (meconium ileus equivalent). There may be RECTAL PROLAPSE in an older child, although cystic fibrosis is not frequently associated with this.

FAILURE TO THRIVE: Blockage of the pancreatic ducts prevents release of enzymes which are necessary for food digestion.

Repeated chest infections: The child has more frequent and more prolonged colds and eventually a frequent, productive cough with thick yellow to green sputum. There may be associated VOMITING. PNEUMONIA and chest infections with certain BACTERIA may require management in the hospital. The child may also develop wheezing and increased shortness of breath when exercising. The area below the finger-nail beds becomes swollen (clubbing). With more severe lung disease a cyst may burst and leak air into the chest cavity and cause partial collapse of that lung (pneumothorax). This causes chest pain and more shortness of breath.

Abdominal problems: The obstruction of the pancreas will lead to fibrosis which, if severe, may also stop insulin production. The child may then develop DIABETES MELLITUS, usually from adolescence onwards. Fibrosis (CIRRHOSIS) of the liver will cause back pressure on the blood in the veins to the liver. This in turn may cause distension of the veins around the esophagus (var-ices) and this can make the child vomit blood. As a result of the liver cirrhosis, the spleen may become enlarged due to the back pressure.

Cardiac complications: Fibrosis in the lungs will restrict the blood flow from the heart. Increased pressure in the lung circulation may lead to heart strain and eventually to HEART FAILURE, which will be associated with increasing BREATHLESSNESS and swelling of the feet and ankles. There may be FAILURE TO THRIVE in the later stages.

Fertility: Most males with cystic fibrosis are sterile because of fibrosis and blockage of the tube that carries sperm from the testes to the penis. Females are fertile but may have thicker than normal cervical and vaginal muscles.

■ INVESTIGATIONS A sweat test can reveal abnormal salt content, giving a firm diagnosis. An X-ray of the chest showing scattered areas of acute and chronic infection may suggest the diagnosis. Raised levels of fat in the stool and excess trypsin in the blood, may be helpful indicators when screening infants. Measuring pancreatic enzymes in intestinal fluids obtained by passing a tube into the small bowel (duodenal intubation), may also be helpful.

■ MANAGEMENT Use of pancreatic enzyme preparations regularly with meals to aid digestion. High calorie diet with VITAMIN supplements.

Appropriate ANTIBIOTIC treatment, possibly long-term.

Special chest physiotherapy to help the child cough up the secretions.

INHALERS and treatment for bronchospasm if the child is wheezy.

For bowel obstruction in an infant or older child, clear away sticky bowel contents, preferably using special fluids either orally, via a nasogastric tube and/or by ENEMAS or surgery.

Treatment for diabetes; appropriate management for cirrhosis and vomiting blood.

Diuretic drugs to help remove extra fluid in heart failure.

Most children in the United States who have cystic fibrosis are cared for in regional clinics that specialize in this disease. Adult clinics are now being developed because of the increased survival of patients with cystic fibrosis.

▓ OUTLOOK Although children with cystic fibrosis are now surviving with normal intellect into adult life, their life span is considerably reduced. Treatment of lung infection and maintenance of good nutrition help to keep them as well as possible. Heart/lung transplantation is now being tried, with some success, in those with severely affected lungs.

Most males will be sterile, but girls can produce normal babies.

If a family has one child with cystic fibrosis, the risk of a further child having cystic fibrosis is one in four. The condition can be diagnosed during pregnancy by sampling tissue from the fetus.

Much research is being conducted to discover the basic defect in this disease and to find better treatments to prolong survival.

CYSTITIS
See *URINARY TRACT INFECTION.*

CYTOMEGALOVIRUS INFECTION
A common VIRAL INFECTION. Older children and adults usually have a mild form that may pass unnoticed. If it occurs during pregnancy it can be transmitted from mother to baby (congenital cytomegalovirus infection), causing serious illness.

▓ SYMPTOMS OF CONGENITAL INFECTION Congenitally infected babies may be asymptomatic at birth if the infection is mild. More severe infection may cause LOW BIRTH WEIGHT, an enlarged liver and spleen, JAUNDICE and ANEMIA.

MENTAL HANDICAP can occur, but if the signs are not marked, this may only be noticed later in childhood. Inflammation of the eye can lead to BLINDNESS. Some babies can carry the virus without it causing significant problems.

▓ SYMPTOMS OF INFECTION ACQUIRED AFTER BIRTH FEVER, COUGH, HEADACHES and muscle pains may mimic infectious mononucleosis, but the infection may also be asymptomatic. Some children, especially those with reduced immunity such as leukemia, may have more severe infections with HEPATITIS and/or PNEUMONIA. Premature babies may develop pneumonia if infected with cytomegalovirus in the new-born period, but they do not have all the serious complications seen in congenitally infected babies.

▓ TESTS URINE and BLOOD TESTS confirm the diagnosis.

▓ TREATMENT None effective.

▓ OUTLOOK In congenital infection, this depends on the severity of the infection. A mother who has had a congenitally infected baby may have problems with another pregnancy, but the next infant usually has a much milder disease.

Most infants and children who are infected with cytomegalovirus after birth have no long-term problems.

D

DARK URINE

The color of the urine varies with its concentration. Urine formed during the night is more concentrated, and therefore looks darker than daytime urine. Urine that has been standing for a while may become cloudy, and this may look similar to the 'smoky' color caused by NEPHRITIS. Red candies, certain antibiotics and sometimes beets make the urine red. Occasionally a viral infection of the bladder causes bleeding into the urine (HEMATURIA).

If you are worried or suspect there is blood in your child's urine, take a sample to your doctor to be tested.

DEADLY NIGHTSHADE

See *POISONING*.

DEAFNESS

The medical description for any loss of hearing, mild or severe. There are two main types of deafness: conductive, when there is obstruction of the outer ear canal or disease of the eardrum or the middle ear that prevent the passage of sound from the outside to the sensitive inner ear; and perceptive, when the problem lies in the inner ear itself, with the nerve connecting the inner ear to the brain or with the hearing-receptive part of the brain.

■ CAUSES Perceptive, or nerve deafness, is commonly present from birth, and may be due to a variety of causes, especially birth injury or congenital RUBELLA. Babies and older children are routinely checked for hearing at well-baby clinics, by their doctor and in school. It may also be caused by certain VIRAL INFECTIONS and bacterial MENINGITIS in childhood, or by certain drugs. Conductive deafness is usually due to an obstruction in the sound pathway, such as MIDDLE EAR INFECTION or GLUE EAR; and, most commonly, by WAX IN EARS.

■ SYMPTOMS vary according to the child's age. Young babies will normally 'startle' at a loud noise. As they get older, normal babies respond in many ways to even the faintest sounds, such as a carer moving quietly round the room, or talking softly; deaf babies, on the other hand, may be startled by suddenly *seeing* someone beside the crib. Once a child is beginning to understand speech – say at two to two-and-a-half years old – you can test his hearing by whispering to him, but remaining out of sight.

Hearing is necessary for the development of speech: deaf children do not learn to speak, while partially deaf children are delayed in developing their speech. Older children who develop deafness may lose interest in school, and may be wrongly labelled 'backward'.

■ ACTION If you suspect your baby

does not hear, tell your family doctor or pediatrician during the baby's check-up visit. Even young infants can be tested for hearing loss. If you suspect that your child's speech is not developing like other children's (see *SPEECH DISORDERS*), you should consult your doctor. He can refer you to an ear doctor or to a hearing specialist. Early detection and treatment are essential to minimize developmental delays. Children who have had repeated middle ear infections should be checked for hearing loss and they should be monitored until they recover. Before school entry any child with speech difficulties should see a hearing specialist for thorough assessment.

■ TESTS If severe congenital deafness is suspected in a baby, audiometric and electrical tests are done to measure how much hearing and at what frequencies (pitch) it is present. These tests are also used to assess what sort of hearing aid will be best for the child. In older children, hearing can be assessed either by pure tone AUDIOMETRY, or by impedance audiometry, or by using spoken words in a specially fitted room.

■ TREATMENT The sooner you help a severely or totally deaf child with his hearing or communication problems, the better. It is essential to try to understand his difficulties. You may have to help him adapt to a hearing aid, and go through special training in sign language and lip reading. Conductive deafness due to glue ear is often temporary, but if it persists, ear tubes may have to be inserted. If the conductive deafness is due to a perforated eardrum, usually following middle ear infection, surgical repair of the drum may be re-

quired after the infection has completely cleared.

■ LONG-TERM MANAGEMENT Hearing aid technology continues to improve, and deaf children now have a better chance than ever before of receiving their education in regular schools.

A child may take time getting used to a hearing aid, but it is worth persevering. It is important that deaf children receive as 'normal' an education as possible, and mix with hearing children to help their integration into society as adults.

For the profoundly deaf child, sign language provides an important tool for learning and communicating. Using sign language may enable many children to progress at a normal rate. Thus, in some cases, special educational help may be helpful and is often available within the regular school system.

DEHYDRATION
Caused by loss of body fluids, as in severe DIARRHEA and VOMITING. The danger is that the circulating blood volume may be reduced, with a fall in BLOOD PRESSURE. This can, if not corrected quickly, result in life-threatening SHOCK.

■ SYMPTOMS to watch for in a child with severe diarrhea or vomiting: thirst – a typical response to early dehydration, but one that is not always obvious in infants, especially if the baby is generally ill and vomiting; passing less urine than usual – a sign that the body is having to conserve fluid; eyes looking sunken; dry mouth and tongue; shallow breathing and general weakness; rapid pulse rate.

■ ACTION Dehydration requires prompt action to replace body

water. See GASTROENTERITIS. With severe dehydration in a child who is unable to drink fluids, hospitalization and intravenous fluids may be needed.

In common gastroenteritis of childhood, dehydration can usually be avoided by giving oral rehydration fluids. These are available from the drugstore or supermarket, or can be made up according to instructions from your doctor. This therapy can succeed, even in the presence of continuing diarrhea and some degree of vomiting.

■ OUTLOOK Given prompt treatment, the child will have no long-term ill effects.

DELIRIUM, DELIRIOUS CHILD

An old-fashioned term for the confusion a child may experience in association with a high FEVER, as in TONSILLITIS and lobar PNEUMONIA. The child may cry out or scream while half-awake and appear highly disturbed. Nowadays, fevers are usually treated quickly and effectively with sponging and antipyretic drugs such as acetamenophen. As a result delirium is uncommon and short lasting.

For action and treatment, see FEVER.

DEPRESSION

Children, like adults, have sad and tearful moods in response to frustration, disappointment or failure. A child may be suffering from depression only if such episodes occur without external provocation, are frequent and long-lasting, and are accompanied by other symptoms (see below). Before adolescence, it is unusual for children to complain explicitly that they are depressed.

■ CAUSES Any big change, especially if this involves losing a valued close relationship (be it a relative, a friend, even a pet), can initiate a period of sadness. Parental unhappiness, worries or discord can also cause unhappiness in a child. However, the term depression implies something deeper and longer-lasting, usually against a background of previous episodes of feeling low.

■ SYMPTOMS Tearful, unhappy moods that seem to arise spontaneously or for trivial reasons; irritability; problems with concentration; a falling off in performance of school work (this can be an effect as well as a cause). Awkward, obstinate and/or bad behavior may also be part of the picture, as may poor sleeping patterns and a change in appetite.

■ ACTION Obviously you will try to identify what may be upsetting your child, and talk to him about it. This is an important step, which may be quite difficult with a teenage child. Young children often feel responsible for things that are not their fault: for example, if a parent has been ill, the child may think he has caused it with his bad behavior. See also *BEREAVEMENT* and *DIVORCE*. However, it is not always clear to the parents or child himself what may have initiated the depressive state. Talk to your doctor if the change lasts longer than a few weeks, or if the symptoms are worsening.

■ TREATMENT Your doctor may feel that the help of a child psychiatrist or psychologist is needed. Such problems are often best dealt with by family therapy, even if only one member appears to be affected. Antidepressant drugs are rarely used, but they can be helpful, even in young children. Your doctor may also want to consider whether the depression could be a symptom of an underlying physical illness.

DERMATITIS
Literally, this means 'inflamed skin'. The term is commonly used when inflammation or irritation of the skin occurs from any cause. ECZEMA and other forms of ALLERGIC skin disease are the commonest causes.

▩ CAUSES There are two main types: irritant dermatitis, and contact dermatitis. Irritant dermatitis is caused by the direct action of chemicals on the skin – a common example is DIAPER RASH, where the irritant is ammonia, formed by the breakdown of urine. Contact dermatitis is an allergic reaction to a substance which has been in contact with the skin. One of the commonest is nickel, the metal found in bracelets, necklaces and watch bands, but there are many other substances that cause this kind of allergic rash.

▩ SYMPTOMS The skin becomes red and feels sore or itchy. In more severe forms, blisters and cracks are seen. The rash is limited to the area in contact with the irritant or allergy-producing substance.

▩ ACTION If the cause can be identified, simply removing it and avoiding further contact may solve the problem. Simple soothing creams, or mild hydrocortisone cream (obtainable from the drugstore) will relieve the itching.

▩ GET MEDICAL ADVICE if the rash persists, or if you cannot identify a cause.

▩ TESTS If a child with contact dermatitis is referred to a dermatologist or allergist, tests can be done to find out what substances might be causing it. Patches containing various chemicals and other irritants are applied to the child's skin. Allergy is shown by a red reaction to the patch.

▩ TREATMENT Once a cause is found, care must be taken to avoid it. Sometimes the allergy is one of the common constituents of skin creams, such as lanolin.

▩ OUTLOOK Children who have allergic rashes after contact with certain substances are likely to have other forms of allergy, and may have some allergic symptoms throughout life. Many, however, will grow out of it.

DEVELOPMENTAL DELAY
See 'NORMAL' DEVELOPMENT.

DIABETES MELLITUS
A disorder resulting from insulin deficiency. Insulin is a hormone produced by the pancreas gland. Its main function is to help glucose enter the body's cells where it can be used for energy and growth. If there is a surplus of glucose in the blood, insulin directs it into the liver for storage.

▩ CAUSES The cause(s) of childhood-onset diabetes is unknown. The current view is that it probably results from an 'insult' to the insulin-secreting cells of the pancreas. The 'insult' may be a VIRAL infection that activates the body's immune system to attack the insulin-producing cells of its own pancreas. These cells then fail to produce insulin, and the child's blood glucose level rises.

▩ SYMPTOMS The excess glucose in

the blood is excreted in the urine, carrying with it an excess of water. Thus the untreated diabetic child passes ever-increasing volumes of urine; he may have to get up during the night (perhaps many times) to urinate or he may wet the bed. He will be excessively thirsty and drink large volumes of water to compensate for the excessive loss of water in the urine, and he will lose weight as energy that should be used to build tissues is lost as glucose is excreted in large amounts in the urine.

He may become tired and irritable; his breath may smell sweet or fruity (due to the presence of acetone); and if the condition remains undiagnosed and untreated, it may progress to a dangerous state in which the child becomes unconscious (goes into coma), dehydrated and begins to breathe heavily and deeply.

■ ACTION If your child develops these symptoms, you must of course get medical advice. Your doctor will do a URINE TEST for glucose (there is normally none present) and a BLOOD TEST for a high glucose concentration. If the result is positive, the doctor will either refer the child to a specialist or arrange his urgent admission to hospital.

■ TREATMENT The basis of treatment of childhood diabetes is replacement of the missing insulin, which must be given throughout life as the body is unable to make its own. Insulin is usually given by injection once or twice a day; it cannot be given by mouth as it is destroyed by intestinal secretions. Most children readily adjust to the daily discipline of their injections. On average they begin to show an interest and ability in managing their own injections from the age of eight to 12

years. Once the family have adjusted to the shock of the diagnosis, the clinical routine is not difficult to adopt: the difficulty is in the permanency of the routine.

Regular blood and/or urine tests are necessary to monitor the blood glucose level. The levels during a particular day can then be charted and used as a basis for assessment of the degree of control by your doctor.

A child with diabetes is advised to eat normal foods as part of a well-balanced diet. Restriction of foods high in sugar (carbohydrate) content (sweets, chocolates) and many high-calorie 'junk' foods is essential, because they cause sudden rises in blood glucose. To balance the effects of the injected insulin, and to keep blood glucose levels steady, the carbohydrate intake is calculated and spread over the snacks and main meals of the day. Carbohydrate should preferably come from whole foods, for example fruit, and foods rich in natural fiber, for example cereals, wholewheat bread and beans. Meals need to be eaten at regular times; it is prudent to keep animal fats to a minimum. Most children usually adjust well to the dietary discipline, at least initially. Great ingenuity, encouragement and support are needed to help the child sustain the diet.

■ PROBLEMS IN DIABETIC CONTROL HYPOGLYCEMIA – a low blood glucose level, which may result from extra exercise, a missed snack, or too much insulin – but sometimes for no obvious reason. The child may display pallor, irritability, hunger, dizziness or sudden loss of consciousness. Treatment includes ingesting extra glucose from a drink or a cube of sugar; or may require the injection of glucagon, an injectable hormone that converts glycogen stored in the body's tissues to glucose. Medical help may be required. After recovery, thought should be given to why the episode occurred. It may be preventable next time.

HYPERGLYCAEMIA occurs if the blood glucose rises too high. The initial symptoms of diabetes return, with frequent passage of urine, thirst and weight loss. Vague lassitude and headaches may have gone before. The condition may arise from too little insulin (or the child outgrowing his previous dose); from eating more than usual; from a change in lifestyle or exercise; from worry over school work; or as a result of infection. In diabetic children, blood glucose tends to rise during infections, even though they are eating less.

The key to coping with hyperglycaemia is frequent thoughtful measurements of the child's blood glucose, judiciously injecting extra quick-acting insulin, maintaining fluid intake and keeping in touch with the doctor.

■ SELF-HELP Always carry an emergency supply of glucose (most conveniently in the form of sugar cubes or a candy bar) to counter an unexpected fall in blood glucose.

Change the site of the injection from day to day. This will help maintain the injection sites in a smooth and supple state, and will help the regular pattern of insulin absorption.

■ OUTLOOK With adequate control of his diabetes, and his blood glucose levels, your child will grow up to lead a near-normal adult life with very few restrictions. The discipline needed to control the diabetes will still be required; and certain jobs may not be open to him such as army service or piloting airplanes. However, diabetes is not a factor in most jobs. There are many actors, athletes, teachers and construction workers who have diabetes.

Childhood diabetes may, in a minority of cases, result in problems and complications in adulthood. These include: changes in the small blood vessels of the eyes, kidneys and feet, with additional problems affecting the nerves and heart in some instances. Such problems are worrisome to parents and children alike, but they are a long way off and should not cloud the life of the diabetic child. It is true that there is some relationship between control of blood glucose levels in childhood and future health. But, in coming decades we can expect improvements in methods to control diabetes; and so it is fair to take an optimistic view of a diabetic child's future health.

DIABETIC PREGNANCY
A pregnancy in which the mother has DIABETES. A woman may have diabetes before she becomes pregnant or develop it during pregnancy. All women are screened for diabetes during pregnancy by testing their urine for sugar. A BLOOD TEST is usually necessary to confirm the diabetic state.

Whatever the type of the mother's diabetes, the health of the fetus may be affected. If the mother's BLOOD SUGAR level is not well controlled, the extra sugar crosses the placenta and may make the fetus large and fat. As a rebound effect, after birth the blood sugar may drop severely (see HYPOGLYCEMIA).

Diabetic mothers run a slightly increased risk of STILL BIRTH in late pregnancy, so many obstetricians advise induction of labor at 38 weeks of gestation.

DIALYSIS
See RENAL FAILURE.

DIAPER RASH
A common and temporary redness with or without raised confluent or discrete spots in the diaper area.

■ CAUSE Urine turns into ammonia after being in the diaper a short time. Ammonia is identifiable by its strong smell. It irritates the baby's skin, making it vulnerable to infection by BACTERIA or yeast. Some babies develop diaper rash as an early manifestation of ECZEMA or PSORIASIS.

■ SYMPTOMS The skin under the diaper becomes red, and later raised areas or raw ulcers may appear. These may be painful, causing the baby to cry. The skin in the folds between the baby's legs and buttocks may be relatively less affected by the rash.

■ ACTION Simple measures often work: **1** Remove the diaper in order to expose the area to open air, for as long as possible. **2** Apply a simple barrier cream containing zinc. **3** Avoid close-fitting diapers, and change the diaper as frequently as possible.

■ GET MEDICAL ADVICE if the rash does not clear in a few days following these simple methods.

■ TREATMENT The doctor will consider the possibility of other skin problems, and may prescribe a cream to clear any yeast or other infection. This may also contain hydrocortisone to relieve the inflammation. Oral yeast infection (CANDIDIASIS) may also be present and require oral antifungal treatment.

DIARRHEA
The passage of frequent, loose or watery bowel movements. Often caused by VIRUSES, more rarely by BACTERIA or PARASITES. Infectious diarrhea, with or without vomiting, is often called GASTROENTERITIS.

Rarely diarrhea may be a sign of a more serious abdominal problem such as APPENDICITIS. Many toddlers are, however, prone to short episodes of non-specific diarrhea which need not cause concern if they last no longer than a day or two. GIARDIA should be considered as a possible cause if the diarrhea is long lasting.

■ ACTION A child with diarrhea may have a poor APPETITE for a few days. This does not matter, except that it is important to ensure sufficient fluid intake in order to prevent DEHYDRATION. Give frequent feedings of clear fluids and water. If you are breast feeding, you should continue supplementing your milk if necessary with clear fluids. Change diapers frequently to avoid soreness of the baby's bottom due to the acid content of the stools – use a protective cream.

Get medical advice if there are any signs of dehydration, if the child is generally sick, or has abdominal pain or vomiting, or if the diarrhea lasts more than two or three days.

■ TESTS A specimen of the child's stool may be sent to the laboratory for culture and microscopic studies for viruses, bacteria or parasites.

■ TREATMENT The only treatment needed in most cases of diarrhea is fluid replacement to avoid dehydration. Oral rehydration fluid can be bought over the counter at your drugstore, and can be used when diarrhea is severe and frequent, to replace fluid and salt loss. Medicines that 'stop' the diarrhoea by reducing bowel mobility should be avoided, especially in babies and children. If a stool specimen shows a parasite such as *Giardia*, your doctor may prescribe a specific medicine. If the stool specimen shows a bacterium such as *Shigella* or *Campylobacter*, ANTIBIOTICS may be prescribed.

DIPHTHERIA
Now rare in most developed countries because of IMMUNIZATION. It is caused by BACTERIA that only infect humans. The infection is highly contagious and is spread from one person to another through the secretions of the nose and throat. The bacteria produce a toxin that can damage the heart, nerves and other organs in the body. The INCUBATION PERIOD is from two to seven days.

▦ PREVENTION Diptheria immunization is safe and efficient.

▦ SYMPTOMS FEVER, HEADACHE and feeling generally sick are early signs. The glands of the neck become very large. A membrane forms in the back of the throat and in the nose, causing difficulty with breathing. Complications include muscle PARALYSIS, PNEUMONIA and HEART FAILURE.

▦ ACTION Get medical advice. Your doctor will arrange hospital admission.

▦ TREATMENT A diphtheria antitoxin injection and ANTIBIOTICS are given.
  If the membrane is obstructing breathing, a tube may have to be passed down the windpipe. If the muscles of breathing are paralyzed, the child may need a ventilator (life-support machine). See the separate entries for treatment of heart failure and pneumonia.

▦ OUTLOOK This illness, now rare, is most severe in younger children. Convalescence is usually long, and complications can occur late in the course of the disease.

DISLOCATION OF A JOINT
A joint becomes dislocated when the 'ball' (see diagram) loses proper contact with its 'socket'. As might be expected, this is almost always caused by injury. Joints commonly dislocated are those of the shoulder, elbow and fingers. One type of dislocation is present at birth: CONGENITAL DISLOCATION OF THE HIP.

DISLOCATION OF JOINT

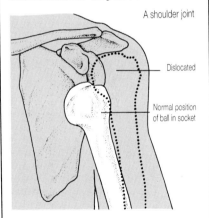

A shoulder joint

Dislocated

Normal position of ball in socket

▦ SYMPTOMS The injury is usually obvious, and there may be exceedingly painful swelling and deformity of the joint. The exception is nursemaid's elbow, seen in young children when the head of the radius is pulled out of its ligament socket. The cause of the 'injury' may be trivial, such as quickly pulling a child by the wrist out of the street on to the sidewalk. There may be only minimal swelling at the elbow, or none at all, but the toddler or young child refuses to use the arm, or may cry when he tries to use it.

■ ACTION Get medical advice or take the child to hospital. An anesthetic may be necessary to correct (reduce) the dislocation, so don't give him anything to eat or drink, otherwise the anesthetic may have to be postponed. For nursemaid's elbow an anesthetic is not needed. The radius slips easily back into place.

■ TESTS An X-ray may be necessary to make the diagnosis. It is usually repeated once the dislocation has been reduced, to make sure that everything is back in place.

■ TREATMENT The joint is manipulated into its normal position. A sling may be used to rest the joint for a few weeks.

It is important to exercise other joints and muscles as usual, otherwise they will become stiff and weak.

■ OUTLOOK is usually good, but if ligaments, tendons and muscles around the joint are badly torn, the joint can be weakened, giving rise to repeated dislocation. Nursemaid's elbow usually heals completely and rarely recurs.

DIVORCE

The sad truth is that in many Western countries, marriage break-up affects one child in six, and that this rate is still increasing. There is no disguising the fact that divorce causes children tremendous distress. And it is hard for parents to cope with this because at the time they themselves are tense and upset.

Recent research shows that, however bad the marriage, children like their parents to stay together. You may know this is impossible, but remember that your child may secretly wish and hope it for years.

Unless the parent who leaves has been violent, most children want and need to keep in contact with that parent. It is important to try to maintain this relationship, and to recognize that the person who has left can be a good *parent* even though not a good *spouse*.

Access to the child or children by the parent who has left (visitation rights) will often be regulated by the court that grants the divorce, but it is in your child's best interest for this to be predictable, planned and (depending on the age of the child) of sufficient length to maintain a meaningful relationship.

■ REACTIONS TO DIVORCE
Pre-school children: Babies and toddlers are unlikely to show specific reactions, but may be upset if the parent is absent. A slightly older child may be concerned about the absent parent's welfare in a practical sense: "Will Daddy have a bed to sleep in?" "Will Mommy have food to eat?" Children at this age may also feel that their own bad behavior has caused problems between the parents and need reassurance that this is not the case.

Five to eight/nine years: Children are still likely to feel responsible for what has happened and they may also worry that the absent parent has died. It is important to reassure them and to encourage communication by cards or brief telephone calls if in-person meetings are a problem. The child may be tearful, upset and wakeful at night and there may be difficult behavior at home or at school. Tell your child's teacher what is happening to the marriage.

Nine to 12 years: The child will probably not feel responsible for the break-up, but may take sides. He may show considerable emotional distress; and his behavior may become very difficult indeed: a challenge, perhaps, for the remaining parent to demonstrate whether he or she can really manage alone.

Teenagers are likely to argue quite vehemently for or against one of the parents. They may well feel strong loyalty to the absent parent and should be given some say in visiting arrangements and, in some instances, where they will live. They need to be kept informed about what is happening. They may be upset for several months, with difficult behavior and worse marks than usual at school. There may be SCHOOL ATTENDANCE PROBLEMS.

■ ACTION Remember that you are bound to be upset and this will make matters even more difficult for your children. Try to keep in contact with the absent parent, maintain the child's or children's routines as far as possible and allow them to miss the absent parent without feeling they are disloyal to you.

Don't let them take sides, and encourage them to keep their own photos of the family group. Try to preserve 'space' for the child or children, even though you will be concentrating on keeping yourself together.

If a child's reaction to separation and divorce is severe and lasts longer than a few months, ask your doctor to refer him to a child psychologist or psychiatrist for help before the problem becomes unsolvable.

DIZZINESS
A sensation that children may describe in a variety of ways, including 'fuzziness', light-headedness, a sense of spinning (also called vertigo). It is a rather vague symptom with many possible underlying causes ranging from MIDDLE EAR problems, side-effects of medication, DRUG ABUSE or OVER-BREATHING. If dizziness is the only complaint, it rarely justifies major investigation or treatment.

DOWN SYNDROME
A relatively common CHROMOSOMAL abnormality. Affected children are born with an extra chromosome in their cells: the children have three number 21 chromosome, rather than two. Approximately one in 700 children are affected, and the likelihood increases in pregnancies among older women. The chance of a woman over 44 having a Down child is one in 40.

■ PRENATAL DIAGNOSIS Down syndrome may now be diagnosed during pregnancy by amniocentesis, which makes analysis of fetal chromosomes possible. A BLOOD TEST performed on the mother before the 16th week of pregnancy can also be useful in making the diagnosis.

■ FEATURES OF DOWN SYNDROME The child's facial features have a characteristic 'Mongoloid' appearance: the eyes slant upwards and outwards, and may be widely separated. The bridge of the nose tends to be flat and the ears small. The tongue may be larger than normal. Other identifying features include a single crease line across the palm of the hand. The baby may be especially quiet and placid, with poor muscle tone. He has a tendency to CONGENITAL HEART-DISEASE, and may be born with a blockage of the upper intestine (DUODENAL ATRESIA).

■ PROBLEMS AFTER BIRTH As

with any other baby, he can be breast or bottle fed. However, he may take longer to feed because he may find sucking difficult. He may also be slow to put on weight at first.

An operation for either the bowel or heart problem may be necessary.

■ PROBLEMS IN CHILDHOOD
During their first few years, children with Down syndrome tend to have minor infections of the eyes and ears particularly OTITIS MEDIA. They are more prone than other children to colds and chest infections.

The main point, however, is that they can and do achieve all the usual childhood skills: the Down child will walk, and talk, albeit at a later age than others. Techniques for assisting development have improved enormously, and with professional help parents can ensure that the Down child reaches his full potential.

Down children are typically affectionate, lovable and sociable. They need to be included, stimulated and treated as normally as possible.

They will have a lower I.Q. than normal, but many, with the proper stimulation, can learn to read, write and do uncomplicated calculations. Educational needs must be individually assessed. Often children can attend and blossom in a regular class if given special help.

■ ADOLESCENCE AND ADULT-HOOD Prior to leaving home as a young adult, all patients with Down syndrome should have a full assessment, including an inventory of job and personal skills. Some Down adults are fully self-supporting in unskilled or semi-skilled jobs and live with parents, friends or in a sheltered group home. Others need

help from an adult training center to develop daily living skills or to gain employment.

The critical time for Down syndrome adults tends to be middle age. With their own parents in old age, and the possibility of serious health problems resulting from congenital heart-disease, the outlook can be uncertain. But provision for this type of handicap is improving, and today's Down patient may well fare better in middle age than parents dared hope in the 1960s and 1970s. Your national association for Down syndrome can offer support.

DROWNING
Most drownings occur in swimming-pools, in rivers, brooks and lakes, or in the bath tub. A young child can drown in a few inches of water. With hindsight, most accidents appear easily preventable by adequate supervision at swimming-pools, beaches and during bathtime; by provision and use of child life jackets in boats; and by fencing off public and private swimming-pools. Additionally, children should be taught water safety and how to swim.

■ IMMEDIATE ACTION Summon an ambulance. Even if the child appears to be dead, start EMERGENCY RESUSCITATION. Try to give the child a few breaths even as you pull him from the water. Be prepared to continue artificial ventilation until professional help arrives, even if this is for several hours. If possible, wrap the child in a blanket (or suitable substitute such as a jacket), since chilling can lead to HYPOTHERMIA.

When the child starts breathing, put him in the RECOVERY POSITION.

■ OUTLOOK Best in those who recover consciousness soonest, but it is always worth attempting emergency resuscitation and persisting until medical help arrives. Even after prolonged periods of UNCONSCIOUSNESS and artificial ventilation, some children recover completely.

DRUG ABUSE
A potentially grave problem. The most common drug abused in adolescence is ALCOHOL. Adolescents may abuse more than one drug.

Illegal 'street' drugs such as heroin, cocaine, hallucinogenics, amphetamines or their derivatives may be sniffed, smoked, injected or taken as tablets. For some social groups drug abuse, particularly of heroin, crack and cocaine is an increasingly serious problem during adolescence. The expense of purchasing the drug may lead the youngster into crime and prostitution. Risks to health include AIDS from shared needles, quite apart from the specter of addiction and the general undermining of a youngster's self-respect and direction.

Taking medication prescribed for a parent is a separate, also dangerous problem which should never be ignored.

■ SYMPTOMS Sudden changes of mood after being out with friends – being suddenly elated, laughing inappropriately, then quickly becoming depressed and withdrawn; hiding parts of the body where drugs have been injected; a sudden need for money; intoxication although there is no smell of alcohol: all are grounds for suspicion. If a teenager has needle puncture marks, typically on the forearms, or if you find needles or syringes among his possessions, take immediate action.

It is unusual for drug abuse to be a teenager's first problem: it usually occurs when there is already trouble with relationships, school work, SCHOOL ATTENDANCE or with the law.

■ ACTION Confronting your child with the evidence is not enough. Get help from your doctor, school guidance counsellor and from local counselling services for drug dependence. Be prepared to undergo family counselling too, as part of a comprehensive management plan.

DRUGS IN PREGNANCY
No drugs are allowed on the market that are known to cause malformations of an unborn baby. However, rare, minor or subtle effects may be associated with many 'drugs' (including aspirin, herbal remedies, alcohol, tobacco and drugs of addiction). So it is prudent to avoid, as far as possible, all drugs during pregnancy. If in doubt, get medical advice.

DRUGS, ALLERGIC REACTIONS TO
Not all unwanted effects of drugs or medicines are allergic in nature; some are the direct effect of the drug itself, often mistaken for an ALLERGY. However, many drugs can produce genuine allergic reactions when given more than once, and occasionally these reactions can be serious.

■ TYPES OF ALLERGIC REACTION Rashes are the best known, and are most likely when the drug – typically an ANTIBIOTIC or an antihistamine – has been used directly on the skin. Any form of skin RASH can be caused by allergy, including: URTICARIA, ECZEMA, DERMATITIS, BLISTERS, and rashes that resemble MEASLES. In general, oral antibiotics only rarely cause skin rash in young children. Allergic reactions are more common in adults.

Drug allergies can also cause ASTHMA and ALLERGIC RHINITIS, various blood disorders such as APLASTIC ANEMIA or, most serious of all, ANAPHYLACTIC SHOCK. However, this last is most unlikely, except when the drug is given by intramuscular or intravenous injection. Emergency remedies are always on hand whenever injections are given.

■ CAUSES The drugs most likely to cause allergic reactions include: penicillin and other antibiotics; sulfonamides; aspirin (now rarely given to children); dyes used to color medicines; vaccines.

■ ACTION If you suspect a child is suffering from an allergic reaction to any drug or medicine, you should report it as soon as possible to your doctor. If the symptoms are severe, immediate treatment should be obtained, but if less severe, such as an itchy rash, there is less urgency.

■ TREATMENT The suspected drug should be discontinued. If anaphylactic shock has occurred, emergency treatment with injections of adrenalin, antihistamine and hydrocortisone will be given. Less severe reactions may be treated with an antihistamine or sometimes by a corticosteroid. Blood disorders will require special investigations and treatment in hospital.

■ TESTS It is not always possible to prove that a reaction is due to a drug allergy, but BLOOD TESTS are available that may help to determine the cause. Skin tests for drug allergy can themselves be dangerous, and are only used under certain circumstances. Patch tests for skin allergies are widely used in dermatology clinics, and are helpful if allergy to an ointment, cream or other contact chemical is being considered. Remember that sometimes the rash attributed to an oral antibiotic is actually part of the underlying infection for which the antibiotic was prescribed. For example, *Otitis media* may sometimes be due to a virus. A rash may develop on the body from the virus, not the drug. Separating out the cause of the rash is often difficult in these cases.

■ OUTLOOK Once an allergy has been demonstrated, it is important for the child to avoid further contact with the drug. However, many so-called allergies, for example to penicillin, are not genuine. Doctors may reasonably test a small dose of the drug by mouth, in order to discover whether a reaction actually occurs.

DUODENAL ATRESIA
An uncommon CONGENITAL ABNORMALITY of the duodenum (the part of the bowel connected to the stomach, and forming the first part of the small intestine). A short section does not develop properly in the fetus and fails to open up at birth, leading to obstruction of the bowel.

Duodenal atresia can be associated with DOWN SYNDROME (a CHROMOSOMAL defect).

■ SYMPTOMS Vomiting bile soon after birth, inability to feed properly.

■ INVESTIGATIONS An X-ray usually shows gas in the stomach and the upper duodenum. However, if there is only partial obstruction, gas may be present in the lower bowel.

■ TREATMENT Surgery to remove the blocked section of bowel and rejoin (anastomose) the normal portions of the duodenum.

■ OUTLOOK is excellent: no further bowel problems need be expected.

DWARFISM
See *SHORT STATURE.*

DYSLEXIA
A controversial term describing severe difficulty in reading or spelling inconsistent with the child's level of intelligence. It is the result of one or more specific aberrations in the complex process of learning to read. A child with dyslexia is now usually described as having a specific learning disorder. In all but the mildest forms of dyslexia, which are in fact quite common, the child will usually profit by specialized help with learning to read, usually in a regular school. See *LEARNING DISORDERS.*

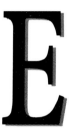

EAR INFECTIONS
See *MIDDLE* and *EXTERNAL EAR INFECTIONS.*

EAR TUBES
Small plastic tubes inserted by an ear surgeon through a child's eardrum. They allow free passage of air in and out of the middle ear. By assisting in the pressure regulation of the middle ear, the accumulation of fluid (and 'glue') is reduced, as is the frequency of middle ear infections. If a child is experiencing partial DEAFNESS as a result of GLUE EAR, insertion of tubes during a minor surgical operation (no painful after-effects) can be very effective, both in improving hearing and the frequently associated BEHAVIORAL DIS-

ORDERS. Tubes often work free from the eardrum after six to 12 months. Follow-up visits to a specialist will establish whether they need to be removed or replaced.

EARACHE
Any pain in or around the ear.

■ CAUSES are MIDDLE EAR INFECTION (*Otitis media*) – especially in association with VIRAL INFECTIONS of the nose and throat – EXTERNAL EAR INFECTION (*Otitis externa*) and EAR, FOREIGN BODY IN. It is commonest in young children, whose Eustachian tubes are short, enabling BACTERIA to travel easily from the back of the nose to the middle ear.

■ SYMPTOMS Infants have non-specific symptoms such as FEVER, crying and VOMITING. Toddlers and older children will hold their ears or complain of earache – which can be *very* painful. See *MIDDLE EAR INFECTION (OTITIS MEDIA).*

■ ACTION If you think your child has an earache, get medical advice. While awaiting medical attention, you could give your child a simple painkiller such as acetamenophen. The urgency depends on the severity of the pain and the degree of general illness, especially in infants, but all children with earache should be assessed. If untreated, middle ear infection may on occasion lead to EARDRUM PERFORATION or serious infection of the mastoid bone, the bone behind the ear. Both conditions may need attention from an ear, nose and throat specialist. Infection of the external ear can usually be treated with ear drops prescribed by your doctor.

EARDRUM PERFORATION

The eardrum may be perforated by direct injury, by extreme changes of pressure, and most commonly by MIDDLE EAR INFECTIONS (*Otitis media*), in which case a discharge may appear in the external ear canal.

■ SYMPTOMS Discharge (see above); pain and/or bleeding.

■ TREATMENT If the cause is a middle ear infection, your doctor may prescribe an ANTIBIOTIC. Perforations usually heal without treatment. Occasionally an ear, nose and throat specialist may be consulted, particularly if there is any suggestion that hearing has been impaired.

EARS, FOREIGN BODY IN

Any object – animal, vegetable or mineral – lodged in the ear canal, where it can cause irritation, swelling and lead to infection.

■ SYMPTOMS Pain, itching or simply a complaint of a blocked ear. If it has been there for some time a foul-odored discharge may be noted.

■ ACTION Many foreign bodies, including insects, can be removed by lying the child on his side and gently pouring warm water into his ear. Make sure the water is not too hot. Some objects will have to be removed by a doctor, who will syringe the ear to wash out the foreign body, or use a special probe or tweezers to pluck it out.

■ TREATMENT If the ear canal is inflamed or infected, ANTIBIOTIC drops may be prescribed.

■ OUTLOOK There should be no long-term problems, but young children who have put things in their ears tend to do it again.

ECG (ELECTROCARDIOGRAM)

ECG

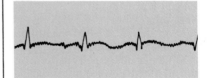

A typical ECG print-out.

A test to measure the electrical function of the heart. The patient is connected to an ECG recording machine by wires pasted to the arms, legs and chest. A recording of the electrical activity of the heart is then obtained.

This is completely painless – there is nothing to feel while the tracing is taken. But the child must be fairly still for a few minutes. The ECG can show whether the heart is beating irregularly, and whether there are signs of strain on the heart caused by HEART-DISEASE.

ECZEMA

In childhood, an itchy, scaling or oozing rash, often associated with other allergic conditions such as HAY FEVER and ASTHMA. It has a tendency to run in families.

▓ SYMPTOMS Childhood eczema usually starts in infancy. Initially it is prominent in the diaper area; later in childhood it presents as a symmetrical rash affecting the hands and wrists, the creases of the arms, ankles and behind the knees, and in more extreme cases the face, neck or trunk. The rash is pink or red, and may be dry and scaly or develop cracks and become wet and oozing. It usually itches.

▓ ACTION Because of the family pattern, many parents recognize eczema when it starts. While treatment is not necessarily urgent, it is wise to get medical advice early on as with the diagnosis and treatment of any skin rash.

▓ TREATMENT It is important for parents to realize that however unsightly, eczema is not contagious, and usually lessens in severity in later childhood, often completely clearing by the teens. It does not cause scarring, although a dryness of the skin may remain in adulthood.

There are four main groups of therapeutic agents employed in the treatment of eczema: 1 Emollients –

creams or ointments to keep the skin soft, supple and moist – should be used freely. Emulsifying agents in place of soap for bathin, play a most important role in the everyday skin care of children with eczema. 2 Steroid creams. These can completely clear the skin, but excessive use leads to side-effects: thinning of the skin, and an increased risk of infection. If too strong a cream is used for too long, there is even a risk of the steroid being absorbed into the body, causing serious side-effects. Thus the weakest steroid cream or ointment that proves effective for your child should be used. One percent hydrocortisone is the weakest, and is often effective in mild eczema. Nothing stronger should be used on the face, except under medical supervision. Stronger steroids may be prescribed for limited use, for localized angry patches and for short periods when the skin becomes particularly troublesome. 3 Antihistamines, given as syrup or tablets, relieve itching and, taken at bed time, will help the child sleep. This may be of particular importance for the child and parents alike in early infancy. 4 ANTIBIOTICS, usually taken by mouth, will be prescribed if there is evidence of infection of the skin. See IMPETIGO.

▓ SELF-HELP Persist with moisturizers – childhood eczema tends to cause a very dry skin, and drying out of the skin tends to make eczema worse. Soaps and detergents can irritate eczema, so avoid them. For affected infants and young children, mittens or gloves may help reduce the effects of scratching, especially at night. Dress the child in cotton. Wool and synthetic fibers may cause irritation if worn next to the skin. Clothes, and bedclothes, should be cool and loose: itching is worse when the body is hot. If a child with eczema has a specific allergy (this is not usually the case), then allergen avoidance is naturally advisable.

■ DIET For some children the removal of certain foods from the diet may improve the eczema: your doctor will advise you about the foods to avoid. The principal foods implicated in eczema include cow's milk, eggs, cheese and chocolate.

■ OUTLOOK Eczema persists through childhood in many children, waxing and waning in severity, so a long-term approach to management may be needed. Children are naturally sensitive about their appearance, and may need moral support, sometimes including professional psychological help. If in real difficulties, ask to be referred to a skin specialist (dermatologist).

Occasionally it is necessary to admit a child to the hospital for a period of intensive treatment. Remember that children with eczema are healthy and normal in other respects, although they do sometimes have the related problems of asthma or hay fever.

EDEMA

Excess fluid retained by the body. Normally fluid is removed from the body in a well regulated fashion as urine produced by the kidneys and, to a lesser degree, as sweat and water in the exhaled breath and in the stools. If these regulatory processes fail, the excess fluid passes from the blood into the body tissues. The legs swell and the eyes become puffy. In a baby, edema may be generalized or show itself as a sudden increase in weight. See also *HEART FAILURE.*

EEG RECORDING (ELECTRO-ENCEPHALOGRAM)

A test of brain function, obtained by placing special electrodes on the scalp. The brain's surface electrical discharges are detected, and through a system of amplification are transcribed on to paper as a wave pattern. The equipment is expensive, and the technique requires specialized training for performance and interpretation.

Recent electronic technology has allowed ambulatory monitoring: the leads from the scalp electrodes are connected to a tape recorder worn on a belt. The child's EEG can then be monitored in this way over several hours as he walks about freely, and the tape can be studied in detail.

EEG is commonly used in childhood to confirm the diagnosis of EPILEPSY, and to characterize its type and source. The diagnostic value of EEG may be enhanced by asking the child to breathe rapidly and deeply, and to look at a flashing light. Sleep recordings may also be helpful. The test is safe and painless, and can be used at any age from birth onwards. With reassurance, children are usually happy to cooperate.

ELECTRIC SHOCK

Electric shock can cause a variety of injuries from superficial BURNS to FRACTURES and widespread internal damage. Electrical mouth burns, from placing a live electrical plug in the mouth, can be very serious. The most immediately serious threat may be that the heart will stop beating. See *EMERGENCY RESUSCITATION.*

■ PREVENTION Cover electrical outlets with safety plugs. Do not leave live (attached to the socket) extension cords lying around. Teach children about the dangers of electricity. Make sure electrical appliances and tools are used properly as directed.

■ ACTION 1 Disconnect or switch off the source of electricity. If this is impossible, don't touch either the child or any conductive surfaces – such as metal – that are in contact with him, or you may also receive a shock. If necessary, use a broom handle or some other non-conductive object (for example, anything made of wood), to dislodge him from the source of electricity. 2 Assess the situation – see EMERGENCY RESUSCITATION. If breathing and pulse are absent follow steps A, B and C. 3 Look for burns at the entry and exit sites of the electric shock. For emergency treatment, see BURNS. All burns caused as a result of an electric shock should be assessed by a doctor, since internal damage may well exceed the extent of the superficial burn.

■ ACTION AT HOSPITAL If necessary, the child will be resuscitated. Burns and internal injuries will then be assessed and treated. A plastic surgeon will usually be consulted if the burn affects the face or hands, or is extensive.

■ OUTLOOK depends on the severity of the shock and the extent of the injuries.

EMERGENCY RESUSCITATION

■ IMMEDIATE ACTION IN A LIFE-THREATENING EMERGENCY 1 Make sure there is no further danger to you or to the child. 2 Call for assistance to help with resuscitation. 3 Call an ambulance.

■ OUTLOOK Best if resuscitation starts immediately and the child responds fairly quickly. But never be in doubt that it is worth trying to resuscitate, even if it seems to you to be too late.

■ ASSESS THE SITUATION What has happened to the child? See DROWNING, CHOKING, BURNS AND SCALDS, SUFFOCATION, POISONING for appropriate first-aid measures. If there could be damage to the neck, only move the child if absolutely necessary. If you must move the child, and no trained person is present, summon help and support the child's neck, head and shoulders at all times. Unless the neck is kept immobile, there is a risk of causing damage to the spinal cord, which might result in paralysis.

Next, look at the whole child and try to observe problems:
– Is the child breathing? Listen for sounds of breathing, look and feel for the rise and fall of the chest. If breathing is noisy and difficult, see CHOKING. If there is no breathing, follow steps A, B and C below.

– Is there a heartbeat or pulse? Listen or feel for the heartbeat over the central and left side of the front of the chest. Try feeling for the radial pulse, at the wrist near the base of the thumb; or the brachial pulse, on the inner surface of the straightened arm at the level of the elbow; or the carotid pulse, felt in the neck, below and inwards from the angle of the jaw. If you cannot quickly detect a heartbeat or pulse, do not waste a long time searching; follow steps A, B and C below.

– Is the child unconscious? If so, turn him on to his side in the RECOVERY POSITION, with his head and mouth tilted downward towards the floor. If the child vomits, it will be

EMERGENCY RESUSCITATION

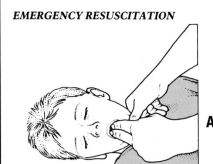

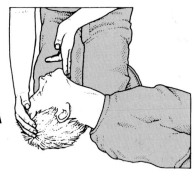

A

*Emergency resuscitation –
see the entry, starting on
the previous page, for full
details.*

Step A: Clear the airway
Step B: Establish breathing
Step C: Establish circulation

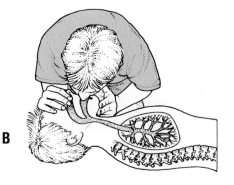

B

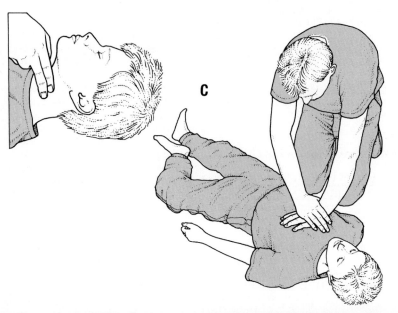

C

more likely to spill out of his mouth and not be inhaled. Contine to check that breathing and pulse remain satisfactory.

– Is the child bleeding? Use firm pressure to control bleeding. See CUTS AND ABRASIONS. Preferably apply a pad of clean gauze or other material, but if unavailable, use firm hand pressure over the wound. Steps **A**, **B** and **C** can best be learned by attending a first-aid course.

Step A: Clear the airway. Lie the child flat on his back, choosing a firm surface. Clear the mouth of vomit and/or other obstructing matter. Tilt the head back and support the chin.

Step B: Establish breathing. If step A does not start the child breathing, begin artificial ventilation. **1** Squeeze the nose shut. **2** Cover the mouth of child with your mouth. **3** Breathe into child's mouth. Take care not to blow; 'breathe' really does mean what it says: gently exhale from the base of your lungs. If the victim is a baby, cover both nose and mouth with your mouth. Breathe four times, then check for the pulse. Check that the chest moves as you breathe into the child. If the chest wall is not moving, repeat step A and consider whether an object has been inhaled. See CHOKING.

Step C: Establish circulation. If no pulse is felt, start cardiac (heart) massage immediately. Make sure the child is on a *firm* surface. If the victim is a baby, use your first two fingers to forcibly depress the sternum (breastbone) + to one inch. Give 100 compressions a minute at a count of "1, 2, 3, 4, 5". Allow a slight pause between compressions. Give a mouth-to-mouth breath (step **B**) between every five compressions.

For older children, you will need to press more forcibly using the base of your hand to depress the breastbone one to 1+ in at a count of "1 and 2 and 3 and 4 and 5". Avoid fracturing a rib by being too forceful, but remember you are trying to squeeze the heart and make it pump the blood to rhe rest of the body.

What to expect at the hospital: The child's vital supply of oxygen to the blood (and hence to the brain) will be enhanced by delivering oxygen through a mask. The hospital staff may also try intubation and mechanical ventilation: a tube is passed through the mouth (or nose) into the wind pipe to deliver a supply of oxygen directly to the airways with the help of a breathing machine (ventilator). Intravenous fluids will be given to supply essential solutions and/or drugs. An ECG will monitor heart function. Defibrillation – an electric shock to the heart – may be needed to restore a regular hearbeat (pulse). When these essential life-support systems are running, attention will then be directed to determine why the heart and lungs stopped functioning.

ENCEPHALITIS
An acute dysfunctional illness of the brain due to inflammation. This may be due to direct invasion by the agent, such as POLIO or RABIES virus, or a reaction to an infection elsewhere two to three weeks earlier. Viruses, fungi and certain bacteria can cause encephalitis.

ENCEPHALOPATHY
An acute (or chronic) dysfunctional illness of the brain that may be due to biochemical abnormalities such as

liver failure, REYE SYNDROME and drug intoxication.

ENCOPRESIS
See *SOILING*.

ENEMA
An enema is a process by which a liquid is passed under pressure through a tube into the lower bowel through the anus. A plastic or metal container attached to a tube and nozzle holds the liquid and the pressure is created by holding the container several feet above the anus. Some small-size enemas are squirted into the rectum by pressing on the plastic container. The fluid usually consists of water containing some salts and stool-softening agents to relieve CONSTIPA-TION but may contain medication, for example paraldehyde for a child who is having a seizure that is not stopping. A barium enema is used as part of an X-ray examination to outline the lower bowel to show, for instance, the extent of inflammatory bowel disease (ulcerative colitis), or to identify and reduce an INTUSSUSCEPTION.

ENURESIS
See *BEDWETTING, WETTING, URINARY TRACT INFECTION*.

EPIDURAL ANESTHETIC
The injection of anesthetic drugs into the epidural space – the space surrounding the nerves of the spinal cord. An epidural anesthetic may be used (in some hospitals more than others) during labor to relieve painful uterine contractions and to anesthetize the pelvis if forceps are to be applied. An epidural anesthetic may also be used in place of a general anesthetic for a CESARIAN SECTION.

The woman either lies on her side or leans forward in a sitting position. A small area of skin on her lower back is numbed with local anesthetic and a needle containing a fine plastic tube is inserted into the epidural space. Small amounts of anesthetic drug are continually infused through the tube.

Epidural anesthesia gives excellent pain relief but it may prevent the woman from contracting her stomach muscles to aid in pushing the baby through the birth canal, and thereby increase the chance of a FORCEPS delivery. Occasionally epidural anesthesia results in a drop in blood pressure; this will require treatment with intravenous fluids and drugs.

EPIGLOTTITIS
A rare, but serious, bacterial INFEC-TION of the epiglottis causing obstruction to breathing.

■ CAUSE *Hemophilus influenzae*, a BACTERIUM.

■ SYMPTOMS The child rapidly becomes unwell and lethargic, with a fever and distressed noisy breathing, with drawing in of the space under the ribs. The throat will be sore, so that he refuses food and drink, and drools saliva. Although the condition is similar to CROUP, the drooling (due to difficulty swallowing saliva) is distinctive. The symptoms differ in several other important ways: the noise is more of a rattle, occurring with every breath, not just with the cough; the child is much more feverish and toxic.

■ ACTION 1 Keep the child sitting up, leaning forward. 2 Summon urgent medical help. *This is an emergency.* If a doctor is not available, send for an ambulance.

■ TREATMENT If there is a danger of obstruction of the airway, an experienced anesthetist will be called to insert a tube into the child's windpipe, through his mouth or nose.

This will be left in place for a few days, allowing him to breathe freely. ANTIBIOTICS (active against *Hemophilus influenzae*) will be given, initially by injection into a muscle or a vein.

■ OUTLOOK If treatment is commenced early, recovery is usually complete with no long-term effects.

EPILEPSY
The experience of recurrent seizures (or convulsions) over a period of months or years. There are many types and most start in childhood. Some only occur in children or adolescents. About eight in 1,000 children compared with five in 1,000 adults suffer from epilepsy.

■ SYMPTOMS depend on the part of the brain from which the seizure discharge begins. In generalized seizures, the onset is sudden with loss of awareness or consciousness (see *GRAND MAL and PETIT MAL SEIZURES*). In focal or partial seizures there may be an awareness of twitching, a feeling of pins and needles, flashing lights, odd smells, abdominal pain, a sense of choking, hallucinations, dizziness, inability to talk or general confusion, even fear. Such seizures may become generalized or remain focal. (But note that these symptoms have many other causes.)

■ ACTION Place the child having a seizure in the RECOVERY POSITION (see *EMERGENCY RESUSCITATION*) and protect him from danger, especially from falling, fire and sharp edges. If you suspect epilepsy, you should of course take your child to your doctor, who will arrange for a pediatric neurologist to see the child. Write down precisely the circumstances under which the seizure began and what happened.

■ INVESTIGATIONS The most helpful information comes from an accurate description of the events by the child and a witness. Provoking factors, for example lack of food or sleep, feeling ill, standing up, watching TV or even just a fright, may help to distinguish between a FAINTING attack and an epileptic seizure. An EEG RECORDING helps to decide between generalized and partial epilepsies. BLOOD and URINE TESTS may be taken to look for chemical causes (rare). A CAT SCAN of the head is only helpful if symptoms, seizure type and an EEG suggest a focal cause, or if other physical findings are present. Skull X-ray rarely shows the cause of epilepsy, but may show signs of uneven growth of the brain in older children.

■ CAUSES Everyone has a seizure threshold. Children with epilepsy have a lower threshold than average, but why one suffers from epilepsy and another does not is often impossible to determine. Two-thirds of children with epilepsy are otherwise normal. The seizure threshold is lowered by structural brain disease associated with mental retardation (see *MENTAL HANDICAP*), CEREBRAL PALSY or HYDROCEPHALUS, and a third of children affected by those problems will have epilepsy (compared with one in 200 children with no neurological disability). Epilepsy does not cause these disabilities to appear – it is a symptom of them. It is not infectious to others. There are some specific genetic causes of epilepsy, but the genetic risk is low – about 3 to 5 percent of children with epilepsy have an affected parent. Genetic risk is higher for generalized than for partial seizures. If no obvious cause is found, the epilepsy is termed idiopathic.

■ TREATMENT Ensure that the child, relatives and teachers understand the problem. Promote a regular and healthy lifestyle and deal with any concerns your child may have about his problem. Your doctor will consider medication if seizures are frequent or prolonged (usually anticonvulsant tablets given twice daily, which may need to be taken for several years). Drugs control generalized seizures in 80 percent of children and partial seizures in 50 percent but the greater the associated disability, the less likely that any drug or combination of drugs will be effective. The minimum amount of a drug that gives appropriate blood levels is used to minimize side-effects.

■ SELF-HELP Regular and sufficient sleep, meals and recreation will probably help. Encourage your child to develop his talents. He can learn to swim under supervision, and ride his bicycle in parks or bike paths. He should wear a medical information necklace or bracelet if seizures are likely to occur outside the home. Check if drugs for other conditions interact with the anticonvulsant drug. Alcohol should not be taken. Join a self-help group or the local chapter of the national epilepsy association.

■ OUTLOOK depends on type and frequency of seizures and associated disabilities. The best chances of recovery are with idiopathic generalized and benign partial seizures, when few seizures have occurred and the child is otherwise well. Altogether, a third of children with epilepsy recover, a third continue with seizures but are treated successfully with drugs, and a third have incompletely controlled seizures in adult life. Social attitudes toward epilepsy are improving slowly. Future employment prospects depend on seizure type, frequency and associated disabilities. Get advice in childhood to avoid unrealistic expectations for employment and independent living. *The Epilepsy Reference Book* by Peter M. Jeavons and Alec Aspinall (Harper and Row, 1985) is useful.

EPISTAXIS (BLEEDING FROM THE NOSE)
See *NOSEBLEED*.

ERYTHEMA TOXICUM
New-born babies frequently have crops of tiny red spots on the face and neck. These come and go rapidly, often appearing and disappearing the same day. Their cause is unknown. They are not painful or sore and do not require treatment.

EXCHANGE TRANSFUSION
The replacement of much of the blood in the body. This is usually performed if a new-born baby has a dangerously rising concentration of bilirubin in his blood (see *JAUNDICE*). A small amount of the baby's blood will be slowly drawn out from a large blood vessel – usually the UMBILICAL vein. The same amount is then replaced by donor blood. This procedure is repeated many times until almost all of the baby's blood is replaced by the donor's blood.

EXTERNAL EAR INFECTION (*OTITIS EXTERNA*)
This is an INFECTION of the skin lining the outer canal of the ear, up to the eardrum. It can be confused with a MIDDLE EAR INFECTION. It is especially

common in children who swim frequently. Hence the name 'swimmer's ear'.

■ SYMPTOMS The ear may be blocked by a mixture of WAX and inflammatory (pus) discharge, leading to DEAFNESS. Itching is often a feature, especially if the child also has ECZEMA. Pain is the main symptom in diffuse *Otitis externa*. The pain is made worse by moving the ear lobe or pressing just anterior to the lobe.

■ ACTION Any child with these symptoms should be seen by a doctor, both to find out exactly what is causing them, and for treatment.

■ TREATMENT The discharge or wax may be gently removed by syringing, although some children find this too painful or frightening. ANTIBIOTIC ear-drops or ointment are commonly prescribed. A cotton wick may be inserted into the outer portion of the ear canal and the drops applied three to four times a day. Dilute vinegar or other solutions may be used to rinse out the ear canal. When pain is severe, dry heat and painkillers such as acetamenophen or codeine may be needed.

■ OUTLOOK If the problem recurs, there might be an underlying skin disorder such as eczema. Usually the infection clears quickly with treatment. For children who swim frequently and are troubled by recurrences, ear plugs or prophylaxis with dilute alcohol or vinegar in the ear may help. Discuss with your doctor.

EYE, FOREIGN BODY IN

See the illustration showing how to examine a child's eye.

If a foreign body, or indeed an eye-

EYE, FOREIGN BODY IN

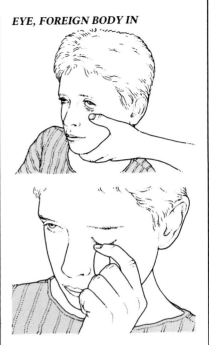

Top, *pulling down lower lid to examine eye and* **above,** *action for object under lower lid.*

lash, is stuck on the white part of the eye, it is worth giving the child's tears (a normal response to the irritation) a chance to wash it out naturally: blinking and blowing the nose may assist the process. Try to dissuade your child from rubbing his eye.

If this does not work, and the particle is not stuck fast to the eye, lift it off using a damp corner of a clean facial tissue.

If the foreign body overlies the colored part of the eye (the iris), don't try to remove it. Cover the child's eye with a clean pad or persuade him to keep his eyes closed, and take him to a hospital emergency department. If an object is embedded anywhere on the eyeball (see *EYE INJURY*), don't try to remove it; take the child straight to the hospital.

If a foreign body is caught under the

upper lid, ask the child to look down. Grip the eyelashes of the upper lid and pull the lid out and down. The lower lid lashes may brush the particle off. If this fails, you may be able to persuade your child to blink his eyes under water; the irritant may then float off.

If this fails, cover the eye with a pad and get medical care.

If in doubt, always get professional advice. Untreated, a minor eye injury may progress to become serious.

EYE GLASSES

Commonly prescribed for children with a variety of eyesight problems including LONG- or SHORTSIGHTEDNESS, LAZY EYE, ASTIGMATISM and STRABISMUS.

Eye glasses are prescribed after an EYE TEST, which needs to be repeated regularly as eyesight changes with age. Glasses will not only improve the accuracy of vision but may also relieve headaches from 'eye strain'.

Children sometimes don't like wearing their glasses, but they should be encouraged to do so. In toddlers and young children, it makes sense to buy inexpensive frames and to have a spare pair as accidents are almost inevitable. Plastic lenses which do not break are universally used in the United States. To help persuade a reluctant toddler to wear glasses, try showing him how much clearer the television screen is while wearing his glasses. Point out the number of heroes and heroines who wear eye glasses. Rewards and constant encouragement for regular wearing are helpful.

In older children, the option of fashionable frames or contact lenses may be a helpful inducement to keep wearing eye glasses. Special lenses and frames for sports activities may help protect the eyes of the young athlete.

EYE INJURY

See the illustration showing how to examine a child's eye at EYE, FOREIGN BODY IN.

Obvious damage or penetration of the eye by an object requires urgent medical treatment. Internal damage may lead to infection and blindness. Cover the eye with a clean pad: this helps to prevent the child moving the eyeball and worsening the damage. If the child will allow it, cover the good eye too: this makes movement even less likely. Alternatively, ask your child to keep his eyes closed.

It may be difficult to know whether an object has actually penetrated the eye. If in doubt, get urgent medical advice.

Chemicals in eye: Act quickly to prevent damage to the eye's surface. Don't let the child rub his eye.

Hold the eye open under running water (from a tap or pitcher). If the eyelid is shut as a reaction to the pain, you should nevertheless try firmly to hold the lids open to allow the water to irrigate it. Cover the eye lightly with a clean pad. Alternatively, ask your child to keep his eyes closed. Take the child to the hospital without delay.

EYELID, SWOLLEN

See *BLEPHARITIS, ALLERGY*.

EYE TESTS

These are important because visual disorders in childhood are relatively common; untreated, they may result in learning difficulties.

Children are more likely to have eyesight problems if there is a family history of STRABISMUS or LAZY EYE, or if they were born very PREMATURELY.

Measuring a child's vision requires patience and skill. A baby's eyesight may be assessed by his ability to follow a moving light or object. A toddler may be asked to identify shapes or toys at a distance. After three years of age, single letters or shapes on cards can be used.

■ TESTS FOR EYE GLASSES On the basis of the above tests, an eye specialist may decide that your child is either FAR- or SHORT-SIGHTED, or that he has a more complex focusing problem, or an eye muscle weakness (strabismus). Further examinations are required to fit the correct EYE GLASSES.

In the rare event of a baby requiring eye glasses, the prescription test may involve giving eye drops and noting the reaction of the lens of the eye to objects.

Tests for older children are the same as for adults. Different eyeglass lenses are fitted into a frame, and the child is asked to look at a chart through the lenses and say which one gives the clearest picture.

As eyesight changes with age, eye tests need to be performed regularly, and the lens prescription of the glasses adjusted accordingly.

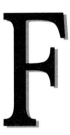

FAILURE TO THRIVE

A medical term used to describe infants and children who, without superficially evident cause, fail to gain weight normally, or actually lose weight. See *GROWTH PATTERNS*.

At WELL-BABY CLINICS or check-ups it is usual for babies to be weighed to check whether they are growing at a normal rate. If a child fails to gain weight normally, or loses weight, this calls for close attention: is this a sign of ill-health or undernutrition? If this is a baby who is otherwise well, you may simply be encouraged to feed your baby more often (breast or bottle), and increase the energy (calorie) content of his diet. If weight gain is still poor, or the child is not developing normally – that is, failing to thrive – then your doctor may want to investigate the reason for this.

■ TESTS It is unusual for a single or simple test to resolve the child's problem. The specialist will want to take a broad view of all aspects of your child's development. You will be asked questions about his birth weight, diet, behavior and development; and about family relationships and the dynamics of your household. Special tests may be performed to rule out particular conditions. Examples might include a URINE TEST to look for urinary INFECTION; a stool sample to search for PARASITES such as GIARDIA in the bowel; BLOOD TESTS for hormonal problems such as an underactive

thyroid gland; à sweat test' for CYS-
TIC FIBROSIS; an examination of the
upper bowel for CELIAC DISEASE.

■ OUTLOOK Many specific causes of
failure to thrive respond well to
treatment. It is often the case, however, that the child turns out to be
essentially healthy but displaying a
pattern of transient slow growth; in
which case, apart from your natural
concern, the outlook is excellent.

FAINTING

A transient form of unconsciousness
equally common in boys and girls,
caused by transient inadequate blood
circulation to the brain.

■ CAUSES Fainting occurs typically
when standing in a warm room, or
when experiencing something unpleasant or after a fright.

■ ACTION Allow the child to lie flat
on the floor. Recovery will follow
naturally and speedily.

■ SELF-HELP If a child is prone to
recurrent fainting when standing,
teach him how to contract his leg
muscles: this will speed the blood
circulation and may prevent fainting
in future.

■ OUTLOOK Fainting is rarely significant. It may require investigation if it occurs during vigorous
exercise, or in association with PAL-
PITATIONS. It can be confused with
EPILEPSY.

FALLOT'S TETRALOGY

See *CONGENITAL HEART-
DISEASE.*

FALLS

See *CLUMSINESS, CONVUL-
SIONS.*

FAMILY PROBLEMS

Almost any family problem will affect
children, even if they are not the cause
of it. Children are sensitive to, and react to, changes or upset feelings in
their parents, whether or not they
know or can understand their causes.

■ PROBLEMS OUTSIDE THE
FAMILY
Unemployment, or the threat of it,
moving to a new home, illness in a
grandparent or family friend,
BEREAVEMENT, money worries,
changes or upheavals in the community or school, racial harassment:
all these may affect your child indirectly through their effect on you,
or directly from what the child
reads, hears or sees. Don't pretend
these things are not happening. Try
to explain in a reassuring way what
is causing the worry and what you
are feeling and doing as a result.
Give what reassurance you can
about what will *not* change: various
routines, your love, affection and
protection for the child.
　Try to consider *his* level of understanding. You may need to spell out
several times everything that will remain normal, and how the child
should cope with any changes that
do occur.

■ PROBLEMS WITHIN THE
FAMILY
Marital unhappiness, separation,
DIVORCE or remarriage, illness or the
need for medical investigation,
problems with the law: all will pro-
duce stress in parents and this will
affect a child. Give a simple and
straightforward explanation, tail-
ored to his age and understanding.
Your child may show ANXIETY or
STRESS SYMPTOMS, SLEEP or FEEDING
PROBLEMS or BEHAVIORAL DIS-
ORDERS, or SCHOOL ATTENDANCE
PROBLEMS. These can all be kept to a

minimum if you explain what is happening and as far as possible avoid disrupting routines.

Sometimes a problem with one child can affect the others. Illness or school difficulties, step families, problems of adolescence are all typical ones. Sometimes you may need to reassure the other children that this problem will not necessarily happen to them, or that you still love them even though you are preoccupied with the child in difficulty. Make special efforts to remember that children who are *not* causing you anxiety need your attention too. The symptoms a child may show in these circumstances will vary with his age.

■ ACTION Discuss problems with all members of the family if at all possible. Talk about it together, read the section in this book that relates to your problem. If it persists see your doctor who may suggest other sources of help.

FAMILY THERAPY
A form of treatment which enables families to sort out problems, usually identified with, or brought to light by, one of the children. It is based on the premise that difficulties in family relationships are associated with psychological problems, and that they can best be helped by involving all members of the family. Such therapy may also help when one family member has a problem, but the family as a whole can be of general help and support. This can be a powerful way of effecting change. It is practiced by a range of professionals including psychologists, social workers and child psychiatrists. Often more than one therapist will be involved. In a broader sense, however, most pediatricians' approach to practice includes an element of family therapy. See also the entries on *FAMILY PROBLEMS* and *BEHAVIORAL TREATMENTS*.

FARSIGHTEDNESS (HYPEROPIA)
The eye sees well in the distance, but has difficulty focusing on near objects. This may be due to the globe of the eye being 'shorter' than it ought to be, or the lens or cornea not bending the rays of light enough. It is the commonest eyesight problem in children, and usually becomes apparent at around three years of age.

It may be associated with STRABISMUS and/or complaints of 'eye strain', HEADACHE, and disinterest in reading. An EYE TEST will determine which EYE GLASSES are needed to correct the child's vision.

FEARS
Fear is a natural and self-protective instinct that all children develop as part of their own self-defense. During the first few years of life all children have frights and develop fears; normally they acquire the confidence to deal with them unaided as they mature. See also *ANXIETY and PHOBIAS*.

FEBRILE CONVULSIONS
Usually generalized (rather than focal) CONVULSIONS of sudden onset in association with a FEVER in susceptible infants and young children from six months to five years, but mostly under three years of age. They need to be distinguished from FAINTING attacks and shaking chills that occur with high FEVER.

They can run in families, and boys appear to be more susceptible than girls.

■ ACTION Place the child in the RECOVERY POSITION. When he recovers, give frequent drinks (typically, half cup of water, cola or juice per hour when he is awake) and acetamenophen to reduce fever. Don't give aspirin – see *REYE SYNDROME*. Future febrile illnesses should be treated in the same way to reduce risk of febrile convulsions. See *FEVER*. Get urgent medical help if a convulsion continues for five minutes or longer. Always get medical advice when a child of any age has a febrile convulsion, in case it is a first sign of MENINGITIS.

■ TREATMENT Anticonvulsant drugs will not prevent recurrences, and the risk of drug side-effects outweighs the risk of harm from febrile convulsions.

■ OUTLOOK Most febrile convulsions are brief and harmless, though alarming to parents who may even think the child has died. If a child has had one febrile convulsion, there is a one in three chance of it happening again. About 5 percent of all children experience at least one febrile convulsion, but only one in 50 of them go on to experience EPILEPSY in later childhood.

FEEDING PROBLEMS
These tend to occur at times of change – see *WEANING*. The baby (or toddler) simply finds the next stage of development tiresome or difficult. For example, VOMITING or regurgitating may be associated with the introduction of solids. In three-year-olds and above, the problems are usually seen as insistence on eating the same food(s) at every meal, poor appetite or over-eating.

■ CAUSES Almost all day-to-day feeding problems have to do with difficult behavior rather than with poor health. They usually arise for a combination of reasons:

The child may be eating enough, despite what his parents think. Particularly for toddlers, food can provide an ideal opportunity to assert independence.

Suspecting a child may not be getting adequate nourishment causes anxiety; anxiety leads to pressure on the child to eat: a battle of wills between parent and child occurs with the child in an ideal position to win. Deliberate vomiting by the child is often associated with this conflict.

Children, like adults, can be conservative in their tastes and may dislike trying new foods. They do, however, become more willing to try out new foods as they grow older.

Meal times in many families provide an opportunity for demonstrating individuality through food choice. Having something prepared especially for your child is both a treat and a useful and comforting demonstration of parental attention.

■ AVOIDING PROBLEMS Have a routine; take meals in a relaxed atmosphere – let the child eat at his own pace; encourage independence, and allow likes and dislikes, without over-indulging.
– Avoid fussing, cajoling, threatening or bribing your child to eat.
– Avoid battles: remove food if it is not eaten after two or three attempts at gentle encouragement. But don't reward the child's refusal with cookies or ice-cream to follow.
– Put very small amounts of food on your child's plate rather than overwhelming him with more than he wants to or could eat. He can always be offered more when the first serving is finished.

■ ACTION If you are really worried

that the child is not eating properly, check with your doctor about whether he is gaining weight at the normal rate for his age and height. Try recording everything that your child eats and drinks, not just at meal times. It may be more than you think.

When weaning a child from the breast or bottle, do not allow him to drink too much milk at the expense of other foods and liquids. Reduce his milk intake and give him other drinks instead. Gradually increase the consistency of his food, offer finger foods, and allow him to do as much feeding of himself as he wants.

Don't feel that you always have to cook alternatives for poor eaters. Discourage eating between meals and always encourage your child to taste a little bit of anything new. The 'two bite rule' is often helpful. The child must east two bites of the food item he does not like on his plate, but is allowed to refuse the rest of it provided he eats all the rest of the food on his plate.

Get medical advice if vomiting seems related to eating and occurs at most meals.

The advice of a clinical psychologist may be suggested if severe feeding problems persist. See also *WEANING, OBESITY, ANOREXIA, FAILURE TO THRIVE, BREAST FEEDING, BOTTLE FEEDING.*

FETAL DISTRESS

As the term implies, the fetus is in a state of distress. This may arise from problems of circulation or oxygenation, usually due to problems of placenta function. If the distress is unrelieved, the health and life of the fetus may be jeopardized.

■ SIGNS Green-brown staining of the amniotic fluid that surrounds the fetus while it is in the mother's uterus (waters) due to the fetus emptying MECONIUM from its bowels as a response to distress: if the waters break at home and are seen to be green-stained, go to hospital immediately. The baby's heart rate changes in response to distress, sometimes rising (to rates greater than 160/min) or, more seriously, falling (to rates below 120/min). Changes in fetal movements may also point to distress, especially if fetal movements become less frequent or stop altogether. If you think your baby has stopped moving, contact your doctor and go to hospital without delay.

■ TESTS The baby's heart rate can be monitored either by listening with a stethoscope or by electronic monitoring (see *BIRTH, PROBLEMS OF*). If fetal distress is suspected, a sample of blood may be taken from the fetus' scalp. In skilled hands, this is harmless to the baby, and a minimally discomforting procedure for the mother. The blood is then analyzed for acidity: the more acidic, the greater the severity of the fetal distress.

■ ACTION Your obstetrician, often in consultation with a pediatrician, will decide whether any immediate action is called for. Often careful observation as pregnancy or delivery progress is all that is needed. At other times, particularly if there are indications of severe distress, the decision may be made to deliver your baby urgently, by forceps or Caesarian section.

■ OUTLOOK In the majority of cases, the baby comes to no harm, and is well at birth and thereafter. Occasionally distress proceeds to asphyxia: if delivered, the baby will then need vigorous skilled resuscitation; if undelivered, the fetus is in danger of dying.

FEVER

A child who has a temperature of more than 100°F or 37.7°C orally, or 101°F or 38.3°C rectally definitely has a fever. Temperatures below this but above 98.6°F or 37°C orally may indicate fever, or may be part of the normal variation seen in some children and adults. The most common causes of fever are VIRAL and BACTERIAL INFECTIONS. However, a fever may also be a sign of a less common underlying general disease, such as inflammation of the joints (ARTHRITIS) or the intestines (CROHN DISEASE). The child feels generally unwell and may appear miserable and irritable. If the temperature is rising rapidly, he may shiver and feel cold; if the temperature is steady or falling, he may sweat, look red and feel hot. Other symptoms may be associated depending on the cause of the fever.

■ ACTION 1 With low-grade fever (oral temperature 101°F or 38.3°C or less), supportive treatment such as fluids, acetamenophen or loosening of the child's clothing may be all that is required.

However, with higher temperatures it is important that the child be assessed by a doctor, since fever is a symptom or sign to an underlying disease which may be mild but also may be serious.

Febrile convulsions or seizures may occur in young children with high fever. In such children, up to the age of six years or so, it is important to bring the temperature down as quickly and effectively as possible. Undress the child and use antipyretics and sponging with tepid (not cold) water.

But remember: fever is not a disease; it is an indication that a disease may be present.

Acetamenophen is the safest and most effective treatment for fever (antipyretic). Aspirin should *not* be given to children under 12 years old, because of the risk of REYE SYNDROME. The dose of acetamenophen will vary with the age of the child, and is shown on the bottle. It may be given up to every four hours. 2 Sponging with tepid water is an effective way of treating fever, but this should not be done for any longer than an hour at a time, and no more often than three or four times daily. If the fever persists after 24 hours, or if other signs and symptoms of illness appear before then, your child should be seen by your doctor. 3 Dress your child in light clothing to make heat loss from his body easier. 4 Encourage your child to drink clear fluids. This is generally comforting and avoids dehydration.

■ GET MEDICAL ADVICE if the fever continues or recurs, or is very high (say over 102.5°F or 39°C), or if your child is irritable or has other symptoms.

The doctor will advise additional treatment or tests depending on the pattern and duration of the fever, and the constellation of associated features. Tests may range from urine culture (for suspect URINARY TRACT INFECTION), to chest X-ray (for suspect PNEUMONIA) to a lumbar puncture (for suspect MENINGITIS).

FINGER INJURIES

Hands and fingers are precious, so injuries need prompt treatment. Don't delay in seeking treatment for anything beyond a small cut – in children as well as adults. The 'pulp spaces' in the fingertips and palms are especially prone to infection, and may need treatment with ANTIBIOTICS. Tendon injuries are another common problem, so get medical advice if the hand doesn't seem to work properly after an injury, or if there is any numbness which may indicate damage to nerves. Your doctor may refer your child to a hand surgeon if the injury is severe or if he suspects that an infection has developed.

FIRE SETTING
Some children find fire fascinating and, if they have the means, will seek to light one. They may do this by copying what they have seen adults do, for instance poking paper into a fireplace and lighting it with a match. Keep matches and cigarette lighters away

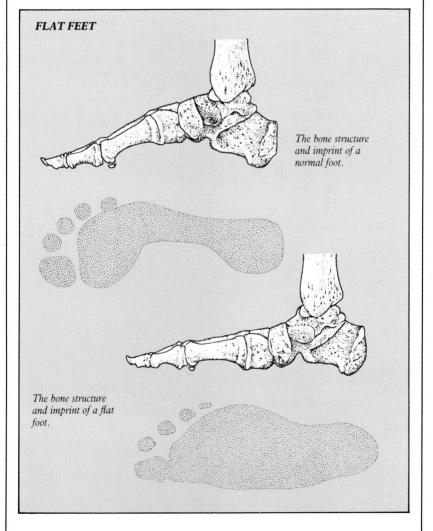

FLAT FEET

The bone structure and imprint of a normal foot.

The bone structure and imprint of a flat foot.

from children. Teach respect for fire by showing and telling them what they should do, and by doing the same yourself. *Never* leave a young child alone with an unguarded fire in a fireplace or wood stove. See also *ACCIDENTS IN THE HOME, BEHAVIORAL TREATMENTS.*

FLAT FEET

Common, particularly in children who are overweight. All babies and young children have flat feet until bone growth gives the necessary modelling. Most older children and adults with flexible flat feet have loose ligaments, allowing their loose-jointed feet to sag when they bear weight. They usually also have hyperextendable knees, elbows and fingers.

■ SYMPTOMS Loss of the normal arch of the foot, so that the sole is in contact with the ground over its whole length. The heel tilts inwards and the front of the foot turns outwards. Shoes bulge inwards and the heels wear down quickly on the inner side. Sometimes the child also has KNOCK KNEES. Most children, however, form a definite arch if they point their toes. This is in contrast to secondary flat feet seen in CEREBRAL PALSY and MUSCULAR DYSTROPHY. Flat feet are not usually painful. Very occasionally the child may complain of sore legs and feet.

■ ACTION In most instances no specific action is required, since flat feet are a variant of normal. Special arch supports or shoes are expensive and are rarely clinically indicated. If your child often complains of sore feet or legs, you may want to discuss this with your doctor. Flat feet are rarely the cause of the complaints.

■ TREATMENT is not necessary.

FLU
See *INFLUENZA.*

FLUORIDE
See *TEETHING.*

FONTANELLES
The gaps or soft areas between the bones of a baby's skull. There are two: one at the front, of about +-one in (15-30 mm) in diameter in the newborn period, which closes when the baby is around 18 months old; and a second, smaller fontanelle at the back of the skull, which closes in the early weeks after birth.

The size of the fontanelles varies greatly. They allow the brain to continue to grow rapidly, as it does in the first year or so after birth.

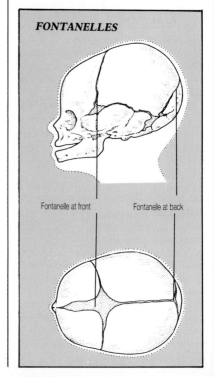

FONTANELLES

Fontanelle at front   Fontanelle at back

FOOD POISONING

Acute DIARRHEA and VOMITING caused by food-borne toxins produced by BACTERIA in contaminated food. Meat that has been inadequately cooked or stored without refrigeration, and insufficiently reheated, or cream and mayonnaise are typical foods that can become contaminated by bacteria. Several members of the family are likely to be afflicted at once.

■ SYMPTOMS Rapidity of onset depends on the bacteria involved. Vomiting, ABDOMINAL PAIN and profuse diarrhea occur two to seven hours after staphylococcal food poisoning, and usually last only one day. Symptoms due to *Bacillus cereus* or *Clostridium perfringens* (botulism) occur seven to 24 hours after eating the contaminated food and usually cause symptoms for several days.

■ ACTION Get medical advice if your child develops acute and severe symptoms (see *GASTROENTERITIS*). Admission to the hospital may well be required. ANTIBIOTICS and other drugs are not usually given.

■ TREATMENT Oral or intravenous fluids to correct DEHYDRATION. Antitoxin injections and machine-assisted breathing (ventilation) may be necessary for the rare peripheral nerve complications of botulism, which affect the mechanisms that control breathing.

■ OUTLOOK Most cases of food poisoning are mild. Even in severe cases, early treatment limits the risk of death. See the entry on *GASTROENTERITIS*.

FOOT INJURIES

Apart from SPRAINS AND STRAINS, the most common injuries to the feet are caused by dropping heavy objects on to them. Symptoms may well include BLEEDING, BRUISING or possibly FRACTURES. The worst of the swelling and pain of the injury will start to subside after two days unless there is a fracture, in which case the child may still be unable to walk on the affected foot. Fractures of the bones of the foot are uncommon in childhood, but you may wish to take your child to the hospital for an X-ray, just in case. Fractures of the small bones of the toes can occur, but are usually treated with strapping or left to heal by themselves. Fractures of the ankle may occur in older children. These need prompt treatment and immobilization in a plaster cast to ensure full recovery.

■ ACTION Use cold compresses for pain at the site of injury. A painkiller such as acetamenophen will also help. If the child is unable to put any weight on the foot after 24 hours, or if there is marked swelling or bleeding, get medical advice to be sure there is no fracture.

FORCEPS

Spoon-shaped instruments placed on either side of a baby's head to aid DELIVERY. Forceps delivery may be used to facilitate the delivery of the baby when there is FETAL DISTRESS, or if the baby has difficulty in descending through the birth canal, or if the mother is judged to need help in the second stage of labor, when she is timing her contractions of her stomach muscles with the contractions of the uterus to aid in pushing the baby through the birth canal. The mother's legs are put in stirrups and she is given a local anesthetic if she has not already had an EPIDURAL ANESTHETIC. An episiotomy is usually performed, the forceps are slipped round the baby's head and pulled gently but firmly as the mother pushes with each contraction. Forceps delivery rarely results in BIRTH INJURY. Sometimes marks are visible on the baby's face, but these usually disappear in 24 hours.

FORCEPS DELIVERY

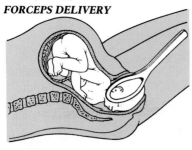

FOREIGN BODY ASPIRATION

Inhalation of a foreign material into the upper airway or lung. The foreign body may be food the child choked on and 'swallowed the wrong way', a small object such as a coin, a peanut, a button or a small piece off a toy.

This problem most commonly occurs in older infants and young children. Aspirated peanuts are a common problem.

■ SYMPTOMS Usually sudden onset of COUGHING, CHOKING and gagging. If the object obstructs the airway tube inside the lung and is not cleared by coughing, the child may develop a wheeze, a cough and possibly PNEUMONIA in that part of the lung.

■ ACTION See *CHOKING*. If you feel the object was inhaled and not coughed up, seek medical advice. Aspiration of food particles, especially peanuts, can lead to inflammation in that area of the lung which may cause local lung damage.

■ TREATMENT Chest X-ray; bronchoscopy – a special flexible lighted tube is passed down the wind pipe (trachea) into the larger airway tubes in the lung (bronchi) to give a picture of the foreign body which is then removed with forceps attached to the bronchoscope. This is done in the operating room under general ANESTHESIA. ANTIBIOTIC treatment may be needed if pneumonia has developed in the affected part of the lung.

■ OUTLOOK If not removed, foreign bodies in large airways can have serious long-term consequences and may even cause death. However, with removal, almost all patients recover completely.

■ PREVENTION Carefully check all toys for small pieces that could come off. Do not give young children small pieces of hard foods such as peanuts or candies.

FOREIGN BODY INGESTION

Children may swallow a variety of objects that can pass through the entire intestinal tract without complications. Occasionally an object gets stuck in the food tube (esophagus), stomach or intestine and may have to be removed surgically.

■ FOREIGN BODY IN ESOPHAGUS Swallowing the object may provoke an attack of coughing and choking. If stuck in the esophagus, there is usually pain in the chest and difficulty swallowing (especially solid foods).

A chest X-ray will reveal radiopaque foreign bodies. If not opaque (meaning the body does not show up on an X-ray), a barium meal may help to outline the object.

The object can be removed by passing a flexible lighted tube down the esophagus (endoscope) and retrieving the object with forceps attached to the endoscope.

■ FOREIGN BODY IN STOMACH OR INTESTINES An object that reaches the stomach will in most instances pass through the intestines without injury. Certain types of objects, however, may cause problems and are potentially dangerous. Needles, hairpins, bobby pins and nails occasionally get stuck in the intestines. If they are large, removal from the stomach by endoscopy may be necessary – see *foreign body in esophagus*, above.

FRACTURES

This is the medical term for broken bones. The pliability of young bones, however, means that they may often bend rather than break, hence the term greenstick fracture.

You may also hear the term undisplaced fracture: one in which the normal line of the bone is not changed by the fracture, and the two ends remain in contact.

■ SYMPTOMS There has usually been an obvious injury, but this is not always so.

There is pain and swelling or other deformity over the point where the bone is fractured. The pain may be severe, and aggravated by the slightest movement.

The child is usually extremely reluctant to move the limb.

Sometimes the pain is not particularly bad because the fracture is stable: there is not much movement at the site of the fracture when the bone is not being used, or indeed on slight movement. Occasionally, the fracture can be so stable that the child continues to use the limb. However, in these cases, there is usually some swelling that does not disappear, or slight pain.

Occasionally, a fracture may be so severe that one end of the bone comes through the skin (an open or

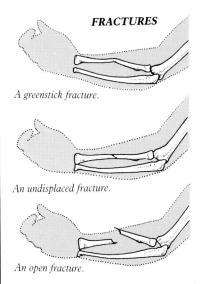

FRACTURES

A greenstick fracture.

An undisplaced fracture.

An open fracture.

compound fracture). This kind of fracture can easily be infected causing OSTEOMYELITIS.

■ ACTION The pain can be relieved by keeping the affected area still. If an arm or leg is affected, a sling or splint will be helpful.

The swelling can be eased by the application of ice or by elevating the limb.

If you suspect a fracture, you should get medical advice or go directly to a hospital where an X-ray can be taken to establish whether the bone is broken or not.

If there is a chance that your child may need an anesthetic for an operation to get the bones back into normal position (reduction or 'setting' the fracture), don't give him anything to eat or drink since this will postpone the use of an anesthetic and starting proper treatment. If in doubt, get medical advice.

■ TESTS X-ray is the common, reliable means of making the diagnosis. It is also useful for checking that the bone is healing properly.

■ TREATMENT A painkiller such as acetamenophen with or without codeine (do not give aspirin – see *REYE SYNDROME*) will ease the pain.

Fractures usually require a plaster cast to keep the bone from moving as it heals.

It is important to keep exercising those parts of the injured limb which are not in the plaster cast. This prevents the joints from becoming stiff and the muscles weak.

A child will usually exercise naturally if it does not cause pain: there is no need to discourage him from doing so.

If his fingers or toes are swollen, encourage him to use them.

Occasionally, a plaster cast becomes too tight because of swelling of the tissue around the fracture after the plaster cast has been put on. This can affect important arteries and nerves, and is the reason why your child may be kept in hospital overnight after having a plaster cast applied. If you notice that his fingers or toes have become pale or blue, or if he complains of numbness, tingling or severe pain, let the nurse or doctor know immediately and make sure that it is carefully checked.

Fractures of the collar-bone (clavicle) usually require a shoulder brace or an arm sling to prevent the ends of the bone from moving and causing pain.

Fractures of the skull need special treatment because of the risk of damage to the brain.

Fractures heal more quickly in children than in adults, particularly the greenstick type. Healing occurs by the natural production of a bridge of bone between the two broken ends. Extra bridging is needed in bones that bear weight, such as those of the leg, and these take longer to heal.

The bone will only regain its normal strength after several months, but this will happen fastest if the bone is used. Physiotherapy may help.

■ OUTLOOK Most fractures in children heal completely without any long-term complications.

FRAGILE (BRITTLE) BONE DISEASE

See *OSTEOGENESIS IMPERFECTA*.

FRIENDS – REAL OR IMAGINARY

Making friends may start as early as the third year, but what the relationship means at this age may of course be different than later on. At this age, or later, when your child's imagination is very rich, he may acquire (or invent) an imaginary friend, whether or not he has real friends. This friend often seems to have characteristics, rights and possessions your child would like to have. Sometimes he, or she, vanishes quickly as a younger brother or sister starts to talk and provides the child with increasingly good company. Having imaginary friends is a phase that usually passes naturally and can be regarded as perfectly normal.

FUNGI AND FUNGAL INFECTIONS

In medical terminology, fungi are organisms such as molds and yeasts. Most fungi are harmless but a few can cause INFECTION, particularly of the skin, hair, nails and the membrane linings of the mouth and vagina. Common fungal infections include CANDIDIASIS, ATHLETE'S FOOT and RINGWORM.

Serious or recurrent fungal infections may represent a complication of extensive antibiotic therapy or, rarely, point to an IMMUNE deficiency.

Thrush and fungal diaper rash, however, are common in infancy.

■ TREATMENT Thrush and fungal diaper rash are usually cured by antifungal medication. Other fungal infections of skin and nails are more difficult to cure and may need to be treated for several weeks or months until all the infected skin, often several layers deep, has been replaced by healthy tissue.

FUNNEL CHEST
See *PECTUS EXCAVATUM.*

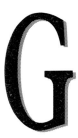

GALACTOSEMIA
A rare condition in which digesting galactose, a form of sugar, results in toxic symptoms because of an inherited deficiency of an enzyme essential for its metabolism.

■ SYMPTOMS usually appear soon after birth and within a few days of the baby starting milk feedings. VOMITING and DIARRHEA, FAILURE TO THRIVE, prolonged JAUNDICE and enlargement of the liver are all common in the first month of life. In severe cases, the abdomen may become swollen with fluid and the child may develop INFECTION in the blood (septicemia). Some children have CATARACTS (opacities of the lens in the eye) and if the condition is not recognized promptly, brain development will be impaired resulting in MENTAL HANDICAP.

■ TREATMENT depends on the elimination of galactose from the diet. Completely avoiding it is the goal, but this may be difficult. There are several milk preparations available that are virtually galactose free, including soy milk.

Dietary advice must be followed closely as the child grows. There are lists of permitted foods available, and it is essential that parents become very familiar with dietary do's and don'ts if treatment is to be successful. If an affected child drinks cow's milk or eats foods containing galactose, vomiting and diarrhea will quickly develop. In the long term, inadequate control of the diet may result in poor growth and mental handicap.

■ OUTLOOK Those children identified in the first month of life (and correctly treated) will have normal INTELLIGENCE, although minor LEARNING DISORDERS may develop later. Close follow-up of intellectual development is advisable: minor problems can be dealt with early, and the child can be motivated to maintain sound dietary control.

Children diagnosed late, or whose dietary control is poor, may be below average intelligence. Girls may be infertile because of poor development of the ovaries.

GASTROENTERITIS

A common condition of infants and toddlers consisting of DIARRHEA with or without VOMITING coming on quite suddenly, and lasting a few days. Usually caused by VIRUSES of various types, occasionally by BACTERIA or PARASITES. Transmission is usually by direct contact with a person with gastroenteritis, through contaminated food/water or via airborne virus-containing droplets.

■ ACTION Keep the child away from others (especially from other small infants) until the signs and symptoms of gastroenteritis have disappeared. Don't worry if the child has no appetite – a few days without solid foods will do him no harm. But it is important to maintain an adequate fluid intake to compensate for the fluid lost through diarrhea and vomiting – see DEHYDRATION. This is the most significant danger of gastroenteritis. Concentrate on encouraging the child to take frequent drinks of clear fluids, despite the vomiting. These fluids are rapidly absorbed, so even if the child vomits soon after a drink, some will have been retained in the stomach.

Traditionally, milk is considered to be poorly tolerated by the bowel in gastroenteritis; however, this is controversial. Thus, for breast-fed babies, it is often preferable, despite gastroenteritis, to continue with breast feeding.

If the symptoms continue for more than a day or so, or if your baby shows signs of illness or dehydration, then get medical advice. The smaller or younger your baby, the sooner you should see a doctor.

■ TREATMENT Most doctors do not give medicines to slow down the bowel; the emphasis is on maintaining your baby's hydration while allowing the body's natural defenses to eliminate the virus. If the gastroenteritis is due to bacteria such as *Shigella* or *Campylobacter*, ANTIBIOTICS may be recommended. In most gastroenteritis cases, however, antibiotics are not useful.

■ OUTLOOK This is a common illness, and recovery is usually complete within a week or ten days. Appetite then improves and the child eats normally and puts on weight. Occasionally, following a severe bout of gastroenteritis, there is a period of intolerance to certain foods which may continue to be poorly absorbed and to cause diarrhea. Complete recovery follows, usually within a few weeks.

GASTROESOPHAGEAL REFLUX (CHALASIA)

When the lower sphincter muscle of the food tube (esophagus) does not develop properly. When the stomach empties, gastric juice passes upwards and leads to inflammation and ulceration of the esophageal lining (esophagitis).

■ SYMPTOMS Excessive VOMITING in infancy starting often in the first week of life and usually related to feeding. The vomiting may occur mostly at night in an older child. There may be mucus (a slimy substance) mixed with the vomited milk.

Brown staining of the vomitus due to blood (hematemesis) and, more rarely, blood in the stools (which are black) can occur after bleeding of the ulcerated areas. The baby or child may be pale due to ANEMIA from acute or chronic BLEEDING. CONSTIPATION is common. There may be CHEST PAIN from the acid reflux. There is often FAILURE TO THRIVE and occasionally the child may become DEHYDRATED.

An infant may have a choking episode from the reflux, or he may wheeze and suffer repeated CHEST INFECTIONS from inhalation (aspiration) of milk into the upper and lower airways; but these occurrences are rare.

■ ACTION Discuss your child's vomiting with the family doctor. Marked symptoms will usually require referral to a pediatric gastroenterologist.

■ INVESTIGATIONS Mild cases: careful clinical assessment may be sufficient. X-ray of the esophagus and stomach is taken after barium is swallowed; in some hospitals, special acid- (pH)- measuring tubes passed into the esophagus may help quantify the degree of acid regurgitation. Other tests are available to investigate reflux up the esophagus and into the lungs.

■ MANAGEMENT Small frequent feedings; feeding and nursing in an upright position for several months may be necessary.

Thickening the feedings with cereal may be recommended although their value has not been proven. The vomiting often improves when solids are introduced into the baby's diet.

The effectiveness of medications, including antacids, is not well proven but they are often used. Antacids help treat the esophagitis but do not improve lower esophageal sphincter function.

Surgery will be necessary only in those children with major problems. These include continuing failure to thrive, persistent bleeding or repeated chest infections. The surgery is not as extensive as that required for a diaphragmatic HERNIA and usually designed to tighten the esophageal sphincter muscle.

■ OUTLOOK Most babies with gastroesophageal reflux improve with time.

GENES

Biological codes containing the inherited characteristics are passed on from parent to child. Every body cell, except the father's sperm cells (spermatozoa) and the mother's egg cells (ova), has 23 pairs of CHROMOSOMES, and each chromosome carries hundreds of genes. Each gene has a matching gene on the other chromosome of a pair. For every inherited characteristic, a child inherits one gene from one parent and another gene from the other parent. Genes responsible for a particular characteristic can be dominant or recessive. If the child inherits one gene for blue eyes and one for brown, then he will, generally, have brown eyes because the gene for brown eyes is dominant over the gene for blue eyes. Deficiencies or abnormalities in the chemical structure of genes can result in diseases that can be passed on in this way from parent to child. These are called INHERITED DISORDERS.

GENETIC COUNSELLING

Genetic counselling is of value if you

have a family history of a particular disease, or if you have a child with an INHERITED DISORDER or CONGENITAL ABNORMALITY. Genetic counselling aims to explain the nature of an inherited disorder – its severity, treatment, complications and likely outcome – as well as the genetic mechanisms that cause the disease; most important, it also aims to define and advise upon the risk of the disease recurring in future pregnancies. The calculation of the risk is based on a variety of factors, including the recognized disease frequency in relatives of the child. Whether or not you decide to embark upon future pregnancies will depend on the severity of the disease and your attitude about the disease; additionally, in the case of a disease that can be identified in pregnancy, you would be helped to form your own opinion about termination of a pregnancy. Specific tests may be used to determine the risk of a particular disease in a family and in a particular pregnancy. Physical examination and BLOOD TESTS may indicate whether relatives are carriers of the disease. Research in this field is expanding rapidly, but we are a long way from being able to test for all genetically inherited diseases in this way.

If the risk of a recurrence of the disease is unacceptably high to you, you will need to discuss such matters as contraception, and the possibilities of adoption or artificial insemination by donor. If you are already pregnant, PRENATAL DIAGNOSTIC tests may ascertain whether or not the fetus is affected, and termination of the pregnancy can then be considered by all persons involved.

GERMAN MEASLES
See *RUBELLA*.

GIARDIA
Giardia lamblia is a PARASITE that in-habits the small bowel (see diagram of intestine at front of book), and interferes with absorption of food (see *MALABSORPTION*). The INFECTION can be contracted in the United States from infected water or food; the risk is even higher in tropical, developing countries. *Giardia* is an important cause of diarrhea in children in daycare.

■ SYMPTOMS may come on gradually, with the child eating poorly, being tired and irritable and losing weight. The stools may be loose, pale and float in the toilet because they contain large amounts of non-absorbed fats. However, the symptoms may be more severe, with nausea, vomiting or stomach ache, as in GASTROENTERITIS. Others in the family may be similarly affected.

■ TESTS *Giardia* may be detected in stool samples examined in a laboratory. However, because *Giardia* is excreted intermittently, multiple stool samples obtained on different days should be examined. Examination of the fluid in the duodenum (first part of the intestine after the stomach) can also detect the parasite.

■ ACTION Make sure everyone washes their hands thoroughly after going to the toilet. (This is, of course, normal good health practice, but especially important if a member of the household has diarrhea.) Get medical advice if your child is acutely ill or the symptoms continue for more than a few days.

■ TREATMENT is only recommended for symptomatic cases. Your doctor may prescribe quinacrine hydrochloride, which has a bitter taste, furazolidine (better tasting but less effective) or metrinidazole (its use in children is limited).

■ OUTLOOK A marked improvement in symptoms should follow in a few days after starting treatment. There is a risk of reinfection; this is best prevented by culinary hygiene and washing hands.

GIFTED CHILD

Children are defined as gifted if they are in the top 2 percent of intelligence for their age. Many experts consider that gifted children have special educational needs: their abilities may make them stand out from their peer group, which can lead to social isolation. However, exceptionally bright children as a whole usually do not have special difficulties in regular schools. It is important, however, to balance academic and social development. If made to feel too special, the child may behave as if he is superior to other children, and his social development may suffer. If you feel that your child is very bright and is not performing as well as expected, or if he seems unhappy at school, discuss the matter with his teacher. If the problem cannot be easily resolved, the teacher may refer your child to an educational psychologist for assessment. Educational and/or social alternatives for gifted children include enrichment programs available through many school boards and special extracurricular programs offered in some communities.

GILLES DE LA TOURETTE SYNDROME

A severe form of TIC which typically takes the form of repeated words, phrases or noises, sometimes rude or even obscene. The child cannot stop these utterances, but may be able to control them for a few minutes. If severe, medication may be required.

GINGIVITIS ('GUM DISEASE')

Gingivitis, or inflammation of the gums, is the first stage of 'gum disease' (periodontal disease): the start of a process which, if neglected, results in tooth loss. In children it is usually just the gums that are affected.

■ CAUSES Plaque (a substance containing bacteria) collects on the teeth and in the crevices between the teeth and gums, as a result of poor cleaning.

■ SYMPTOMS Soreness and bleeding from the gums, often during toothbrushing, and foul breath.

■ TREATMENT The process is easily reversed by regular and effective removal of the plaque by brushing and flossing or by the dentist with special scaling instruments. Regular checkups with the dentist are important for assessment of the problem. If bleeding is excessive and persistent, consult your dentist or doctor to check that there is no underlying cause.

GLANDULAR FEVER

See INFECTIOUS MONONUCLEOSIS.

GLOMERULONEPHRITIS

See NEPHRITIS.

GLUCOSE 6-PHOSPHATE DEHYDROGENASE DEFICIENCY

An INHERITED DISORDER that can cause a HEMOLYTIC ANEMIA. There are slightly different incidences of occurrence of this deficiency among various ethnic groups around the world.

■ SYMPTOMS JAUNDICE can occur in new-born babies and may be severe enough to require EXCHANGE TRANSFUSION. If a baby or child has the condition, acute INFECTIONS, exposure to moth balls and certain drugs can trigger a marked breakdown of red blood cells resulting in severe ANEMIA and jaundice. The drugs include some ANTIBIOTICS and anti-malarial drugs, and a few other medications seldom given to children.

Between episodes, the child is usually well. But in some children the breakdown of red blood cells continues at all times. This results in increased red blood cell production in the liver, spleen and bone marrow; if this does not compensate fully, a mild anemia can result.

■ ACTION The child should wear a bracelet stating he has G6-PD deficiency, to ensure that he is not given inappropriate medication.

A BLOOD TEST can reveal the diagnosis, and if there is a family history this testing should not be neglected.

■ TREATMENT Infections require immediate action: get medical advice. A BLOOD TRANSFUSION can be given to treat severe episodes.

■ OUTLOOK Usually good, once the disease has been diagnosed and the drugs to which the child is sensitive are identified.

GLUE EAR (SERIOUS *OTITIS MEDIA*)

The accumulation of sticky fluid in the middle ear behind the eardrum.

■ SYMPTOMS Partial deafness is the main symptom. The child may say his ear feels 'full'. The symptom may first arise following a MIDDLE EAR INFECTION.

■ ACTION Any suspicion that a child has hearing problems should be raised without delay with your doctor – see *DEAFNESS*.

GLUE EAR

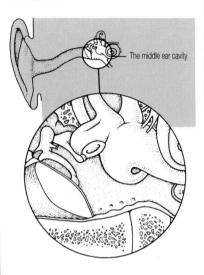
The middle ear cavity

Sticky fluid accumulates here.

■ INVESTIGATIONS If examination confirms any degree of deafness, you will be referred to a specialist for full-scale hearing tests – see *AUDIOGRAM*.

■ TREATMENT Glue ear often clears up in two to three months without treatment. Your doctor may suggest a course of oral ANTIBIOTICS. It is usual to wait three months, then re-check the child's hearing, before considering the insertion of small plastic EAR TUBES through the eardrum to help drain the remaining fluid and to prevent another middle ear infection.

■ OUTLOOK Hearing may vary in infancy and may affect early LANGUAGE DEVELOPMENT. In the long term, however, the outlook for health, hearing and speech is normally good.

GLUE SNIFFING
See *SOLVENT ABUSE, ADDIC-TION.*

GOITER
A swelling in the neck caused by an enlarged thyroid gland. This can signify HYPERTHYROIDISM, HYPOTHYROIDISM, or result from a deficiency of iodine in the diet (now rare in the United States since all salt contains added iodine). The goiter itself usually requires no treatment (other than occasionally for cosmetic reasons) unless it is so large that it causes obstruction to the airway. In such cases, surgical removal or thyroidectomy is indicated. Treatment is directed towards the underlying cause of the goiter.

GONORRHEA
A SEXUALLY TRANSMITTED DISEASE due to BACTERIAL INFECTION. If a mother is infected when giving birth, it can give her baby severe CONJUNCTIV-ITIS. If this is not treated with injected ANTIBIOTICS, damage to the eyes can result.

Older children can catch the infection from an adult carrier through SEX-UAL ABUSE. Gonorrhea is not caught from toilet seats. Gonorrhea is now a major problem among sexually active adolescents in North America.

Vaginal infection in young children as well as in adolescents may be asymptomatic or it may cause a vaginal discharge. In adolescents, this may be associated with abdominal pain if the infection has spread from the vagina. In boys, asymptomatic infection is common but discharge from the penis and burning with urination may occur.

The diagnosis is confirmed by culturing gonorrhea from swabs taken from the infected area. Treatment with antibiotics, once rapidly effective, has become increasingly less so, such that various kinds and combinations of antibiotics may be required to irradicate the infection.

GRAND MAL SEIZURE
The most florid form of EPILEPSY in which the child loses consciousness and may be variously rigid, or jerk some or all parts of the body. As with other seizures, it may also be described (loosely) as a fit, seizure or CONVUL-SION.

■ SYMPTOMS There is stiffening of the whole body ('tonic phase'), followed by generalized shaking ('clonic phase'), followed by deep sleep. The child may bite his tongue, lip or cheek during the attack, and produce frothy saliva around the mouth; he may also pass urine or have a bowel movement. Rarely, on recovery, the child may have a temporary loss of speech or temporary paralysis of an arm or leg, or one side of the face ('Todd's paralysis'); he commonly feels groggy and may have a headache.

■ ACTION See *EPILEPSY.* Place the child lying on his back on a flat surface (floor, bed or couch), and loosen his collar and belt. *Take the child to hospital immediately* if the convulsion lasts more than ten minutes, or if the child has not had previous convulsions.

■ TREATMENT A prolonged convulsion can be brought to an end by an intravenous injection of an anticonvulsant drug.

■ OUTLOOK See EPILEPSY.

GROWTH PATTERNS
The weight of a baby together with his maturity (gestational age) at birth re-

present the first measurements against which early postnatal growth and development are judged. Most babies lose weight in the first few days after birth, and regain their birth weight within ten days. They should then increase in weight month by month throughout childhood. The greatest increases are in the first year, with the additional major growth spurt occurring in the years leading up to and around the time of PUBERTY.

Growth charts display the normal range of children's weight and length according to age. An individual baby or child's growth will depend on many factors: maturity and weight at birth, the mother and father's height, illnesses, family relationships, and diet or nutritional intake.

WELL-BABY CLINICS willor checkups are used to follow your baby's growth and development through the first years of life. Your doctor can advise you if you are worried about your child's growth – see *FAILURE TO THRIVE.*

GUILLAIN-BARRE SYNDROME
Also known as infectious polyneuritis.

■ SYMPTOMS Progressive weakness and numbness often following two weeks or so after a VIRAL illness.

■ CAUSE Inflammation of the nerve roots where they emerge from the spinal cord.

■ TREATMENT There is no specific treatment and management is supportive in the acute phase, with attention to rehabilitation and physiotherapy in the recovery phase. The most serious complications, which are rare in childhood, are breathing difficulties and disturbances of heart rhythm or BLOOD PRESSURE, which may require intensive care including artificial ventilation.

■ OUTLOOK The majority of patients are ill for only a few weeks and their recovery is complete.

H

HALITOSIS

This is not a medical term, but it is nonetheless commonly used by doctors to describe foul-smelling breath.

■ CAUSES **1** INFECTIONS of the mouth or throat, such as TONSILLITIS. Even a severe COMMON COLD can cause halitosis for a short time. **2** 'Gum disease' (GINGIVITIS), tooth decay (dental caries) and chronic SINUSITIS can cause a more persistent unpleasant odor from the mouth.

■ ACTION For a short-term infection a mouthwash and thorough tooth brushing will help. However, if the problem persists and your child appears to be brushing his teeth properly, consult your doctor or your dentist.

HALLUCINATIONS

May be defined as seeing, hearing or smelling things that do not exist in reality, but which the individual perceives to be real. In young children, it may be hard to distinguish hallucinations from figments of a vivid imagination. Children are prone to hallucinations when they have a high temperature; when the temperature drops, the hallucinations cease. In older children, hallucinations in the absence of fever, particularly if they occur in the daytime, may be symptomatic of a serious underlying emo-tional disease; if in doubt discuss the matter with your doctor. See also *NIGHT TERRORS, EPILEPSY, SCHIZOPHRENIA and SOLVENT ABUSE.*

HAY FEVER

A group of symptoms in susceptible individuals due to ALLERGY to various pollens, especially from grass and trees, occurring through the summer months. It is perhaps the commonest form of allergic rhinitis and CONJUNC-TIVITIS (irritation, congestion and secretion from the linings of the nose and surface of the eyeballs).

■ SYMPTOMS Sneezing, blocked running nose, itchy or watery eyes. In some children, this may be accompanied by wheezing – ASTHMA.

■ CAUSE Many airborne pollens, because of their very small size, are capable of being inhaled and react with the lining of the nose and eyes in an allergic way. The tendency to this type of allergy runs in families.

■ TESTS Skin and BLOOD TESTS can identify particular pollen allergies. However, this is hardly ever necessary, since the connection between the symptoms and exposure to pollens is usually obvious.

■ ACTION **1** Take common-sense

precautions: beware of the particular pollen and take note of the day-to-day pollen count; when possible, avoid exposure to freshly mown grass or hay (if they aggravate your child's symptoms). As far as possible and when appropriate, keep your child out of the 'fresh pollenated' air. Places where pollen is likely to be minimal include air-conditioned rooms, boats on lakes and swimming-pools. Dark glasses don't help the conjunctivitis: they don't keep pollen out of the eyes. **2** Get medical advice if symptoms are sufficiently troublesome to disrupt the child's life and make him miss school.

■ TREATMENT Antihistamines are usually some (limited) help in relieving both rhinitis and conjunctivitis. Astemizole and terfenadine are relatively new antihistamine drugs that do not cause drowsiness. Chlorpheniramine is cheaper to buy over the counter, but does cause drowsiness. Antihistamines are usually recommended for use over a few days. They may be used for longer periods of time if medically advised.

Both rhinitis and conjunctivitis can be treated with preventive drugs, given by nasal spray or drops daily throughout the pollen season. These drugs are available by prescription only.

■ SELF-HELP Anticipating, if possible, the pollen season and starting preventive treatment before the pollen count rises. Desensitizing injections are usually not recommended: they carry a risk of adverse reaction in children, and they are often not particularly effective.

■ LONG-TERM MANAGEMENT There is no effective way of 'curing' hay fever, but regular use of preventive treatment can keep the misery of summer at bay.

■ OUTLOOK Better and safer treatments are being developed each year. Many children grow out of hay fever.

HEAD BANGING
Repetitive banging of the head against walls, furniture, and other objects. This is a COMFORT HABIT which some toddlers display while settling to sleep. It may also occur during TEMPER TANTRUMS, or as a result of frustration or boredom. It may constitute an effective means of attracting parents' attention. Although it is disturbing to witness, it is physically harmless; your best strategy is to ignore it. However, it is prudent to cover sharp corners or objects adjacent to the bed. During the daytime, attempts should be made to distract the child's attention if you can anticipate when head banging might start. Consider whether this habit indicates that your child has worries that can be addressed. If in doubt discuss the problem with your doctor.

HEAD INJURY
Caused by a direct blow to the head or by rapid movement of the head forwards or backwards. Among the commonest causes of severe head injury in childhood are automobile accidents. See *SEAT BELTS*. All children bump their heads at times with no serious consequences. Moderate head injury may result in CONCUSSION.

■ SYMPTOMS of head injury will depend on the severity and location of the brain injury. Minor head injuries usually only cause a mild headache. More severe injuries may result in symptoms such as UNCONSCIOUSNESS, PARALYSIS, loss of speech, abnormal eye movements, uncoordination and/or CONVULSIONS. There may be loss of memory for events immediately preceding, as well as following, the incident in proportion to the severity of the injury, with a tendency for improvement over time.

■ ACTION See *ACCIDENTS IN THE HOME*. Minor head injuries usually do not require medical attention. However, if a child is unconscious from a head injury for more than a few seconds, take him to hospital for assessment and observation. Bleeding inside the head may occur following the injury and cause a deterioration in the child's condition within a few hours. If the doctors judge it safe to allow a child home after a head injury, instructions on observing the child over the next few days will be given.

■ TREATMENT The child's overall neurological state is the most useful guide to the nature and severity of the intracranial injury. Minor head injuries may not require any specific therapy. An ice-pack to the area may minimize the bump. The presence of a fracture does not affect management unless the fracture is depressed, or causing leakage of cerebro-spinal fluid. A blood clot causing raised pressure inside the skull may need surgical removal.

■ OUTLOOK Most children with minor head injuries make a full recovery. With more serious injuries the long-term outlook depends upon the severity and location of the brain injury. Brain damage may occur at the site of injury, or on the opposite side if the brain was compressed against the skull bones ('contre coup' injury) following rapid forward or backward movement, or as the result of bleeding. Personality changes, including increased impulsiveness and irritability, and loss of inhibition may occur but are often temporary. Recovery is usually progressive over many weeks or months, and rehabilitation involves many disciplines. HEADACHES are a common sequel for months after serious head injury.

HEADACHE
Pain in the head, which may be sharp, tight or thumping, is common in children. One child in 20 has one headache per month. One in 100 has one a week.

■ CAUSES Commonly these are the result of worries, tiredness, FEVER, the COMMON COLD, hunger and tension. Most children who have regular headaches have a family history of the problem. Periodic headaches can occur for weeks or months after a mild or moderate HEAD INJURY. See also *MIGRAINE IN CHILDHOOD*.

Diet and eye problems are often blamed for headaches, however such factors are uncommon as causes of headache. SINUSITIS can cause acute headaches, but is not a common cause of chronic or recurrent headache in children, whose sinuses are relatively undeveloped compared with those of adults.

Headaches are rarely an indication of grave disease. (The rare, serious type of headache is completely different from a run-of-the-mill headache, much more severe and disabling. Typically, raised pressure in the head causes sudden onset of brief, bursting pain associated with vomiting first thing in the morning.) See also *MENINGITIS*, in which severe vomiting, fever and headache may occur, and BRAIN TUMORS.

The longer a child has been experiencing headaches and the longer they last, the less likely it is that there is a serious underlying cause. They are more likely to reflect tension and fatigue in the scalp muscles or migraine.

■ SELF-HELP Occasional headaches respond to a drink and a cookie and sitting or lying down quietly. Acetaminophen syrup or tablets will probably help the headache that fails to disappear quickly. Aspirin is not suitable for children – see REYE SYNDROME. If your child has frequent headaches, try to identify and resolve the underlying causes of ANXIETY. Encourage regular eating and sleeping habits and methods of relaxation, especially at bedtime.

Distract him: headaches hurt less when the child is preoccupied with pleasant thoughts.

■ OUTLOOK Headache is a very common symptom, tending to come and go: headaches are more frequent during school time than during holidays, on weekdays than weekends, especially for children who are under stress as school.

HEART-DISEASE

One child in every hundred has some form of heart-disease. The range of conditions involved are described in detail under CONGENITAL HEART-DISEASE, HEART FAILURE, ARRHYTHMIA, MYOCARDITIS or CARDIOMYOPATHY. It is essential to read this entry in conjunction with the entries listed above. RHEUMATIC FEVER, once a leading cause of heart-disease in children, is now rare in much of the Western world. However, there have been several recent localized outbreaks in the United States.

■ SYMPTOMS See the separate entries listed above. The most general symptoms of heart-disease in childhood are breathlessness and blueness (cyanosis), the latter especially in the lips.

■ ACTION If your child is breathless or blue, or has any of the symptoms described in the entries listed above, get medical advice. You will probably be referred to a pediatric cardiologist.

■ TESTS include ECG, X-ray of the chest and an ULTRASOUND SCAN of the heart (echocardiogram). Admission to the hospital may be necessary for other tests such as cardiac catheterization.

■ TREATMENT See the entries listed above. Recent advances in heart surgery have led to a much lower risk for all types of operation, particularly in very young children. Operations are now being performed for heart problems that were previously considered inoperable. In some cases, more than one operation will be necessary.
  Make sure you thoroughly understand your child's treatment by discussing all aspects of it with the doctor. You should understand the risks of any operation, and what is likely to be achieved.

■ LONG-TERM MANAGEMENT The severity of heart-disease is very variable. Some abnormalities are so mild that they only require a check-up every few years. Sometimes medical treatment is needed and is continued for many years. Heart surgery may be indicated but not performed until your child is older.
  Make sure that any specialists who see your child write to your

doctor and keep him or her fully informed. Your doctor is likely to be the person you will turn to if you need to discuss difficult decisions. He or she can only advise you with all the facts at hand.

If your child has a severe heart problem, he may gain weight more slowly than normal. He may also be slow to sit and walk. Such great restriction of activity and developmental delay may not improve until after successful surgery. However, even in extreme cases, the child usually makes normal intellectual progress, although his range of experience may be constrained by physical limitations. A child with heart-disease will instinctively rest when he is tired, so activities need not be limited (with the exception, for some children, of most competitive sports, which demand great physical exertion or stamina). His greater need for rest should be made clear to teachers. (The degree of disability will, of course, vary enormously depending on the heart problem in the individual child.) Discuss this with your doctor.

Your child should be IMMUNIZED at the normal times.

Children with many types of heart-disease should have an ANTIBIOTIC when they have dental treatment, and also for some other operations, to prevent INFECTION. Discuss this with your doctor.

▓ OUTLOOK Heart-disease in childhood sounds grave, but in most cases the outlook is surprisingly good; depending as ever on the nature of a particular child's problem, the odds are your child will lead a more or less normal life.

HEART FAILURE
The heart is unable to pump the blood around the body to meet its needs effectively.

▓ CAUSES HEART-DISEASE of any kind, if severe, can result in heart failure.

▓ SYMPTOMS include BREATHLESSNESS, caused by blood pooling in the lungs: this makes the lungs stiff and breathing becomes more difficult and more rapid than usual. In a baby, this is most noticeable during feeding. He may not be able to finish his feedings (and may be noted to perspire with the effort) and fail to gain weight at the normal rate (see FAILURE TO THRIVE). An older child may become more breathless than expected during exercise, and may spontaneously limit his activities. If heart failure is severe, he may be breathless while resting. EDEMA is also a feature. Sluggish circulation leads to fluid leaving the capillaries and collecting in the soft tissues of the body. This results in swelling, most noted in children as a puffiness around the eyes. In a baby, heart failure can result in a sudden increase in body weight due to fluid retention. Enlargement of the liver may also occur as a result of back pressure of blood from the heart. This can cause abdominal swelling.

▓ TREATMENT Digoxin and some other drugs will help the heart muscle to beat more strongly.

Diuretics such as furosemide will help the kidneys remove the excess water from the circulation.

▓ LONG-TERM MANAGEMENT will depend on the cause of heart failure. If it is due to CONGENITAL HEART-DISEASE, surgery may be necessary. If the cause is an ARRHYTHMIA, this must be treated with drugs. If there is muscle damage as in MYOCARDITIS or CAR-DIOMYOPATHY, drug treatment is usual. If medication is not effective, and an operation will not help, a heart transplant may be considered.

■ OUTLOOK has improved over the last few decades because of advances in both medical and surgical treatment.

HEART MURMURS
Noises made by the heart in addition to the normal heartbeats. Murmurs are usually caused by defects in the structure of the heart. However, 'innocent murmurs' can be caused simply by the turbulence of blood passing through the heart. This type of murmur can be heard in about half of all children at some time or other, especially when they have a FEVER.

■ SYMPTOMS See *HEART-DISEASE.* If your child has an innocent murmur, he will have no symptoms related to his heart. The murmur is only detected when he has a routine check-up, or is examined for another illness.
   Innocent murmurs usually have characteristics that make them easy to distinguish from heart-disease. Occasionally this is not the case, and your doctor will refer your child to a cardiologist.

■ TESTS include an X-ray of the chest, an ECG (electrocardiogram) and occasionally an ULTRASOUND SCAN of the heart (echocardiogram).

■ TREATMENT An innocent murmur requires no treatment. It usually becomes softer with time and may eventually disappear. If the murmur is due to heart-disease, the exact abnormality will be deter-

mined and appropriate treatment given.

HEAT EXHAUSTION (SUNSTROKE)
A relatively common condition in its less extreme forms due to loss of salt in sweat in a person not acclimatized to high temperatures. This can be seen in young children in very hot weather who are given inadequate salt and fluids, and are too young to ask for them. Occasionally seen in children with CYSTIC FIBROSIS, since the salt loss in their sweat is already high.

■ SYMPTOMS Tiredness, muscle cramps, fever, vomiting. If untreated, collapse and SHOCK may occur.

■ TREATMENT For mild heat exhaustion give plenty of fluids and salty foods such as crackers and potato chips. Children with cystic fibrosis may be given salt tablets during very hot weather.
   For severe cases, urgent medical attention is needed. Intravenous salt and water can correct the shock.

■ PREVENTION During very hot weather ensure that babies and toddlers are given liberal amounts of fluids. Wearing hats, playing in shaded areas and cooling off in water may help decrease the amount of sweating and, therefore, high salt loss.

HEAT RASH
Transient redness of the skin attributed to overheating. This is not a disease, rather the natural effect of sweat and heat on the skin.

■ SYMPTOMS The redness is especially evident in skin folds, such as those on a baby's neck and groin.

▓ ACTION Careful washing and use of talcum powder may help. It is easy to dismiss a RASH as a heat or sweat rash. If in doubt, especially if your baby is not feeling well, get medical advice.

▓ TREATMENT None is necessary.

HEAT-STROKE AND MALIGNANT HYPERTHERMIA

A rare condition more likely to occur in the very young, very old or those debilitated by disease. The heat-regulating mechanism fails. The infant or child does *not* sweat (in contrast to HEAT EXHAUSTION). The skin is dry, fiery red and hot. The body temperature rises rapidly. Seizures and coma will be followed by death unless cooling is started quickly.

This condition occasionally occurs as a reaction to certain ANESTHETICS in patients with an underlying inherited defect (malignant hyperthermia). If there is a family history of this, warn your doctor before your child receives any anesthetic.

▓ TREATMENT This is a medically urgent problem – take the child immediately to the nearest hospital. Cool him as best you can during transport. Treatment is aggressively cooling with cold water, cold baths, cold water-bed, sponging, fans and ice-packs. Intravenous fluids, corticosteroids and sedations may be required.

HEMATURIA (BLOOD IN THE URINE)

This is rare in babies but more common (though still rare) in older children. It can be a symptom of a URINARY TRACT INFECTION, NEPHRITIS, or injury to the kidneys or bladder, WILM TUMOR or HENOCH-SCHONLEIN PUR-

PURA. If the number of red cells in the urine is enough to give it color, it will appear pink or brown. Other substances can cause red or DARK URINE, and these may be confused with blood. Get medical advice if you suspect blood in your child's urine. Treatment will depend on the cause.

HEMOLYTIC ANEMIA

ANEMIA caused by increased breakdown (hemolysis) of red blood cells.

▓ CAUSES There are many, but the most common include THALASSEMIA, SICKLE-CELL ANEMIA and GLUCOSE 6-PHOSPHATE DEHYDROGENASE DEFICIENCY (G6-PD deficiency).

▓ SYMPTOMS Similar to anemia from other causes, but there are some additional features:

JAUNDICE occurs because hemoglobin released from the red blood cells is changed into bilirubin, a pigment that, when deposited in the skin, turns it yellow.

The child's body has to manufacture extra red blood cells to replace those broken down. If the bone marrow is unable to replace them adequately, the liver and spleen will help, but they become enlarged as a result. This may cause a chronic, dull ABDOMINAL PAIN.

▓ ACTION Some of the causes of hemolytic anemia are INHERITED DISORDERS. If there is a family history, tell your doctor.

Folic acid is lost when red blood cells are broken down, and this needs to be replaced. Your child may have to take a vitamin syrup or tablets containing folic acid.

For details of treatment and outlook see entries on *THALASSE-*

MIA, SICKLE-CELL ANEMIA and *GLUCOSE 6-PHOS-PHATE DEHYDROGENASE DEFICIENCY.*

HEMOPHILIA

An INHERITED DISORDER causing a lack of Factor VIII in the blood. Factor VIII is needed for normal clotting; deficiency results in a tendency to uncontrolled bleeding.

■ SYMPTOMS may be mild or severe. In the mild form, bleeding only occurs after a definite injury. In the severe form, symptoms begin soon after birth and bleeding can occur for no apparent reason.

In milder cases, the first sign may be bruises that appear when the child starts to crawl or walk. Bleeding into the joints and muscles starts as an ache and then develops into severe pain in the affected areas. The joint or muscle is swollen and movements are limited. NOSEBLEEDS are common. ABDOMINAL PAIN can be caused by bleeding within the abdomen. Bleeding from the kidneys and bladder results in urine that is very dark in color.

■ ACTION If you have a family history of hemophilia, consider GENETIC COUNSELLING before becoming pregnant. It is possible to detect whether a woman is a carrier of the abnormal gene that causes the condition, and PRENATAL DIAGNOSIS can confirm whether the fetus has hemophilia.

If your child starts to bruise easily, get medical advice.

A bracelet stating that the child is hemophiliac can be life-saving in an emergency.

Pain associated with bleeding can be treated with acetamenophen. Aspirin should not be used – it can aggravate the bleeding.

Activities may need to be limited, depending on the severity of the disease. Some sports can be played by children with mild hemophilia.

Care of the teeth is important: having a tooth pulled can lead to prolonged bleeding. A child with hemophilia should never be given an injection into a muscle.

■ TREATMENT Factor VIII, derived from human blood, can be given as a small transfusion into a vein at the first sign of bleeding. Prompt treatment is essential as it prevents further bleeding and pain, and minimizes permanent damage to the joints. A BLOOD TRANSFUSION may be needed if blood loss has been excessive.

Sometimes home treatment with Factor VIII is practical, so that treatment is started early and fewer trips to the hospital are needed.

When there is bleeding into a joint, it needs to be rested until the bleeding has stopped. After this, physiotherapy is essential to ensure that the joint does not stiffen.

Severe nosebleeds are treated by packing gauze into the nose to put pressure on the bleeding area. Factor VIII infusions may also be necessary for the child.

Cuts should not be stitched until Factor VIII has been given. Excessive pressure on areas of bleeding can also cause further injury. Factor VIII must be used before and during any surgical procedure to prevent excessive bleeding.

Factor VIII, in the past, may have contained HEPATITIS B and the AIDS VIRUS. In Western countries, all blood is now tested for these viruses so that spread by transfusion is no longer a problem: hemophiliac children should avoid travel in countries where there is any question of blood stocks being contaminated or bring their own, uncontaminated Factor VIII.

■ COMPLICATIONS Bleeding into joints can cause severe damage, resulting in deformity of joints and chronic ARTHRITIS, but this can often be prevented by prompt treatment with Factor VIII. Bleeding into the brain is a rare complication.

■ OUTLOOK depends on severity. Recent advances in treatment have resulted in a much better quality and duration of life.

HENOCH-SCHONLEIN PURPURA
Inflammation of the tiny blood vessels (capillaries) of the skin and other organs of the body, particularly the kidneys. The cause is unknown.

■ SYMPTOMS A RASH, beginning as URTICARIA, with raised welts, mainly on the arms and legs and the buttocks. This is followed by tiny, pin-point hemorrhages into the skin. These too are found mainly on the arms and legs, but they can occur on the trunk and face. There may be pain and swelling of the joints.

ABDOMINAL PAIN can be caused by tiny hemorrhages into the bowel wall. This is usually an intermittent pain similar to that of COLIC, and it may be associated with vomiting.

The kidneys are often affected, but this usually causes no symptoms. Tests will reveal blood in the urine; occasionally the child's urine looks dark because of the excess blood.

■ ACTION Any rash associated with bleeding should be checked by a doctor.

Pain in the joints or abdomen can

be treated with acetamenophen. Aspirin should not be used without consulting a doctor because of the risk of REYE SYNDROME.

While the rash is severe, the child should probably be in bed: activity seems to make the rash worse.

■ TREATMENT is confined to alleviating the symptoms, but if inflammation of the kidneys is severe, it will be the same as for NEPHRITIS.

■ OUTLOOK is generally good, except in a few cases where the kidneys are severely affected.

HEPATITIS
Inflammation of the liver caused by a number of VIRUSES, certain drugs and non-infectious diseases. Viruses are the most common cause in children. See also *CHRONIC HEPATITIS*.

Viral hepatitis is particularly common in developing countries and occurs at any age.

The viruses (known as hepatitis A, hepatitis B and non-A non-B hepatitis) spread in different ways, such as contaminated water and food for hepatitis A, and through blood or sexual contact for hepatitis B.

■ SYMPTOMS Young children may be infected but not have symptoms. If symptoms do occur, ANOREXIA, ITCHING, NAUSEA and VOMITING, and possibly DIARRHEA and FEVER are common initially. Several days later JAUNDICE develops, together with the passage of DARK URINE and pale BOWEL MOVEMENTS. There may also be a RASH and painful joints. There is often ABDOMINAL PAIN below the right lower ribs. There may be BRUISING due to damage to the liver which decreases the production of substances required for clotting.

There may be a history of contact with a person who had jaundice; or the illness may follow a BLOOD TRANSFUSION.

Some illnesses mimic viral hepatitis and several infections and toxic effects of certain drugs and poisons on the liver can give similar symptoms; a doctor must consider them all when trying to make the diagnosis.

■ PREVENTION Control of hepatitis A requires high standards of personal hygiene and proper sewage disposal, since the virus is spread by contact with infected feces. Outbreaks have occurred in day-care centers through this route.

Injection of human immunoglobulin (specific protein ANTIBODY) can be given to persons in high risk situations, for example, travel in countries where the condition is common, or early after exposure to the infection. This should prevent hepatitis A.

Hepatitis B virus is primarily transmitted at birth from an infected mother to the new-born by contact with infected blood or by sexual transmission. Prevention of hepatitis B infection requires vaccination, (three doses over a period of six months) and blood screening. Babies born to infected mothers can be protected by receiving hepatitis B immunoglobulin at birth as well as the hepatitis B vaccine at birth, one month and six months.

■ INVESTIGATIONS Physical examination for jaundice, an enlarged, tender liver and sometimes an enlarged spleen. BLOOD TESTS; tests for the virus involved.

■ TREATMENT Most children can be treated at home and are not very ill. For hepatitis A, the patient is infectious for up to ten days after the appearance of jaundice. During this time extra care must be taken with hand-washing after diaper changes or using the toilet. The child with major symptoms such as persistent vomiting, general tiredness, bruising and ascites (fluid in the abdomen), which occasionally occurs with hepatitis B, will need to go into the hospital. The child has to be cared for by staff immune to this infection.

Improvement is usual by the end of the second week, but full recovery may take months. In some children, the infection never completely clears and they become chronic carriers of hepatitis B virus and thus capable of passing it on.

■ OUTLOOK Most children with hepatitis A and hepatitis B, and a large proportion of those with non-A non-B hepatitis, recover completely. Hepatitis A rarely causes serious disease. Hepatitis B may cause CHRONIC HEPATITIS, but this is rare. Severe hepatitis with liver failure is rare but dangerous, and needs full support in a special hospital unit (see *CIRRHOSIS*). Long-term infection with hepatitis B does lead to an increased risk of liver cancer as an adult.

Infection with non A non B hepatitis virus is usually mild and there is no specific treatment other than general supportive care.

HERNIAS

Protrusions of organs through openings occurring at points of muscular weakness, either internally between the chest and abdomen, or externally through the abdominal wall. There are several different types:
– Inguinal hernia arises from a canal formed by the muscles of the groin through which the testes or female

ligaments migrate during fetal development. The canal normally closes off. Premature babies are prone to this type of hernia. There will be an intermittent swelling in the groin, which can become firm and tender. The bowel and its lining will have protruded through the muscular gap and become trapped (incarcerated) in the inguinal canal, in some cases limiting the blood supply to the bowel. An infant with an incarcerated inguinal hernia may be irritable, with ABDOMINAL PAIN and VOMITING.

– Umbilical hernia occurs in infancy and is especially common in black babies. It is characterized by a soft prominent, swollen umbilicus (belly button or navel), which may contain a portion of bowel. Rarely, this can become trapped and incarcerated in a similar way to an inguinal hernia. Most umbilical hernias disappear by age one. Even very large ones usually disappear by age five or six. Thus surgery is rarely indicated. If the bowel is irreducible (cannot be pushed back into the abdomen easily) or the hernia is becoming progressively larger after the age of one or two years, then surgery may be considered.

Supra-umbilical hernia (ventral hernia, epigastric hernia) a hernia located above the umbilicus in the upper part of the abdomen) may become painful, and usually requires an operation.

– Diaphragmatic hernia is a protrusion of the intestinal contents through the diaphragm (the muscular partition between the chest and abdomen). It occurs mostly on the left side of the chest and can have grave consequences in new-born babies, but is, fortunately, rare.

A new-born baby with this type of hernia will have difficulty with breathing, that will not respond to oxygen administration.

The baby's abdomen may be flat and bowel sounds can often be heard in the chest through a stethoscope, indicating that the bowel is in the chest cavity. The heart may be pushed to the right and all or part of the left lung is severely compressed.

Artificial ventilation may be necessary, and also measures to keep the bowel empty of gas. Emergency surgery is essential to repair the diaphragmatic hernia and to replace the bowel in the abdomen. The outcome depends on how well the lungs work afterward. The lung may be poorly developed (hypoplastic) on the side of the hernia and thus may not function effectively.

This can be a fatal condition, either immediately after birth, or after operation; but babies whose lung hypoplasia is not too serious can do well. See also *HIATUS HERNIA*.

▮ ACTION Any suspicious swelling in the groin, scrotum (the sac containing the testes) or labia (the female genital area) should be reported to a doctor.

▮ TREATMENT An inguinal hernia will be operated on in infancy, especially if symptoms such as vomiting and pain suggest an incarceration. The operation is simple with no major risk unless there has been delay in diagnosing an incarcerated hernia, and the bowel is seriously damaged. Simple repair requires only a short stay in the hospital. For the treatment of other types of hernia, see above.

HERPES INFECTIONS
See *COLD SORES, CHICKEN POX*.

HICCUPS (HICCOUGHS)
Sudden, involuntary, jerky contractions of the diaphragm muscle, occurring in bouts, often after eating. Usually trivial, but often a nuisance,

hiccups are of course common in children of all ages. They are usually caused by stretching or irritation of the stomach, either by too much food eaten too quickly, or by a specific food or drink. Sometimes they occur spontaneously.

Very very rarely, they may be a symptom of serious disease, in which case they tend to be persistent.

■ ACTION Hiccups usually stop of their own accord, but simple measures such as breath holding or blowing the nose may help.

HIP, DISLOCATION
See *CONGENITAL DISLOCATION OF THE HIP.*

HIRSCHPRUNG DISEASE
Narrowing of the large bowel due to lack of ganglion (nerve) cells in the intestinal wall (aganglionosis). It may involve a short section of the rectum (large bowel), or it may extend throughout the large bowel into the small bowel, but this is rare. The incidence is approximately one in 5,000 births.

■ SYMPTOMS Delayed passage of MECONIUM in infancy. CONSTIPATION in infancy which may be associated with ABDOMINAL SWELLING and VOMITING. DIARRHEA and enterocolitis (severe diarrhea mixed with blood) may occur and should be evaluated by your doctor immediately.

■ INVESTIGATIONS Abdominal X-ray may show an obstructed bowel. A barium ENEMA reveals dilated bowel above a narrowed section. Studies conducted after a balloon attached to a tube and pressure measuring device is passed through the anus into the rectum (monome-

try) may detect a characteristic pattern of bowel contractions. A biopsy of the rectum shows an absence of ganglion cells.

■ TREATMENT Surgical removal of the affected area of bowel with joining of normal bowel ends (anastamosis).

■ OUTLOOK Good if there is only a short segment of the bowel involved. Poor if there is extended aganglionosis into the small bowel. Hirschprung disease carries a small chance of occurring in relatives, principally siblings or children of the individual with the condition.

HIVES
See *URTICARIA.*

HOARSENESS
See *LARYNGITIS.*

HODGKIN DISEASE
See *LYMPHOMA.*

HOLE IN THE HEART
See *CONGENITAL HEART-DISEASE.*

HOSPITALIZATION
Going into the hospital is a worrying thing for most adults. For children, to whom the presence of family and familiar things is essential, and who have less understanding of illness and pain than do adults, it can be a very frightening experience. A child may show his fears through difficult behavior either in the hospital or on his return home. It is quite common for children between 18 months and five years of age to show the effects of separation,

even after they go home, if a parent has been unable to stay with them in the hospital. These usually take the form of increased dependency and clinging behavior, needing extra attention and perhaps reverting to bedwetting. Unpredictable resentment or anger may surface.

▓ HOSPITAL – THE PROBLEMS

– Separation from parents: Studies in the 1950s confirmed that short parental visits simply could not compensate for being left alone at the hospital. Nowadays, many children's hospital wards allow parents to stay with their child at all times, even sleep on a cot in the child's room.

– New and frightening procedures: Children over seven years are likely to have greater worries about medical procedures than the younger child. In fact, children can have strange ideas about how their bodies work until well into their teens. They may even suffer from terrors about investigations and operations. Out-patient investigations are no exception.

– Children are very sensitive to their parents' anxieties: any you express can worsen their own.

▓ ACTION
Since many hospital admissions are planned ahead, take advantage of the waiting time to prepare your child for the experience.

Tell him a couple of days before admission that he is going into the hospital. This is a sensible time lapse – not too long, not too short; you will have several opportunities to go over it together. You might play some hospital games to explain routines and introduce the idea of doctors and nurses; or you might show him a 'going to the hospital' book designed for children. Some hospitals have special preadmission programs to help young children prepare for elective surgery or medical admission. Many children find this very helpful. Give the child familiar objects to take to the hospital, so that he is reminded of home. If you are unable to stay with the child, tell the nurses about any routines he is used to, and any special words he used to indicate his needs, for instance going to the bathroom.

It is generally best to warn, without giving it undue emphasis, that a painful procedure will hurt for a little while but it is important to put the pain in context. For example, the pain of a blood test is like a mosquito bite. Do not dwell on pain or it will become exaggerated and a major cause of anxiety. See also *SEPARATION ANXIETY, BLOOD TESTS, X-RAYS.*

HYDROCELE

A soft, non-tender swelling in the scrotum caused by fluid from the abdominal cavity entering via a channel leading to the sac in which the testicle rests (scrotum).

A hydrocele does not damage the testicle, and causes no long-term problems. The channel that connects the abdominal cavity and scrotum normally closes during the first year of life; if it remains open, a small operation may be needed to close it.

HYDROCEPHALUS

A condition in which there is an accumulation of the fluid within the brain (cerebro-spinal fluid) due to an imbalance between its production and absorption. This can result in intermittent or persistent raised pressure that may cause destruction of the brain tissue and enlargement of the head.

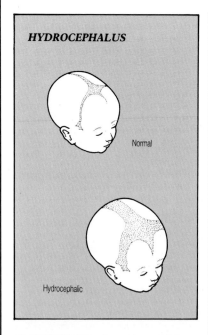

HYDROCEPHALUS

Normal

Hydrocephalic

■ SYMPTOMS In older children, hydrocephalus causes HEADACHES or loss of vision. In infancy, when hydrocephalus is most common, the softness of the skull allows expansion, and leads to an abnormal rate of growth of the head, before causing signs of raised pressure inside the brain.

■ CAUSES Excessive fluid production in the ventricles (fluid chambers in the brain); obstruction to the flow of cerebro-spinal fluid within or outside the ventricles; failure of reabsorption of the fluid. But the commonest cause is obstruction to the escape of fluid.

Narrowing of the canal between the third and fourth ventricles (aqueduct stenosis) is usually the cause, especially in boys.

Many children with SPINA BIFIDA have some degree of hydrocephalus. Other causes include the consequences of MENINGITIS, brain hemorrhage and HEAD INJURY. There is an inherited sex-linked form affecting half the sons of women who are carriers.

■ TREATMENT Some cases resolve of their own accord. If pressure is raised persistently, fluid can be drained from the ventricles through a valved tube (a shunt) into the abdomen. This prevents undue head enlargement or death from excessive pressure, blindness from stretching of the visual pathways in the brain, and even death.

■ OUTLOOK depends on the degree of hydrocephalus and the associated disabilities, for example spina bifida or mental handicap. Most children with hydrocephalus go to regular schools and are often developmentally normal. Intelligence can range from high to low – see *MENTAL HANDICAP* and *LEARNING DISORDERS*. Many children with hydrocephalus lead normal lives as adults provided they do not have associated severe physical and developmental difficulties.

HYPERACTIVE CHILD
An abnormally and excessively active child with poor concentration, restlessness and impulsiveness, often accompanied by a minimal requirement for sleep. He is easily distracted and often disruptive. The more severe degrees of this state are sometimes called hyperkinetic syndrome or attention deficit disorder.

■ INCIDENCE Ten percent of boys show some degree of hyperactivity; hence, to some extent, it is a variant of normal behavior, influenced by the family environment and the tolerance of the parents. Less than 1 percent of children have something approaching hyperkinesis. It is very rare in girls.

■ CAUSES In otherwise normal children no cause is usually identified. Serious degrees of hyperactivity may be seen in children with established BRAIN DAMAGE, EPILEPSY and severe MENTAL HANDICAP. Most research on FOOD ALLERGY, preservatives and ADDITIVES shows *no* link with hyperactivity.

■ SYMPTOMS Many young children are extremely active and may be difficult to control, but the behavior of the truly hyperactive child will be noticed by all his different care givers at all times, in all settings, and will distinguish him from his peers. He may have difficulty relating to other children, a difficult temperament generally and learning problems. Occasionally sleep problems are the dominant feature (INSOMNIA). AGGRESSION and other BEHAVIORAL DISORDERS often accompany hyperactivity.

■ ACTION Give a pre-school child clear instructions, but only when you are sure you have his attention. Praise him when he has concentrated well. Active play out of doors whenever possible will help to use up some of the excess energy. If the problem interferes with the child's learning, friendships and family relationships, ask professionals at nursery school or your doctor for help. Help from a psychologist, pediatrician, social worker or child psychiatrist may be needed.

■ TREATMENT For most hyperactive children BEHAVIORAL TREATMENT will be suggested. If the child is on medication for a condition such as epilepsy, changes in the dose or the drug may be suggested. For very severe cases, stimulant drugs may be prescribed, of which methylphenidate is currently the most commonly used. This drug may speed up the heart rate but reduces the hyperactive behavior to some degree. Loss of appetite, depression and slowing of growth are possible side-effects that cease when the drug is stopped, but require careful monitoring. Most drugs, such as tranquillizers, make the symptoms worse and hinder learning.

■ OUTLOOK Many hyperactive children improve when they start school, although for the severely affected school poses new difficulties. Fortunately, almost all degrees of hyperactivity diminish considerably during adolescence.

HYPERGLYCEMIA
See *DIABETES MELLITUS*.

HYPERLIPIDEMIA
A high level of fat (lipid) in the blood. This can result from a diet high in animal fat, or from the body's inherited inability to remove fats efficiently from the blood. Cholesterol is one of these fats: persistent lifelong high blood cholesterol levels are associated with an increased risk of CORONARY ARTERY DISEASE in later life. If an individual child is shown to have a particular type of hyperlipidemia, then an adjustment to daily diet may be of benefit. Animal fats (found in red meat, eggs, butter and cream) should be kept to a minimum in the child's diet. This is especially important if there is a history of coronary artery disease among young to middle-aged members of the family. Blood fat levels can be measured by a series of complex BLOOD TESTS. This is not usually necessary during childhood, unless there is a

history of young members of the family developing coronary artery disease.

HYPERTENSION

BLOOD PRESSURE above the normal for a particular age. This is relatively uncommon during childhood, but can be due to kidney disease or COARCTATION OF THE AORTA.

HYPERTHYROIDISM (GRAVES DISEASE)

Over-production of the hormone thyroxine, the function of which is explained under HYPOTHYROIDISM. Rare in children.

■ CAUSES The body's immune system may produce ANTIBODIES that stimulate the thyroid. The reason for this is not clear. It may occur at any age during childhood and is more common in girls. A mother who has hyperthyroidism may pass antibodies to her fetus during pregnancy. The new-born baby may then have hyperthyroidism which will be transient, lasting up to three months.

■ SYMPTOMS include restlessness, weight loss, palpitations and poor concentration. The child may have grown rapidly and be tall for his age. Some children have a tremor and some a GOITER.

■ TREATMENT A BLOOD TEST will confirm a high thyroxine level, and the child will usually be given anti-thyroid drugs initially. If drugs fail to control the condition, or the goiter itself is troublesome, surgical removal of part of the thyroid gland may be recommended. If complete removal of the thyroid is performed, the child will need thyroid replacement therapy (thyroxine tablets) lifelong.

HYPERVENTILATION

See *OVERBREATHING, STRESS SYMPTOMS.*

HYPOGAMMAGLOBULINEMIA

See *HYPOIMMUNOGLOBULINEMIA.*

HYPOGLYCEMIA

A low level of glucose in the blood.

■ CAUSES Hypoglycemia may occur when a baby is born to a DIABETIC MOTHER, is PREMATURE or SMALL-FOR-DATES. In older children hypoglycemia may be a symptom of underlying hypopituitarism, certain ADRENAL DISORDERS, or serious failure of liver function. More commonly it occurs in children with DIABETES when their dose of insulin is too high relative to their intake of food and exercise, a condition described as hyperinsulinemia.

■ SYMPTOMS A new-born baby becomes 'jittery', feeds poorly and, if the blood sugar level is very low, may develop CONVULSIONS. An older child may behave abnormally or aggressively, and appear pale and sweaty. Very low levels of blood glucose lead to loss of consciousness or coma.

■ TREATMENT The aim is to raise the blood glucose level. This must be done without delay – as soon as symptoms are recognized – to prevent unconsciousness. A high-sugar food or drink is given to the child or, if that is not effective, glucose is given by intravenous injection or infusion. Glugogon, a hormone derived from the pancreas, can be given by intramuscular injection in emergent situations when the hypoglycemia is the result of hyperinsulinemia.

HYPOIMMUNOGLOBULINEMIA (HYPOGAMMAGLOBULINEMIA)

The term covers a range of diseases, usually congenital in origin, caused by a complete or partial lack of all or just some subtypes of immunoglobulins. These are proteins (also called antibodies) which play a vital role in the body's defences against INFECTION. A transitory form of hypogammaglobulinemia occurs in some infants. They suffer from delayed onset of normal production of these antibodies but eventually have normal levels. This is in contrast to the other types of the disease which are permanent.

■ SYMPTOMS Some patients with congenital deficiency remain surprisingly free from symptoms until later in life. Others may suffer repeated infections such as CONJUNCTIVITIS, SINUSITIS, chest infections and BRONCHIECTASIS. Skin disorders are very common in this condition, typically ECZEMA, skin abscesses and coarse skin. DIARRHEA may occur as a result of either GIARDIA infection, SUGAR INTOLERANCE or MALABSORPTION. Fatal ENCEPHALITIS due to infection with certain viruses may occur. There is also a slightly increased frequency of cancer in this group of children.

Auto-immune illnesses (conditions where the body's defences attack their own cells, for example, JUVENILE RHEUMATOID ARTHRITIS) are strongly associated with complete deficiency, and also partial deficiency of one particular immunoglobulin called IgA.

■ TESTS are easily performed by measuring the level of fetal and specific subtypes of immunoglobulins in the blood. Results must be interpreted with caution in the baby's first year of life because of the high levels of certain types of antibodies passed to the baby from the mother, and of barely detectable levels of other types of antibody. The baby with this problem also tends to suffer an unusually large number of infections in the first year of life.

■ TREATMENT None may be needed if symptoms are mild. Intravenous infusions of immunoglobulin given roughly once a month will usually provide adequate protection against infections. Monitoring of blood levels will show the best interval between infusions.

Children with this problem should have their lung function monitored regularly because of the risk of lung disease. In some cases, continuous ANTIBIOTIC therapy may be necessary. In transient hypogammaglobulinemia, the child outgrows the problem.

HYPOSPADIAS

A condition in which the opening of the urethra is on the under-surface of the penis, instead of at its tip. Sometimes there is also a downward curvature of the penis. A mild degree of hypospadias is common, and may run in families. It requires no treatment. An operation to correct the abnormality is necessary when the opening of the urethra is far from the tip of the penis. This may be done in two stages, usually after the child is out of diapers, but before he starts school. Circumcision is not done in most cases of hypospadias.

HYPOTHERMIA

Low body temperature – 95°F or 35°C. This is a particular risk for all newborn babies, especially those of LOW BIRTH WEIGHT. The condition has been described as neonatal hypothermia. Hypothermia immediately after birth increases the chances of a baby developing RESPIRATORY DISTRESS SYNDROME. Cold stress may also cause the baby to use up calorie reserves to produce heat, with the risk of developing HYPOGLYCEMIA. Since heat is lost rapidly from the skin if the baby is wet, naked and in a cold environment, the labor room needs to be kept as warm as possible. Immediately after birth the baby should be dried with a warm towel, and kept wrapped in a blanket. A small baby may need to be cared for under a heater or in an INCUBATOR (see *INTENSIVE CARE*).

HYPOTHYROIDISM

Low production of the hormone thyroxine, which is produced by the thyroid gland located in the neck. Thyroxine controls the rate of energy production by the body's tissues. It is also involved with growth and mental development. Iodine is needed for its synthesis by the body. Hypothyroidism in babies may be called cretinism.

■ CAUSES The condition may be congenital – a baby may be born without a thyroid gland or with one that is unable to produce enough thyroxine. This sometimes causes a GOITER (enlargement of the thyroid gland). Deficiency of iodine may also cause a goiter.

Some children manufacture ANTIBODIES that act against the thyroid, causing it to function poorly (autoimmune thyroiditis). A much rarer cause is hypopituitarism: underfunction of the pituitary gland in the brain, which has control over the thyroid gland's activity.

■ SYMPTOMS Cretinism can be recognized in the first few weeks of life. The baby may have a dry skin, coarse hair, a hoarse cry, CONSTIPATION, JAUNDICE and be tired all the time (lethargy). He may be slow to

HYPOTHYROIDISM

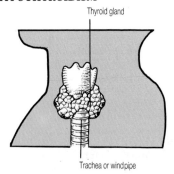

Thyroid gland

Trachea or windpipe

feed. If the problem is not diagnosed, he is likely to suffer retarded development. All states have screening programs to detect hypothyroidism in new-born babies using blood taken from the baby's heel during the first day or two of life.

Symptoms of hypothyroidism developing later in childhood are poor growth (the child becomes short for his age), dry skin, coarse hair, a general inactivity, and a tendency to feel cold. A goiter may or may not be present.

■ TESTS A BLOOD TEST will be taken to measure the level of thyroxine in the blood. Also to test whether there is a high level of the pituitary hormone, Thyroid Stimulating Hormone (TSH), produced by the body in an attempt to induce the thyroid gland to make an adequate quantity of thyroxine. Occasionally, a scan of the thyroid is useful in confirming the diagnosis.

■ TREATMENT Thyroxine tablets are given.

■ OUTLOOK Provided treatment is started in the first weeks after birth and continued throughout life there is a reasonable chance that growth and mental development will be normal.

I

IDIOPATHIC THROMBOCYTOPENIC PURPURA

A blood disease of unknown (idiopathic) cause – although it often follows a VIRAL INFECTION. It is most common in children between two and eight years of age, and involves a decrease in the number of platelets (thrombocytes) in the blood (thrombocytopenia). Platelets are important for normal blood clotting, so the condition may cause uncontrolled bleeding.

■ SYMPTOMS A RASH, consisting of tiny hemorrhages into the skin, mainly of the trunk.

There is also bleeding from the nose and gums, into the bowel and bladder and, in rare instances, into the brain. In most children the illness is mild, and the bleeding is not severe.

■ ACTION Any rash with bleeding should be seen by a doctor.

Try to prevent any injury likely to cause bleeding. It may be necessary to keep your child out of school if minor injuries are causing bleeding.

If the symptoms are severe, your doctor may recommend that the child be admitted to the hospital for a short stay.

■ TESTS include a BLOOD TEST and possibly a bone marrow examination.

■ TREATMENT In mild cases, no treatment is necessary. If the number of platelets in the blood is low, or if the bleeding is severe, intravenous gamma globulin and/or a steroid can bring marked improvement. However, relapses may occur when treatment is stopped. Severe bleeding may require a platelet and/or BLOOD TRANSFUSION.

■ OUTLOOK is usually good. Recovery takes three to six months. Attacks occasionally recur, but with decreasing frequency. The only real hazard is hemorrhage into the brain in the early stages.

IMMUNITY

A defense mechanism of the body that combats the effects of invasion by foreign substances. When an infecting organism enters the body, large molecules in the wall of the organism (called ANTIGENS) stimulate the body to produce ANTIBODIES and/or specific cells directed to remove the antigen (cytotoxic cells). The antibodies react with the antigens or specific cells, thereby potentially neutralizing their effect or assisting other cells in destroying the invading organism, thus fighting the INFECTION. This response is usually of benefit, but occasionally the reaction leads to undesirable side-effects. ALLERGY is one such instance when the antigen (such as pollen) stimulates the production of antibodies, interaction with which leads to a chemical sequence with discomforting clinical effects. Another harmful result of cell-mediated immunity is the rejection of a TRANSPLANTED organ unless special anti-rejection drugs are given.

Immunity is specific. An antibody or sensitized cell will only react with one particular type of antigen. These antibodies and cells remain in the body, or can be produced very rapidly again, so subsequent infection by the same organism will induce a rapid defensive response. Unfortunately the COMMON COLD and INFLUENZA are caused by a number of different VIRUSES and although the body develops an immunity to one, other organisms may still lead to similar patterns of illness.

Babies acquire a degree of immunity passively from antibodies transferred from the mother across the placenta before birth, and via breast milk after birth. This passively acquired immunity decreases over the first six months after birth; as this wanes, the child actively has to build up his own immunity. This happens as a result of natural exposure to antigens and infections, and by IMMUNIZATION.

IMMUNIZATION

Protection against INFECTIOUS disease, achieved by giving the child a killed, weakened or altered strain of a VIRUS or BACTERIUM either by injection or by mouth. This stimulates the body to produce ANTIBODIES and/or cell-mediated immunity against that organism without the child becoming seriously ill. It is sometimes necessary to have more than one dose of a vaccine to gain full immunity, especially if a killed vaccine is used.

All children should be immunized against POLIOMYELITIS (POLIO), TETANUS and DIPHTHERIA. The risk of ENCEPHALITIS from PERTUSSIS immunization is far less than the risk to a child

from the illness. Your doctor can provide information on the benefits and minimal risks of these vaccines.

■ TRIPLE VACCINE of diphtheria, pertussis and tetanus (DPT) is a combination given by injection in three doses during the child's first year followed by a booster dose at 18 months. The first injection is usually given at two months, whether the baby was born as term or prematurely, and the second and third injections are given at about two-month intervals thereafter. Giving the baby acetamenophen at the time of the injection and again four hours later decreases the incidence of post-injection fever and irritability. The injection site may be red, and a small lump may remain for several weeks.

■ A PRESCHOOL BOOSTER INJECTION of diphtheria, pertussis and tetanus is given at four to six years. After this a diphtheria and tetanus booster are advisable every ten years.

■ LIVE ATTENUATED POLIOMYELITIS (POLIO) immunization is given by mouth at about two, four and 18 months of age. It is usually given at the same time as the triple vaccine. There is a theoretical chance that breast milk may inactivate the vaccine, but this has not been found in practice. Side-effects include fever or diarrhea. Live virus is excreted in the stools, so adults caring for the child should be immunized. A booster is given at four to six years.

In some countries a killed or inactivated poliovirus vaccine is given by injection, combined with the triple vaccine to form the quad vaccine (DPTP) instead of giving separate oral polio vaccine. Side-effects of the killed polio vaccine are minimal.

▓ COMBINED MEASLES, MUMPS, RUBELLA VACCINE (MMR) Measles remains a serious illness and can cause death from PNEUMONIA and encephalitis. Measles vaccine is recommeded to be given in combination with MUMPS and RUBELLA vaccine at about 15 months of age. A booster measles vaccine injection given just prior to school entry is required in some states and is likely to be recommended for all children by 1990. Side-effects of the measles vaccine include fever and a rash – these may occur about a week after the injection is given.

▓ RUBELLA vaccine should be given in combination with measles and mumps vaccine to prevent *Rubella* infection occurring in the future during pregnancy – see *RUBELLA*. Side-effects of *Rubella* vaccine given alone (without measles and mumps) in older children may include fever, rash and swollen glands, occurring about two weeks after the injection. This is rare in infants.

▓ MUMPS vaccine should be given to infants in combination with measles and *Rubella* vaccine. Side-effects of the mumps component of the vaccine are minimal.

▓ TUBERCULOSIS (BCG) vaccine is no longer recommended as a routine immunization in the United States. See *TUBERCULOSIS*. In some parts of the world where tuberculosis is a significant problem, BCG may be given soon after birth. (BCG stands for Bacille Calmette Guerin, the French scientist who developed the vaccine.)

▓ HEMOPHILUS INFLUENZAE VACCINE is currently recommended for children at age 18 months to decrease the risk of MENINGITIS, EPIGLOTTITIS and septic ARTHRITIS due to the bacteria. Side-effects are minimal. New *Hemophilus influenzae* vaccines, currently being tested, may be effective in preventing these diseases when given as early as three months of age.

▓ SMALLPOX vaccine is no longer necessary since the disease has been eradicated.

▓ HEPATITIS B VACCINE All infants born to mothers who are carriers of hepatitis B virus should: **1** be carefully bathed at birth to remove all blood; **2** receive hepatitis B-immunoglobulin by injection at birth; **3** receive three doses of hepatitis B vaccine, one within seven days of birth and then at one month and six months. This prevents transmission of hepatitis B to the baby. Side-effects from the vaccine are minimal.

▓ WHERE TO GET YOUR CHILD IMMUNIZED Your child may be immunized by your doctor, at a hospital outpatient clinic or through a local community immunization clinic. Many states require proof of full immunization before a child can attend school.

▓ WHICH CHILDREN SHOULD NOT BE IMMUNIZED? Contraindications to immunization are few and many children remain unnecessarily vulnerable to preventable diseases because their immunizations have been delayed for no good reason.

If your child has a high fever, wait until he is better. A cold, or snuffly nose, is no problem.

If he has a chronic medical condition, discuss immunization with your doctor. Most of these children need all the protection from immunization they can get.

Pertussis or whooping cough vaccine is usually avoided if a child has an unstable neurological condition or has had a serious reaction with the previous injection. Discuss this with your doctor.

ALLERGY to eggs or egg products is no longer considered a contra-indication to measles vaccine unless the child has had a very severe allergic reaction.

Rubella and live polio vaccines are not recommended to be given to pregnant women.

Children who are HIV (AIDS) positive should be immunized as usual because of their increased vulnerability to infection. However, those with lowered immunity may be given a killed or inactivated form of polio virus vaccine.

IMPERFORATE ANUS
See *ANUS, IMPERFORATE.*

INCUBATION PERIOD
The time between contact with an INFECTIOUS disease and the onset of the symptoms of the illness. After an infecting organism (such as a VIRUS) has entered the body, it multiplies. During this process, the child remains well. But during the few days before the symptoms develop, the child may be shedding live viruses and thus can pass the infection on to other people.

The incubation period varies for different infections; details are given under individual entries.

INCUBATOR
If you have a PREMATURE baby, the chances are that he will spend time in an incubator in the hospital's neonatal intensive care unit. The incubator (a crib completely enclosed by plastic glass) helps keep the baby warm by keeping the environmental temperature constant. It allows the baby to be without blankets so he can be observed easily. Some units use overhead radiant heaters for very ill infants to allow maximum access to the baby for the many treatments and tests he requires.

Even if your baby is very ill, you may be able to touch him or hold his hand through circular openings on each side of the incubator. Most units strongly encourage physical contact between mothers and fathers and their premature babies because it helps bonding or attachment to occur. Spending time watching and touching your baby in his incubator will help you get to know him.

INFECTION
Illness associated with an invasion of the body by micro-organisms such as VIRUSES, BACTERIA, PARASITES or FUNGI.

■ SPREAD OF INFECTION How this happens depends on the type of infection. It can be by direct contact (touching the sick person or something he has touched), by aerosolized droplets (from sneezing or coughing), or by contact with infected blood, urine or stools. Infection can also occur when organisms are swallowed.

After invasion there is a period when the organism multiplies in the body: the INCUBATION PERIOD. The child appears well, but may himself be spreading the infection. Hence it is often impossible to prevent many of the common childhood infections from spreading within the family, the school and the community.

Occasionally, a child may be invaded by an organism, but never become ill from it. This child is termed a carrier who can pass on the infection to others.

■ SIGNS OF INFECTION vary according to the type of disease, but many infections have similar symptoms. These may include FEVER, skin RASH, DIARRHEA and general malaise (feeling sick). Swollen glands are an indication that the body is reacting to an infection.

■ RESISTANCE TO INFECTION is achieved by the body in various ways. The skin, nose and tonsils are natural barriers to infection; and intestinal barriers including stomach acid help to exclude swallowed organisms. The body also develops IMMUNITY to infection. ANTIBODIES, specific cytotoxic cells and white blood cells help to destroy the organisms. The lymph nodes and spleen play a part in this process. Immunity can also be stimulated by immunization. BREAST FEEDING enhances a baby's resistance to infection, as antibodies are passed to him in the breast milk.

Resistance to infection can be diminished by diseases that affect the body's ability to develop immunity such as MALNUTRITION and AIDS (AQUIRED IMMUNE DEFICIENCY SYNDROME).

INFECTIOUS MONONUCLEOSIS (GLANDULAR FEVER)

A VIRAL illness caused by Epstein Barr virus (EB virus) that occurs most commonly in older children and adolescents. It is only mildly INFECTIOUS. The INCUBATION PERIOD is estimated to be 30-50 days.

■ SYMPTONS Onset is gradual. There is a low-grade FEVER and loss of APPETITE, and the child feels generally unwell; some of the lymph glands enlarge and become tender. These may be in the neck, under the arms or in the abdomen. ABDOMINAL PAIN is caused by enlargement of the lymph glands or spleen. A sore throat is common and the tonsils are usually enlarged.

Occasionally a RASH occurs, either as little red spots or big blotchy ones. Petechiae (tiny blood spots in the skin) due to minor problems with blood clotting are sometimes present.

The fever and enlargement of the glands can last for several weeks.

■ ACTION There is no specific treatment. Symptoms can be relieved with analgesics such as acetamenophen. ANTIBIOTICS do *not* help and some such as ampicillin may cause a severe skin rash.

The malaise and tiredness may persist for many months, particularly in adolescents. Occasionally, this is severe enough to interfere with school work and other activities. Understanding and support from the family, together with plenty of rest and a balanced diet should be encouraged.

■ TESTS The diagnosis can be made on a BLOOD TEST if there is any doubt.

■ COMPLICATIONS Serious problems are rare, but if the spleen is very enlarged, sports involving physical contact should be avoided because of the risk of rupture of the spleen and internal bleeding.

Rarely, inflammation of various organs can cause MYOCARDITIS, HEPATITIS, PNEUMONIA and MENINGITIS.

▓ OUTLOOK The long-term outlook is usually good, but the feeling of vague ill-health, lasting for months, can be troublesome.

INFECTIOUS POLYNEURITIS
See *GUILLAIN-BARRE SYN-DROME.*

INFLUENZA
The acute, highly INECTIOUS illness caused by the influenza VIRUS. There are many different strains of the virus, and infection by one does not give IM-MUNITY to the others. The virus is spread by direct contact, large droplets (sneezed or coughed into the air) or articles contaminated by nasal discharge. 'Flu' tends to occur in epidemics because infectious carriers are generally feeling well in the days immediately before developing symptoms and continue their usual activities, exposing those who come in contact with them..

▓ SYMPTOMS include FEVER, HEAD-ACHE, shivering, muscle pain and a dry hacking cough. Loss of APPE-TITE, nausea, VOMITING and listlessness can occur. They usually last between two and seven days.

Complications include PNEUMO-NIA, EAR INFECTIONS and SINUSITIS, which result from secondary BACTE-RIAL infection. Rare complications in children include severe MYOSITIS (inflammation of muscles) and EN-CEPHALITIS.

▓ ACTION The fever, headache and muscle pain can be treated with a simple analgesic such as acetamenophen. Aspirin should not be used because of the risk of REYE SYN-DROME. A tepid (not cold) bath is also a helpful way to bring down the temperature – see *FEVER.*

Vomiting is not usually severe, but encouraging your child to take plenty of clear fluids will help to prevent DEHYDRATION, which could be aggravated by the fever.

The child may feel more comfortable in bed while the fever and muscle pains persist.

Get medical advice if the fever does not respond to treatment or if there are any symptoms that worry you.

Your child may start to feel better after three or four days, but you may find that he tires easily.

▓ TREATMENT ANTIBIOTICS will only be necessary if pneumonia or any other secondary bacterial infection occurs.

Management of the other complications are discussed under individual entries.

▓ IMMUNIZATION against influenza is recommended for children suffering from certain chronic diseases (such as CYSTIC FIBROSIS, severe ASTHMA or serious HEART-DISEASE, in whom the complications are likely to be serious. The injection given each autumn contains strains of influenza virus most likely to cause epidemics that particular year. It protects against about 70 percent of infections, and is effective for about 12 months. Side-effects include redness at the injection site, fever, malaise and muscle pain beginning six to 12 hours later, lasting for one to two days.

If your child has a chronic disease, discuss with your doctor whether influenza immunization is indicated.

▓ OUTLOOK after influenza is generally good; there are few serious complications.

INHALERS

Devices used in the treatment of ASTHMA, which deliver small doses of various drugs directly to the small air passages in the lungs.

■ HOW THEY WORK All forms of inhalers create a fine spray of tiny particles, either as powder or as liquid droplets, which is carried by the air flow into the lungs. (Some of the spray is deposited in the throat, where steroid inhalers occasionally cause unwanted soreness due to CANDIDIASIS.) There are three types of drugs commonly used in inhalers: bronchodilators, which open up narrowed air passages; steroids, which help to prevent attacks of asthma; and cromoglycate, which also helps to prevent ALLERGIC asthma.

■ HOW TO USE THEM It is essential that children who have been prescribed inhalers know how to use them effectively. A health professional should ensure that the child is

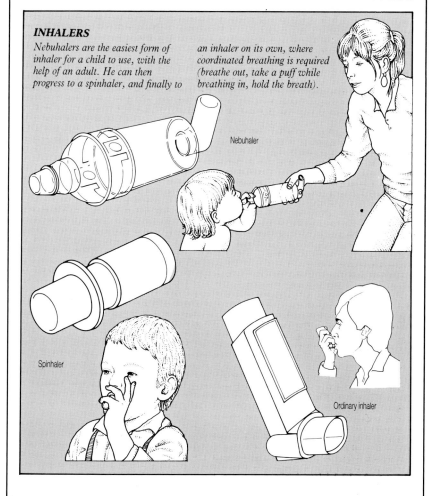

INHALERS

Nebuhalers are the easiest form of inhaler for a child to use, with the help of an adult. He can then progress to a spinhaler, and finally to an inhaler on its own, where coordinated breathing is required (breathe out, take a puff while breathing in, hold the breath).

Nebuhaler

Spinhaler

Ordinary inhaler

taught, but you should always check that the child is still using his inhaler properly. There are several varieties of inhaler, some designed specifically for younger children, so if your child cannot manage one it is worthwhile trying a different type.

INHERITED DISORDERS

These are caused by abnormal GENES or CHROMOSOMES that are passed on from parents. They can also develop for the first time when a gene or chromosome is altered as it is passed to the child. This is called mutation. The abnormality may then be passed on to future generations.

Genetic disorders may be inherited from the genes of one or both parents. Single gene disorders are due to one abnormal gene. This may result in a dominantly or recessively inherited genetic disorder. If one parent has a dominantly inherited disease (as in ACHONDROPLASIA) and the other does not, each of their children will have a one in two chance of inheriting the disease. If both parents have the disease (and therefore the dominant gene), each of their children will have a three in four chance of inheriting it. If an abnormal gene is recessive, a child will have to inherit two abnormal genes, one from each parent (both of whom are carriers of the abnormal gene), in order to develop the disorder. Such diseases include CYSTIC FIBROSIS and THALASSEMIA. If a child inherits only one abnormal recessive gene, he will usually have no signs of the disease, but will be a 'carrier'. If both parents are carriers, each of their children has: a one in four chance of inheriting both abnormal genes, and showing signs of the disease; a one in four chance of receiving no abnormal genes; a two in four chance of receiving one abnormal gene, and becoming a carrier.

If one parent has the recessive disease (and therefore two recessive genes for it) and the other does not have the disease and is not a carrier, none of their children will have the disease. If the parent without the disease is a carrier, each of the couple's children will either inherit the disease (a one in two chance) or be a carrier (also, a one in two chance). If both parents have a recessively inherited disease, all of their children will inherit the disease.

It is usually not possible to test whether a person is a carrier. If parents are related, there is a greater chance of inheriting abnormal recessive genes from a common ancestor.

Abnormal genes can be carried on the sex chromosomes (usually the X or female chromosome). These sex-linked inherited disorders are usually recessive, so if the child is a girl (XX) there will be no signs of the disease. This is because the normal gene on the other X chromosome overrides the effect or the deficiency arising from the abnormal gene. The chromosome make-up of the male is XY. Thus boys have only one X chromosome; if the abnormal gene is on this chromosome, the smaller Y chromosome does not carry a paired normal gene and hence does not counter the effect of the abnormal gene. Common examples of such conditions are HEMOPHILIA and Duchenne MUSCULAR DYSTROPHY. For each son born to a mother who is a carrier of such an abnormal gene there is a 50 percent chance that he will inherit the abnormal gene and develop the disease. If he does not inherit the gene – 50 percent chance – he will not have the disease, or be a carrier for it. Similarly, for daughters born to such mothers, 50 percent will inherit the abnormal gene. They will be carriers, but they will not have the disease.

Chromosomal abnormalities present in the ovum or sperm may be incorporated at the time of conception. Such abnormalities may cause spontaneous abortion early in pregnancy or result in a CONGENITAL ABNORMALITY, such as DOWN SYNDROME. Study of the chromosomes of the affected fetus or child may, depending on the particular abnormality, help in predicting the risk of a similar problem in a future pregnancy.

There are many diseases that have no clear pattern of inheritance, but are nonetheless more common in some families than others. These include DIABETES, CONGENITAL HEART-DISEASE and CONGENITAL DISLOCATION OF THE HIP. Environmental factors are presumed to play a major part in the causation of these disorders.

Parents who have a family history of a particular illness and who plan to have further children should consider seeking advice or GENETIC COUNSELLING. This also applies to parents who are related, since there is a greater chance of them both carrying similar abnormal recessive genes. Tests can often be carried out to determine the risk of an inherited disorder (see *PRENATAL DIAGNOSIS*).

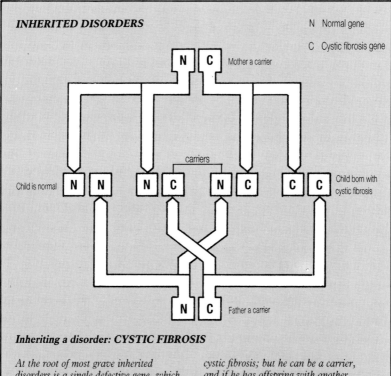

INHERITED DISORDERS

N Normal gene

C Cystic fibrosis gene

Mother a carrier

carriers

Child is normal

Child born with cystic fibrosis

Father a carrier

Inheriting a disorder: **CYSTIC FIBROSIS**

At the root of most grave inherited disorders is a single defective gene, which is usually recessive. This means that only if both parents contribute the gene at conception is the child born with the disorder. If a child inherits one C gene and one N gene, he will not suffer from cystic fibrosis; but he can be a carrier, and if he has offspring with another carrier, there is the chance but not the certainty that they will have a child with cystic fibrosis. About one in 20 people are carriers of this defective gene without knowing it.

INSOMNIA

Spending much of the night awake, unable to fall asleep. Young children are rarely troubled by insomnia (although their pattern of waking and sleeping at night may not meet with their parents' expectations, and thus be a concern for the parents). Older children may suffer from insomnia when worried or upset. See *SLEEP PROBLEMS*.

INTELLIGENCE

Of course, there are many definitions of intelligence, just as there are many forms of it. Here, we use the conventional one for the context of child development: the ability to absorb and remember information and then to use it to solve problems.

Intelligence is partly inherited, but also influenced by the environment in which a child grows and learns. The most important environmental factors are good antenatal conditions, loving care, suitable stimulation of language, encouragement with play and later, support at school. Children from very deprived backgrounds suffer intellectually as well as emotionally and socially.

Long-term exposure to high atmospheric levels of lead seems to cause children to achieve less well. There is some controversial evidence that extra vitamins can improve intelligence slightly in children; however this is not a serious consideration for children on a balanced diet.

Children pass through a number of stages on the way to developing the adult form of intelligence in mid-adolescence.

Up to about two years, a baby understands the world in terms of the here-and-now – what he can do with objects, how they feel, sound, look and taste. Objects are forgotten as soon as they disappear.

Towards the end of this stage, with the acquisition of language, the toddler has some idea of objects when they are not present, and begins to understand how objects can be mentally sorted into groups with similar characteristics. Primitive reasoning now begins and the child develops pretend play and enjoys surprisingly complicated games.

During the infant school years, the mental capabilities increase, so that, for instance, the child begins to manipulate numbers without relying on physical counting. He begins to understand that liquid in different vessels, or indeed modelling clay, may change its shape but remains the same in quantity. However, he still sees the world strongly from his point of view.

In early adolescence, children start to manipulate ideas as well as events and objects. They can imagine things that they have not experienced, organize things systematically, think deductively and see both sides of an argument. From now on they are developing the adult's ability to solve complex problems: a process that must continue with experience.

See also *I.Q., LANGUAGE DEVELOPMENT, LEARNING DISORDERS, DEVELOPMENTAL DELAY*.

I.Q. (INTELLIGENCE QUOTIENT)

A number or score obtained from an intelligence test, which compares an individual child's score with the scores from a large number of children of the same age. The I.Q. represents a composite result from tests of a range of skills. The average I.Q. is 100; 68 percent of people have I.Q.s between 85 and 115. I.Q. scores are limited in their value as predictors of future academic success, because many other factors, such as interest and motivation, are important in learning. Intelligence

Quotient tests are particularly unreliable for pre-school children, because of the wide variation in rates of development at this age. They can be useful predictors of performance in skills such as reading. Nowadays, educational psychologists concentrate on the overall range of a child's abilities, rather than just on I.Q. scores, and aim to diagnose the individual child's strengths and weaknesses, so that teachers and parents can plan for the child's education. See *INTELLIGENCE*.

INTENSIVE CARE

Continuous detailed observation and care of an ill baby or child, by specialist staff. Intensive care of new-born babies (see PREMATURITY and LOW BIRTH WEIGHT) takes place in a neonatal intensive care unit (NICU) or in a special care nursery. In NICUs babies are usually cared for in INCUBATORS or under heaters, to keep them warm while allowing close observation.

Older children who need intensive care (for example after a serious accident or major operation) will be admitted to a pediatric intensive care unit (PICU). In addition to close observation, specialized equipment may be used to assist breathing and feeding, and to monitor the child's condition.

The child may be supported by a ventilator until he can breathe for himself. A tube is passed through his mouth or nose into the trachea (wind pipe), and is connected to the ventilator that expands his lungs in a regulated fashion with air enriched with oxygen to meet his exact needs. The tube will be cleared by suction to remove lung secretions. A child who is ventilated may need sedation.

Most children in a NICU or a PICU need an intravenous drip or infusion, because they are unable to drink or eat normally. Total parenteral nutrition (TPN) consists of fluids enriched with nutrients such as fat and amino-acids that are given into a vein in the arm or leg or through a plastic tube inserted

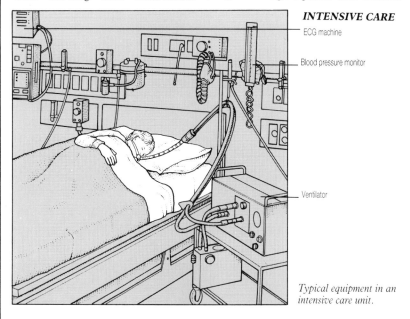

INTENSIVE CARE

ECG machine

Blood pressure monitor

Ventilator

Typical equipment in an intensive care unit.

into a large vein in the chest.

Other equipment used in a NICU or PICU includes monitors of heart rate, breathing rate, blood pressure and temperature. Many children, but more particularly premature babies, will also have their blood oxygen levels monitored, either by an electrode attached to the skin, or by BLOOD TESTS.

Parents are encouraged to be with their children and to help look after them in intensive care units. Stay with your child and talk to him as much as possible. It is helpful to understand your child's condition and the equipment that is being used. Ask the staff anything you want to know. You may feel upset about your child's illness or anxious that he will be left damaged or weak. Try to share your fears and worries with your partner and the staff. It is helpful if you both take part in any discussions. Your other children may also be worried and upset, so try to involve them in the care of their sibling.

INTESTINAL OBSTRUCTION

The intestinal tract (gut) consists of a long continuous tube running from the stomach (or, strictly, from the back of the mouth) to the anus. Obstruction at any point will sooner or later block the passage of food through the intestine. This occurs in childhood most commonly in INTUSSUSCEPTION and VOLVULUS.

■ SYMPTOMS will vary with the nature of the blockage. If this is sudden in onset, as with a volvulus, severe pain or even shock may be present initially, rather than the signs of obstruction. If it is more gradual in onset, as with PYLORIC STENOSIS, then the signs of upper intestinal obstruction will predominate – VOMITING. Unrelieved complete obstruction of the intestine will

INTESTINAL OBSTRUCTION

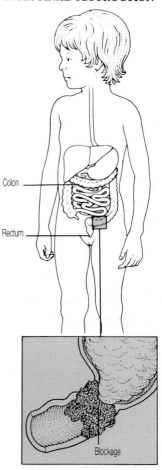

Colon

Rectum

Blockage

lead to ABDOMINAL SWELLING and absence of bowel movements, proceeding to perforation of the intestine and PERITONITIS.

■ TREATMENT depends on the cause, but the usual procedure, once in the hospital, is to give fluids intravenously and to drain the stomach through a tube placed within it through the nose or mouth to reduce vomiting. Then the blockage is treated, usually by surgery.

INTUSSUSCEPTION

The bowel inverts into itself (like the finger of a glove). This may lead to IN-TESTINAL OBSTRUCTION. The problem is uncommon and most often occurs in the last half of the infant's first year. The cause in most cases is unknown. The condition may complicate GAS-TROENTERITIS.

INTUSSUSCEPTION

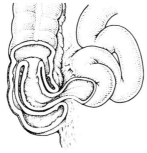

■ SYMPTOMS ABDOMINAL PAIN, COLIC, VOMITING, rectal BLEEDING.

■ ACTION If these symptoms occur, get medical advice. Your doctor will usually have the child admitted to the hospital for tests and observation.

■ INVESTIGATIONS/MANAGE-MENT 1 Examination: the doctor may feel a swelling (the mass caused by the intussusception) in the abdomen. 2 Intravenous fluids may be required if the child is DEHYDRATED. 3 X-ray of the abdomen may show abnormal intestinal gas patterns. 4 Barium ENEMA: this diagnoses the intussusception, which appears as an obstruction. Gentle pressure created by the barium within the bowel below the obstruction usually reduces the intussusception by pushing the inverted portion of the bowel back to its normal position. If this fails, or there is evidence of PERITONITIS, an abdominal operation will be necessary to reduce the intussusception or to cut it out altogether.

■ OUTLOOK Once an intussusception has been reduced either by barium enema or surgically, there is only a 5 percent chance of it recurring.

IRON

See POISONING, ANEMIA.

IRON DEFICIENCY

See ANEMIA.

IRON-DEFICIENCY ANEMIA

ANEMIA caused by a deficiency of iron, which is needed to make hemoglobin, the blood's oxygen carrier.

■ CAUSES It is usually due to an inadequate diet, but poor absorption (as in CELIAC DISEASE), or blood loss, can sometimes be to blame. Premature babies, twins and triplets, who have not built up stores of iron in their bodies before birth, are particularly at risk. Babies born at full-term have iron stores to last until about six months. Thereafter, they need adequate iron in their diet. Breast and cow's milk do not contain as much iron as formula milk. Many diets during the first year of life have insufficient iron. For all these reasons, iron deficiency anemia is most likely to occur between six months and two years.

Foods that contain iron include red meat, wholewheat flour, brown rice, apricots, green leafy vegetables (typically spinach) and iron-enriched cereals. Most infant baby formulas are enriched with iron. Folic acid and vitamin B12 are also needed to make hemoglobin. Lack of them without lack of iron as well, however, is uncommon. Premature babies or those with MALABSORP-TION can be at risk for deficiencies of folic acid and vitamin B-12, as can adults and children who are vegetarians (eat no animal products).

■ SYMPTOMS Similar to other causes of anemia. It usually begins gradually, and is difficult to recognize.

Iron-deficiency anemia can be caused by blood loss (for example during surgery). This may not be severe enough to require a BLOOD TRANSFUSION, but extra iron may be needed to replace that lost.

■ ACTION If your baby was premature, or one of twins or triplets, discuss with your doctor whether iron supplements are necessary.

Ensure that your child has a balanced diet. See *NUTRITION*. If he does not have a good appetite, make sure that what he does eat is nutritious. Don't be tempted to fill him up with 'just anything'. This will further decrease his appetite. Discuss with your doctor the need for giving iron supplements.

If you suspect iron-deficiency anemia, always get medical advice.

■ TESTS A BLOOD TEST will show whether there is anemia, and what has caused it. Occasionally, it is necessary to test for unnoticed bleeding of the bowel as a cause of iron-deficiency anemia.

■ TREATMENT Iron can be given to infants and young children in a syrup and in tablets to older chidren and adolescents. Iron can cause constipation, diarrhea and nausea in children. If the anemia is not severe, it may be possible to simply increase the amount of iron in the child's everyday diet. Iron syrup and tablets can cause serious poisoning if taken in overdose, so keep the bottle away from children and don't tell the child the iron tablets are candy. Treatment begins to show improvement in the anemia in about a week. The body's iron stores can be replenished within a few months.

■ OUTLOOK This is an easily treated form of anemia, usually causing no long-term problems.

ITCHING

Not all itching is due to skin disease: normal skin will itch when certain chemicals or materials come into contact with it. Some babies and young children will find wool unpleasantly itchy, and will not wear it. Important medical causes of itching include: ECZEMA, URTICARIA, INSECT BITES, SCABIES, HEPATITIS, JAUNDICE and DIABETES. Dry skin, particularly in winter when the humidity is low, can be itchy. Summer prickly heat or heat rash can also be itchy.

■ ACTION If the cause is known, and the itching not severe, as for example with some insect bites – see *BITES AND STINGS* – no action is needed. If the cause is dry skin, bath oil and a skin lotion can help. For prickly heat, a cool or tepid bath and talcum powder usually relieve the itch. If necessary, an antihistamine can be given by mouth without consulting a doctor for minor but persistent itching when the cause is known. Promethazine or chlorpheniramine are suitable. Otherwise, get medical advice and your doctor will consider the various possible causes.

■ TREATMENT This depends on the cause: most of those listed above have specific treatments, in addition to which an oral antihistamine medicine may be prescribed. For long-term management and outlook, see the separate entries.

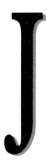

JAUNDICE IN BABIES

The yellow discoloration of the skin and eyes, which occurs to some degree in up to 50 percent of normal new-born babies. It is usually most noticeable between the third and sixth day after birth, and may be slightly more common in breast-fed babies.

■ CAUSES The yellow color, known as bilirubin, is a pigment produced in the body by the breakdown of red blood cells. It is normally disposed of by the liver as bile, which drains into the bowel, and is excreted through the feces. In the new-born this process is 'overworked' because of especially rapid breakdown of red cells, and the relative immaturity of the disposal system of the baby's liver. The bilirubin level in the blood rises, and can be seen as a yellow discoloration of the skin. Most jaundice in the new-born period is harmless and normal. More severe jaundice may be caused by INFECTION, HYPOTHYROIDISM and the rapid destruction of red blood cells that occurs in RHESUS or BLOOD GROUP INCOMPATIBILITY.

■ ACTION In most babies no investigation or treatment is required. Jaundice usually disappears by the tenth day after birth.

Investigation and possible treatment may be required if the jaundice is severe, or the baby is otherwise ill; or if the jaundice appears during the first 24 hours of life, suggesting Rhesus or ABO blood group incompatibility; or if it persists beyond two weeks of age.

■ TESTS A BLOOD TEST can determine the level of bilirubin in the blood; other tests may be used to determine the underlying cause.

■ TREATMENT Adequate feeding is necessary, because dehydration may worsen the jaundice. If the bilirubin level is high, PHOTOTHERAPY is required. For dangerously high bilirubin levels and for babies not responding to phototherapy treatment, EXCHANGE TRANSFUSION is required.

■ OUTLOOK is usually excellent, providing there is no serious underlying cause.

JAUNDICE IN CHILDREN

The symptoms (and underlying process) causing jaundice in children are similar to that of JAUNDICE IN BABIES.

■ CAUSES of jaundice in childhood range from an inflammatory infection in the liver (HEPATITIS), to the destruction of abnormal red blood cells which releases their bilirubin into the blood circulation (hemolytic ANEMIA), to an obstruction of bile drainage.

■ INVESTIGATION AND MANAGEMENT See HEPATITIS and CIRRHOSIS.

JEALOUSY

The only antidote to jealousy is learning to share: to share not only possessions, but attention and affection. Sharing is a social skill, learned rather than inborn, though affected to a degree by the individual's personality and temperament. Any new situation (new baby, new school, new parent) will increase a child's need for attention; with parental skill (and some luck), attention and love can be distributed without engendering jealousy in one or other child. See also *SIBLING RIVALRY, DIVORCE, FAMILY PROBLEMS*.

JELLY FISH STINGS

Jelly fish are equipped with tentacles that have a venom apparatus. The stings vary from mild to very painful. The local signs are redness and swelling. Generalized signs include weakness, fever, chills, nausea and vomiting. The intensity of the symptoms depends upon the length of time the tentacles are allowed to remain in contact with the skin.

■ ACTION Remove tentacles as promptly as possible and wash the area in salt water. If extensive swelling is present get medical advice. Antihistamines and steroids can help.

■ PREVENTION is best accomplished by caution when swimming in tropical waters. Watch for signs warning of jelly fish in the area. Beware of damaged tentacles and 'dead' jelly fish washed up on the beach in a storm. These are still capable of stinging.

JOINT PAINS

See *ARTHRITIS*.

JUVENILE RHEUMATOID ARTHRITIS (JRA)

The term describing a group of illnesses responsible for repeated episodes of ARTHRITIS. One form of this is called Still's disease. Its causes are unknown.

■ SYMPTOMS Painful swelling of certain joints, particularly those of the hands, wrists, elbows, ankles and knees. The neck and hip joints may also be involved. You may find that your child has stiff, painful joints in the morning, which improve later in the day. He may also have a pale pink RASH that comes and goes, mainly on the trunk, face, arms and legs.

A slight FEVER is often present and in some cases may be very high, last many days or weeks, and may be the only sign of JRA early in the course of the disease. There may be small swellings under the skin (subcutaneous nodules).

The lymph glands may be enlarged, noticeably so in the neck or under the arms. The child may also be pale and have ANEMIA.

■ ACTION The joint swelling gives reason for an early visit to the doctor. Diagnosis is not always easy, or made quickly. Tests are necessary (usually BLOOD TESTS and X-rays), and the pattern of the illness needs to be watched for a few weeks and, often, months before a diagnosis can be made.

■ TREATMENT The aim is to let the child lead as normal a life as possible. To achieve this, the pain must be controlled and damage to and deformity of the joints kept to a minimum. Muscles must be kept active to prevent them from becoming weak. Your doctor may refer you to a rheumatologist and/or a clinic specializing in juvenile rheumatoid arthritis.

During the episodes of severe joint pain, rest is necessary. Wrist and knee joints can be kept in splints at night to prevent them from becoming fixed in positions that make them difficult to use.

Pain relief is important. Your doctor may prescribe aspirin: one of the few occasions when it is used in children (see REYE SYNDROME). It is highly effective at relieving joint pain and in allowing joints to function normally again. Aspirin should always be given with food, and never in more than the dose prescribed by the doctor.

Alternative anti-inflammatory drugs may sometimes be used and occasionally steroids are necessary when all other treatment fails.

Once the pain and swelling improves, a physiotherapist needs to teach the child exercises to strengthen muscles and to loosen joints that have become stiff. Some of these can be painful, but they are essential to prevent deformity. This can develop rapidly if the joints are not kept moving. Exercising in a warm swimming-pool can be particularly useful and fun.

An occupational therapist can help the child with games and activities that keep joints mobile: if an exercise is a game, the child needs little motivating.

If deformity has already occurred, the occupational therapist can help with appliances and modification of the home.

Children with this condition may also suffer from anxiety and DEPRESSION. Ask for medical help with this: it is part of the illness.

Some patients with juvenile rheumatoid arthritis have associated inflammation of parts of the eye. The doctor will check regularly for this since it can cause loss of vision if not treated.

ALTERNATIVE TREATMENTS
Acupuncture, homeopathy, specialized diets and many other remedies have all been recommended to relieve the symptoms of juvenile rheumatoid arthritis. None of these have any proven effect, and may do harm if medical recommendations are abandoned and joints are allowed to become stiff and useless.

OUTLOOK is variable, but in most children the symptoms gradually improve during adolescence and the arthritis does not continue into adult life. Thus, if damage to the joints is kept to a minimum, the outlook is usually good. Children with chronic arthritis rarely suffer educationally.

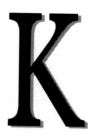

KELOID
See *SCAR*.

KIDNEY FAILURE
See *RENAL FAILURE*.

KIDNEY TRANSPLANT
See *RENAL FAILURE*.

KLINEFELTER SYNDROME
A rare chromosomal abnormality in males where there are three sex CHROMOSOMES (XXY) instead of the normal two (XY). Babies born with Klinefelter syndrome have normal male features at birth, but at PUBERTY tend to be tall without the sequence of development of normal male sex characteristics. Instead, affected boys may develop breasts and a feminine body shape. The testicles remain small and do not produce sperm, resulting in infertility. There may be a minor degree of MENTAL HANDICAP.

If you have one child with Klinefelter syndrome, there is little risk of having another affected in the same way. You will, however, want to discuss this with your doctor and possibly see a geneticist for further information and counselling.

KNOCK KNEES
The child's knees tilt inwards. When he stands, his knees touch and the ankles remain apart. For the majority of cases there is no cause, apart from the fact that the ligaments which support the knee are more lax than usual. The problem is commonest in OBESE children and those with FLAT FEET, and can occur with RICKETS.

■ SYMPTOMS, apart from the knock-kneed appearance, don't really exist.

■ ACTION In most cases, particularly in children under six years, no treatment is necessary. However, it is advisable to encourage your child to sit cross-legged on the floor.

If your child is overweight, a return to a normal weight for his height will usually cure the problem.

■ TREATMENT rarely indicated. In the most severe cases, it may be necessary to raise the inner border of the heel of the shoe slightly to correct the tilt.

■ OUTLOOK Knock knees usually recover without treatment.

KOPLIK SPOTS
See *MEASLES*.

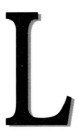

LACTOSE INTOLERANCE

Impaired absorption of the sugar lactose, caused by a deficiency of the enzyme lactase in the bowel lining. There are two types, primary and secondary.

■ SYMPTOMS Watery DIARRHEA from birth in the primary type or after GASTROENTERITIS in the secondary form, which is much commoner. Primary lactose intolerance is an INHERITED DISORDER. Small bowel biopsy (as in CELIAC DISEASE) will reveal low lactase levels. Secondary lactose intolerance occurs in association with many gastro-intestinal disorders, particularly after an episode of GASTROENTERITIS.

Lactase deficiency may also be associated with protein MALNUTRITION and COW'S MILK ALLERGY, and is more common in PREMATURE infants.

■ SYMPTOMS Watery diarrhea, starting when normal feedings are reintroduced after recovery from simple gastroenteritis. The BOWEL MOVEMENTS are passed forcefully, with gas, and there is irritation of the buttocks. There may be excessive fluid loss and DEHYDRATION.

■ INVESTIGATIONS Stool tests; trial with lactose-free milk. The feedings may be changed back to ordinary milk after recovery, but if the diarrhea recurs lactose-free milk may be needed for several months.

■ OUTLOOK Primary lactose intolerance is lifelong and will require continual avoidance of lactose-containing foods. Secondary intolerance may be brief, or last for some months, but full recovery is the rule.

LANGUAGE DEVELOPMENT

The road to speech starts well before a baby's first words. Babies communicate with familiar adults from birth, responding and being responded to as in conversation. Interacting with their mothers, all babies use complex sequences of facial expression and movement. A mother responds by copying the expressions or talking to the baby; in turn, the baby responds. This fine-tuning of responses continues naturally through the period of language development. By about four months, most babies make some sounds during these 'conversations' and soon after will start discriminating among familiar voices.

The babbling which develops from six to 12 months involves word-like sounds with varying pitch and is often used as if in conversation. During this period, the baby's understanding of names of people, objects and actions is increasing. Many babies will be saying their first words at around 12 months, although this can vary substantially, even in 'normal' children. The vocabulary of single words increases slowly at first, then rapidly. The toddler than starts to string these together in two-word sentences from about 18 months.

Over the next three or four years, language develops as a social tool and is encouraged and influenced by opportunities to hear and use it. However, the process is essentially innate and follows similar patterns, though at varying rates, in all children except those with severe MENTAL HANDICAP.

Children who are born deaf babble normally until about eight months, then stop. At this stage they can learn some signs for objects, or, if hearing can be restored, continue to develop language normally. Children brought up hearing two languages may take longer to increase their vocabulary for the obvious reason that they have to learn two names for everything.

Delay in language development tends to run in families and is more common in boys than in girls. It is rarely a cause for concern, but your child should have regular development checks by your doctor up to school entry. Seek advice as soon as you are worried – there may be a simple remedy.

See also *DEAFNESS, LEARNING DISORDERS, INTELLIGENCE, SPEECH DISORDERS, DEVELOPMENTAL DELAY.*

LARYNGITIS

Inflammation of the larynx, or voice-box. See the illustration.

■ CAUSES VIRUSES, more rarely BACTERIA. The problem may be part of a widespread INFECTION, such as CROUP, LARYNGO-TRACHEO-BRONCHITIS, INFLUENZA, or even a COMMON COLD.

■ SYMPTOMS Hoarseness and a SORE THROAT, often with a fever and cough. The illness is usually mild

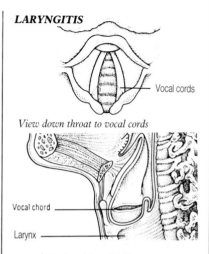

LARYNGITIS

Vocal cords

View down throat to vocal cords

Vocal chord

Larynx

and starts with cold-like symptoms.

■ ACTION For younger children (under five years), see *CROUP*. Above this age there is much less risk of obstruction to the breathing because the air passage is larger. The sore throat can be relieved by suitable doses of acetamenophen. Cool drinks and moist air from a humidifier may be soothing. Talking may be uncomfortable and may make the hoarseness worse.

■ GET MEDICAL ADVICE immediately if the child has any difficulty in breathing or a high temperature. See *EPIGLOTTITIS*.

■ TREATMENT Most laryngitis in children is due to viral infections, which have no specific treatment. Antibiotics are not usually required.

■ OUTLOOK Complete recovery in one to two weeks.

LARYNGO-TRACHEO-BRONCHITIS

The medical term for CROUP. It primarily affects babies and young children. The lining of the air passages from the larynx to the lungs may be infected.

■ CAUSES The so-called para-influenza VIRUSES, and some others.

■ SYMPTOMS The cough sounds like the bark of a seal (once heard, never forgotten). The cough is often worse at night. The child may have a runny nose, sore throat and hoarse voice or cry; this may be accompanied by noisy breathing or STRIDOR. Some children also have a FEVER and are generally sick. This may progress to difficulty in breathing, with a heaving chest and indrawing of the space under the ribs.

■ ACTION 1 You may find that your child gains some relief from sitting in a steamy atmosphere. 2 Get the child to drink plenty of fluids. 3 If he appears unable to swallow, and/or breathing appears difficult or the child is very distressed, get urgent medical advice, even in the middle of the night. Take him to the nearest hospital emergency room.

■ TREATMENT Milder cases may be treated at home. As the condition is due to a viral INFECTION there is currently no specific ANTIBIOTIC that is effective. Fluids and acetaminophen are comforting. More severe cases, especially in younger children, are treated in hospital, where an oxygen tent may be used. An inhaled drug such as racemic epinephrine may be given. Occasionally, if there is severe obstruction to breathing, a tube may be inserted into the trachea through the nose or mouth, and artificial breathing is initiated.

■ INVESTIGATIONS A chest X-ray and BLOOD TESTS will be done in hospital for severe cases, but are unnecessary for milder cases.

■ OUTLOOK Complete recovery, with no long-term effects.

LAZY EYE
See *STRABISMUS*.

LEAD POISONING
Less of a hazard nowadays than it used to be, because many countries now ban lead containing paint. However, old buildings may still contain lead paint on woodwork and walls. Lead is also sometimes used in making pottery and may dissolve into acid fluids such as orange juice kept in these containers.

■ SYMPTOMS Lead poisoning can cause ANEMIA. The most worrying effects are on the nervous and digestive systems: spasmodic ABDOMINAL PAIN, a metallic taste in the mouth, VOMITING, DIARRHEA and CONSTIPATION are associated with lead poisoning. So are headaches, irritability, convulsions, coma and even death. Long-term exposure to lead is a cause of DEVELOPMENTAL DELAY and LEARNING DISORDERS.

■ TESTS BLOOD TESTS to measure the amount of lead in the body, and X-rays, may be made to confirm the diagnosis.

■ TREATMENT in hospital will include ensuring a high fluid intake to protect the kidneys; anticonvulsants if there is a danger of convulsions; and specific treatment with a 'chelating agent' that removes the lead from the blood and tissues of the body. Frequent tests will be necessary to monitor the success of the treatment.

■ PRECAUTION If you are unsure of the glaze on any pottery, use it as a decorative piece and not as a container for fluids.

LEARNING DISORDERS

These are suspected when, despite adequate teaching, a child acquires skills or knowledge at a rate that is much slower than expected for his age and INTELLIGENCE. The problem may be general or specific (limited to one area, such as reading, spelling or arithmetic). Specific disorders are not usually identifiable until the age of seven or eight. This is because of the wide variation in children's learning capacity, particularly for reading, and it is not until this age that slowness becomes a cause for concern. See *LANGUAGE DEVELOPMENT, DEVELOPMENTAL DELAY.*

■ CAUSES General learning problems may result from a short attention span, easy distractability or emotional disturbance. A child gains encouragement from success or the mastering of a skill; persistent failure discourages and may further impair learning. A sudden slowing of progress is frequently the result of emotional distress, but may be the first sign of a serious physical disorder.

There is no consensus as to the cause or causes of specific learning disorders. They are more common among boys than girls and often run in families. Such children appear to have a particular inborn difficulty with one or more fundamental processes, for instance that required to deal with symbols in sequences, match sounds to symbols or memorize from sight. The problem may be compounded by repeated experience of failure.

■ ACTION Meet the child's teacher to discuss progress and your concerns. In general, aim to boost your child's confidence and to reward successes.

■ INVESTIGATIONS Thorough assessment of the nature of the difficulty by an educational psychologist or specialist teacher is a necessary first step. Alternatively, your doctor may suggest referral to a child psychiatrist.

■ TREATMENT depends on the specific nature of the problems identified. Special teaching methods may address a particular difficulty and classroom programs help set the scene for learning (see *BEHAVIORAL TREATMENTS*). Remedial teaching in small groups is provided in some schools, but withdrawing the child from normal class activities may create other problems. In a minority of cases, you may be advised that your child's best interests will be served by attending a special school.

■ OUTLOOK Provided the child's self-esteem and behavior do not suffer, he should respond well to appropriate teaching methods.

LEFTHANDEDNESS

A preference for using the left hand, most evident during specific activities such as eating, writing or participating in sports. Up to the age of five years, uncertainty about hand preference is common. One in three children will demonstrate cross laterality – the ability to use both hands for many common activities.

■ CAUSES More than 90 percent of children of two right-handed parents are right-handers. Only half the children of left-handers are left-handed. In Western countries it is typical for 10-12 percent of children to be left-handed for writing.

■ OUTLOOK There is no essential

disadvantage in being left-handed. Left-handed children may have difficulty with certain manipulative skills since so many tools (for example scissors) are designed for right-handers. When writing, the left hand covers what has been written, unless the child is taught to rotate the page clockwise.

About one in 20 left-handed children are exceptionally poor at right-handed activities. Some reports suggest an excess of left-handers in special classes and remedial services. These children may have suffered a disturbance of the left cerebral hemisphere, having been genetically programmed to be right-handed.

LEGG-PERTHES DISEASE OF THE HIP

Disease of the upper end of the thigh bone (the femur) where it forms the hip joint with the pelvis. The cause is unknown, but it is commonest in boys, usually aged five to nine years.

■ SYMPTOMS A LIMP is usually the first symptom. The child will complain of pain in the groin, thigh or knee – it may be mild or severe. The symptoms can start abruptly, or appear gradually over days, even months.

Occasionally both hip joints are involved. The child appears healthy otherwise.

■ ACTION A limp or joint pain should never be ignored. See your doctor without delay.

■ TESTS An X-ray is needed to make the diagnosis, and this will be repeated often to measure progress. A scan of the bone can reveal early signs of the disease.

■ TREATMENT The goal of treatment is to retain the normal spherical head of the femur. The child is allowed to bear weight, but the leg is held in such a way that the head of the femur is positioned well in the joint. This is done with casts, braces or splints.

Surgery may be necessary if the joint becomes deformed.

■ OUTLOOK Some children continue to have pain or stiffness of the joint once the disease has run its course. A small number will require a hip replacement in later life. Improvement in treatment has resulted in more children with this disease ending up with normal hip joints.

LEUKEMIA

Cancer of the white blood cells. The child's bone marrow produces large numbers of abnormal white blood cells that cannot effectively fight INFECTION. The normal production of red blood cells and platelets is also reduced, leading to ANEMIA and a tendency to bleed.

The cause of leukemia is unknown, but there is an association with exposure to radiation and also with certain genetic disorders such as DOWN SYNDROME. The disease has a tendency to run in families.

There are different types of leukemia, depending on which kind of white blood cells are involved. Acute lymphoblastic leukemia is the most common type in children, and responds well to modern treatment.

■ SYMPTOMS The child is usually pale, with the other symptoms of anaemia. He may bruise easily and have a RASH consisting of tiny bleeding spots on the skin. He may develop a severe infection. FEVER can occur, not always in association with infection. Occasionally the child complains of pain in the bones. The doctor may find that the liver, spleen and lymph glands are enlarged, as they try to produce normal white blood cells to counteract the overgrowth of abnormal cells.

▦ ACTION If you suspect anemia, or find that your child bruises or bleeds too easily, get medical advice. Don't ignore symptoms because you feel that you could not face up to a serious disease. Early diagnosis (see below) gives the best chance of cure: nowadays, the majority of children who develop leukemia *are* cured.

▦ TESTS are necessary to make the diagnosis. A simple BLOOD TEST usually shows a large number of abnormal white blood cells. The number of red blood cells and platelets is reduced. To confirm the diagnosis, a bone marrow examination is necessary: a needle is inserted into bone under local anesthesia and a tiny portion of the bone marrow is drawn out. Other tests such as X-rays and ULTRASOUND SCANS may be necessary; and sometimes a LUMBAR PUNCTURE too. The tests are also used to try to determine which treatment is most likely to be successful.

▦ TREATMENT This has been one of the greatest medical success stories during the past 20 years. Previously, the disease was incurable.

The aim is to destroy all the cancer cells. Unfortunately, anticancer (cytotoxic) drugs damage normal as well as abnormal cells, and this gives rise to side-effects. For this reason, a number of drugs are used in combination to minimize the side-effects of each drug. Another reason for using different drugs is to insure against the abnormal cells developing resistance' to a single drug.

Side-effects include loss of hair, anemia, a bleeding tendency and decreased resistance to infection. Some drugs cause nausea, vomiting and diarrhea: these can be treated with other drugs.

Another problem with treatment is the need for repeated tests to assess whether the drugs are working effectively.

Treatment is given in phases: **1** Inducing a remission: this means clearing the body of all detectable cancer (leukemia) cells. Three or four drugs are usually used over a period of weeks, given either as tablets or by injection. If there is a risk of the disease occurring in the brain, radiotherapy to the head and injection of drugs into the spinal cord are done as preventive measures. **2** Maintenance therapy is continued once a remission has been achieved. The object is to destroy any undetected leukemia cells that may start to multiply and cause further disease. This treatment is usually continued for about three years. **3** During maintenance treatment, and for many years later, tests are done to look for signs of a relapse. If this occurs, further treatment is given. **4** During the whole period of treatment, the specialist will be on guard against anemia, infection and NUTRITIONAL problems. **5** If the leukemia is resistant to treatment, it is sometimes possible to give a bone marrow transplant. If a suitable donor (usually a brother or sister) is found, large doses of drugs and radiotherapy are given to destroy all the leukemia cells. It also destroys all the normal bone marrow cells, which are then replaced by cells from the healthy donor through the transplantation.

▦ SELF-HELP It will sometimes be hard for you to be positive in your feelings about your chld having leukemia, but you must try. If the child feels that you have doubts, he may not trust the treatment. Reassure him that the treatment is necessary to make him well, and that all the family are involved with him in fighting his illness.

Psychological support is available for families going through the ordeal of childhood leukemia. Don't feel that your problems cannot be shared with the doctors, nurses and social workers who staff the children's cancer (oncology) unit treating your child. They are there to help in all ways, not just medically.

Treatment of childhood leukemia tends to change quite rapidly as new developments occur – and also as a result of the child's response. So don't worry if treatment is different from what you have heard or read about – you will soon become an expert in how leukemia is treated.

Ensure that your child's teeth and gums are clean and healthy during treatment to minimize infection.

Alert schoolteachers to the child's condition: he ought to avoid contact with CHICKEN POX or MEASLES, as much as possible. Tell the doctor immediately if he does encounter other children with these infections. Routine immunizations with live virus vaccines such as measles, mumps, *Rubella* and oral poliovirus are usually avoided during treatment.

When the child's blood count is low, keep him away from crowds and social gatherings. On the other hand, he should carry on with school and other routine activities whenever possible. Don't over-protect him, despite the potential seriousness of the condition – to do so will make life even more difficult in the long run.

If your child is old enough, encourage him to ask questions too. He may have worries that have not occurred to you.

■ OUTLOOK At times the discomfort of tests, the side-effects of treatment, and the stress of the illness can seem unbearable. Remember that in most cases, the result of modern treatment is a long-lasting or permanent cure.

LICE OR NITS

These are tiny insects that feed on blood. Head lice are common in children, often being recognized by their eggs, also called nits. Body lice are rather uncommon; symptoms and treatment are similar to those described below for head lice.

■ CAUSE The head louse, *Pediculus capitis*, spreads from person to person as a result of direct contact with infested individuals or indirectly by contact with contaminated objects such as combs, brushes, hats. The bite itself causes no symptoms initially, but with time the child may become ALLERGIC to the saliva injected by the insect and develop an itchy reaction. This leads to scratching, and sometimes to secondary INFECTION (IMPETIGO).

■ SYMPTOMS Itching and scratching of the head are the major symptoms of lice. Inspection of the child's hair will reveal the characteristic oval eggs, firmly fixed to the hairs. Live eggs are brown, and not easily seen; white nits are actually empty egg cases, and signify past infestation. Since the eggs are fixed to the hairs at their roots, the distance of the nits from the skin shows how long the eggs have been there. Hair grows at about + in (1.25 cm) per month. It is sometimes possible, by

LICE

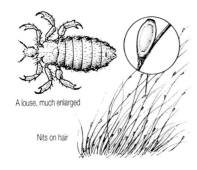

A louse, much enlarged

Nits on hair

parting the hair quickly, to see the insects moving on the scalp.

■ ACTION Effective treatment is easily obtained at the drugstore. Children should be allowed to return to school or day-care centre the morning after their first treatment. Contacts, including family members, should be examined and treated if they are infested. Bed mates should be treated anyway.

■ GET MEDICAL ADVICE if there are sore patches on the scalp, or painful lumps in the back of the neck – both signs of impetigo.

■ TREATMENT There are several effective treatments: lindane, permethrin or natural pyrethrine-based products. Pyrethrine is available without prescription. This is applied as a ten-minute shampoo and requires a second treatment seven to ten days later. Careful removal of nits with a fine tooth comb is recommended. Shampooing with vinegar may also speed up the removal of nits by combing. Permethrin (ten-minute rinse) requires only a single treatment.

If impetigo has developed, your doctor will prescribe an ANTIBIOTIC. Clothing or bedding used in the

48-hour period before treatment can be disinfected by machine washing or drying (using hot cycles). Dry cleaning or simply storing clothing in tightly closed plastic bags for ten days is also effective.

■ OUTLOOK Head lice are common in schoolchildren, and do *not* indicate deprivation or poor personal hygiene. Treatment is easy and safe, and may be repeated from time to time if necessary. Only body lice can carry disease. Infestation with head lice is a nuisance but is *not* serious.

LIES AND FIBS

Until their teens children do not fully understand, in the adult sense, the meaning of right and wrong. Up to the early school years, a child may tell a story that represents what he would have preferred to have happened without necessarily intending to deceive. At this age, it is quite common for children to indulge in vivid fantasies about their own activities, and this is not a cause for concern. As children grow older, they begin to understand the difference between fantasy and reality. All older children, like adults, distort the truth at times to try to protect themselves or others. Generally they will learn to value truthfulness to the same extent as their parents. Persistent lying is often a sign of problems with interpersonal relationships and self-esteem. This often goes with other worrying behavior and parents should seek advice, in the first place, from the family doctor or pediatrician. He or she should have a clear idea of whether the problem needs referral to a child psychiatrist.

LIFE SAVING

See *DROWNING, EMERGENCY RESUSCITATION.*

LIMP

An uneven walk, in which the weight is carried more on one leg than on the other. This is usually caused by pain in one leg, but a painless limp also occurs.

■ CAUSES A painful limp can have many causes including: – Injury to the leg (most commonly the foot).
– A badly fitting shoe.
– A WART on the sole of the foot.
– ARTHRITIS or INFECTION of one of the joints of the leg.
– LEGG-PERTHES DISEASE of the hip.
– OSGOOD-SCHLATTERS DISEASE of the knee.
– A sprained ankle.
– Other more rare conditions such as BONE TUMOR.
A painless limp is usually caused by a problem in the muscle or nerve to the leg, as in
– POLIOMYELITIS (POLIO);
– CEREBRAL PALSY; or
– if one leg is shorter than the other, due to injury or OSTEOMYELITIS.
– CONGENITAL DISLOCATION OF THE HIP.

■ SYMPTOMS The child takes his weight on the 'good leg for as long as possible while walking. This makes him tilt towards the good leg.
There is usually pain, which may help to indicate where the problem lies. However, the pain does not always occur exactly in the place that is causing the limp. In addition, muscles can be strained as a result of the limp, causing even more pain.

■ ACTION If a limp persists for more than a day, and if you cannot find a simple cause, see your doctor.

■ TESTS including X-rays may be necessary.

■ TREATMENT and OUTLOOK

depend on the cause: see separate entries mentioned above.

LOCK-JAW
See *TETANUS*.

LOW BIRTH WEIGHT

This is defined in the Western world as weight at birth of less than 5 + lb (2.5 kg). Low birth weight babies are either premature – see *PREMATURITY* – or born small in relation to the duration of the pregnancy, SMALL FOR DATES BABIES. Some babies may be both premature and small for dates.

LUMBAR PUNCTURE

A medical investigation in which cerebro-spinal fluid is obtained by passing a needle, under aseptic conditions, through anesthetized skin on the lower back, into the spinal canal.

LYMPHOMA

CANCER of the lymph glands, which may also involve the liver and spleen. It usually starts in one group of glands and spreads to others nearby. The cause is unknown. There are various forms of the disease in adults; one that occasionally occurs in older children is known as Hodgkin disease or Hodgkin lymphoma. It is very rare under the age of three years.

■ SYMPTOMS Swollen glands, especially those in the neck, are usually noticed first. Some children have weight loss, FEVER and sweating at night. There may be a decreased resistance to INFECTION.

■ ACTION Glands in the neck may be enlarged for many reasons, including scalp or EAR INFECTION, TONSILLITIS and INFECTIOUS MONONUCLEO-

SIS. If there is no obvious cause, get medical advice and explain why you are worried.

■ TESTS If your doctor finds no simple explanation for the enlargement of the glands, he or she may recommend a BLOOD TEST and possibly a biopsy of the lymph gland. This involves removing a piece or all of the gland under ANESTHETIC and examining it for abnormal cells. If the biopsy reveals lymphoma, further tests are necessary to find out the extent of the disease. These include X-rays, ULTRASOUND SCANS and further blood tests.

Special scans may be done to determine the exact spread of the disease within the glands of the abdomen, the liver and spleen. These measures are called 'staging' the disease; accurate staging enables the selection of the most appropriate and effective treatment plan. These scans have replaced the need for surgical staging of the disease in many cases. Surgical staging involves an operation on the abdomen to determine directly which glands within the abdomen are affected. If surgical staging is done, the spleen is often removed during the operation.

■ TREATMENT Largely due to careful staging, results of treatment have recently improved significantly. If it is known exactly which lymph glands and organs are involved, the correct treatment can be directed at all affected areas at once.

Anticancer (cytotoxic) drugs are used in combination to destroy the cancer cells. See *LEUKEMIA* for an explanation of the technique, and for side-effects.

Radiotherapy (X-ray treatment) is also used, depending on the findings of the staging tests. The side-effects are similar to those of the drugs; growth, fertility and the thyroid gland may be affected.

If the spleen has been removed, there is an increased risk of BACTERIAL infection. ANTIBIOTICS are used to prevent this and a vaccine to prevent infections by *Pneumococcus* bacteria is usually given.

Occasionally, a bone marrow transplant can help in treatment. See *LEUKEMIA*.

The cancer is most likely to return in the first two years after treatment has been started, so blood tests, X-rays and ultrasound scans are done regularly. If necessary, further treatment is given.

■ SELF-HELP Unpleasant tests and treatment put a great strain not just on the child, but on the whole family. Staff in specialized centers that treat conditions such as lymphoma are well aware of this and have considerable experience of helping. Use the support they offer. Discuss any worries that you have and encourage your child to do the same. See also *LEUKEMIA*.

■ OUTLOOK varies a great deal, depending on how far the lymphoma has spread at the time of diagnosis. But the cure rate has improved greatly in recent years, as has life expectancy in those whose disease cannot be entirely eradicated.

M

MALABSORPTION

The child has large, pale, frequent foul smelling BOWEL MOVEMENTS, ABDOMINAL SWELLING and poor growth (FAILURE TO THRIVE). Adequate digestion of food requires a sufficient length of bowel, correct movement of digested food through it (peristalsis), the right enzyme-containing digestive secretions from the pancreas and bile duct system, normal bowel BACTERIA, normal bowel lining (villi), and the absorption of digested food products into the bloodstream.

Disturbances of any of these essential mechanisms may result in an abnormal bowel pattern, usually indicated by DIARRHEA and malabsorption, which is either generalized or limited to certain foods.

▓ CAUSES There may be an abnormality in the lining (mucosa) of the bowel. This can be associated with MALNUTRITION or with CELIAC DISEASE (permanent or temporary); it can occur after prolonged GASTROENTERITIS or infestation with GIARDIA; COW'S MILK ALLERGY; or previous drug therapy.

There may be a rare abnormality of lymph drainage or inadequate enzyme production (see *SUGAR INTOLERANCE*); or the cause may be one of a number of unusual biochemical deficiencies causing defective uptake of minerals and VITAMINS. Malabsorption in CYSTIC FIBROSIS occurs because of inadequate digestive secretions from the pancreas.

BILIARY ATRESIA, HEPATITIS, CIRRHOSIS and bacterial overgrowth may also affect absorption. Previous bowel operations, especially if segments of bowel were removed, are another possible cause.

Toddler diarrhea or 'irritable colon syndrome' may be due to rapid transit in the intestine leading to incomplete digestion; undigested food is found in the bowel movements. Occasionally, inflammatory bowel disease, including ULCERATIVE COLITIS or CROHN DISEASE, have malabsorption as a symptom.

▓ INVESTIGATIONS A clear case history is essential. Plotting the child's GROWTH PATTERN; physical examination to detect poor growth or abdominal swelling; observation and investigation of the bowel movements for infection; BLOOD TESTS to determine ANEMIA and VITAMIN DEFICIENCY; sweat test (see *CYSTIC FIBROSIS*) or jejunal biopsy (see *CELIAC DISEASE*) may help. A barium meal X-ray may be needed to exclude an abnormality of the bowel following surgery, or due to a CONGENITAL ABNORMALITY.

▓ TREATMENT depends on cause. It may include improving the diet (as in malnutrition) or exclusion of food that cannot be tolerated, as in celiac disease, cow's milk allergy, or food intolerance. ANTIBIOTICS may be required to fight *Giardia* to control bacterial overgrowth. Replacement of vitamins, pancreatic enzymes (cystic fibrosis) or other drug treatments may be necessary.

▨ OUTLOOK depends on the underlying condition, but children usually grow out of toddler diarrhea and cow's milk allergy in the first few years of life.

MALARIA

A common tropical INFECTION caused by a PARASITE transmitted via mosquito bites. The parasites multiply in the liver and red blood cells.

▨ PREVENTION Any child going to a part of the world where the disease occurs must be protected by taking anti-malaria tablets before, during and after his stay. The type of tablet will depend on the area, and may change from time to time because the parasite tends to develop resistance to anti-malarial agents. The treatment should continue for at least six weeks after leaving the area. Some anti-malarial drugs may be unsuitable for children, but finding a safe one is usually no problem. Breast-fed babies must also be treated because although drugs taken by the mother pass to the baby through breast milk, the amount is too variable to be relied upon to protect the baby.

Mosquito nets, repellants and protective clothing, especially during late afternoon and early evening when mosquitos appear in great numbers, are also essential preventive measures. Don't put too much faith in these – they are not a guarantee against bites and may give a false sense of security.

The INCUBATION PERIOD is nine to 30 days and the first symptom is usually FEVER with chills, sweating and headache. The vomiting and diarrhea that follow can cause DEHYDRATION and the child is usually drowsy and listless. He may become pale as ANEMIA develops. Treatment usually results in rapid improvement if the diagnosis is made early enough, so get medical advice quickly if you suspect infection.

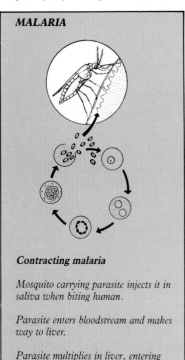

MALARIA

Contracting malaria

Mosquito carrying parasite injects it in saliva when biting human.

Parasite enters bloodstream and makes way to liver.

Parasite multiplies in liver, entering bloodstream periodically, invading red blood cells.

When parasite matures, red blood cells rupture, causing fever and malaria symptoms.

MALIGNANT HYPERTHERMIA

See *HEAT-STROKE AND MALIGNANT HYPERTHERMIA.*

MALNUTRITION

Generally taken to mean undernourishment – see also *FAILURE TO THRIVE*. Undernourishment is associated with poverty, insufficient food supplies, psychological disturbance or insufficient food intake due to loss of APPETITE or ANOREXIA NERVOSA, recurrent VOMITING and CHRONIC ILLNESS (this may reduce appetite and/or cause a 'wasting' process). Overeating and diets consisting largely of low-fiber 'junk food' with a high energy density (as sucrose and fat) lead to *over*nutrition, the leading *mal*nutrition in the industrialized Western world.

■ SIGNS of undernutrition: **1** Weight loss, or failure to gain weight, resulting in a thin body shape (in infancy, undernutrition in the chronic and extreme form is known as *Marasmus*). This chronic process needs to be distinguished from sunken eyes and WEIGHT LOSS associated with acute DEHYDRATION. **2** Apathy, listlessness and irritability. **3** Poor hair growth, dry skin. **4** Changes in distribution of fluid in the body: chronic undernutrition from protein-deficient diets results in puffiness (EDEMA) of feet, hands and face (*very* rare in the United States, but known as kwashiorkor in Africa, where the condition was first identified). **5** See *VITAMIN DEFICIENCIES*.

■ ACTION Malnourished children and their families may need intensive care and rehabilitation from a team of different professionals, including dieticians and doctors. If the origins of the condition are social rather than medical, then the professional skills and leadership of social workers will be of paramount importance. Malnutrition due to *Anorexia nervosa* and chronic disease requires treatment of the underlying problem(s) as well as a balanced diet.

■ OUTLOOK Malnutrition due to inadequate intake with no underlying problems such as *Anorexia nervosa* or chronic illness has a good outlook once the diet is corrected.

MARFAN SYNDROME

A rare INHERITED DISORDER that tends to run in families. Bones, ligaments, eyes and the heart are affected.

■ SYMPTOMS The child is unusually tall and slender with long legs, arms, fingers and toes. He may develop a SCOLIOSIS and the breast bone may be prominent and stick out ('pidgeon breast') or underdeveloped and caved in ('funnel chest'). See *PECTUS EXCAVATUM*. Joints have a greater range of movement than normal. FLAT FEET are common.

Abnormalities of the eye can occur. Most children with Marfan syndrome are SHORT-SIGHTED, and there may be other eye problems such as CATARACTS and dislocation of the lenses.

There may also be weakening of the walls of arteries, and possibly HEART FAILURE may result.

These features may be mild rather than severe, and not all of them occur in every case. In addition, early detection and treatment can substantially lessen their effect.

■ PREVENTION If there is a history of the condition in the family, consider GENETIC COUNSELLING before getting pregnant. If either parent carries the gene, there is a 50 percent chance of each child being affected.

■ ACTION If your child has Marfan syndrome, he will require regular examination to look for the abnormalities mentioned.

■ TREATMENT Scoliosis and short-sightedness are treated in the usual ways.

If there is evidence of heart valve involvement, the child may need an antibiotic before dental treatments and heart surgery.

■ OUTLOOK is improving. Most symptoms can be treated, and the recent advances in heart surgery have greatly improved the prospects for those with significant heart-disease.

MASK FOR INHALATION
See *NEBULIZING MASK.*

MASTOIDITIS
A serious infection of the mastoid bone (the bony prominence behind the ear). It is a rare complication of MIDDLE EAR INFECTION.

■ SYMPTOMS The child becomes very ill, feverish and irritable. The mastoid bone is tender with overlying swelling and redness.

■ TREATMENT ANTIBIOTICS; uncommonly an operation is required, a mastoidectomy, to drain the infected bone.

MASTURBATION
Handling genitalia to gain pleasurable sensation. Children become aware of their genitals from about two, and discover in time that fondling them leads to a pleasurable feeling. Children use masturbation, as adults do, to soothe and relieve tension. Though most do not experience sexual excitement, children are capable of achieving orgasm,

and those who discover this may well repeat the experiment. A child who is found flushed and panting in bed may well have been doing this.

Most children masturbate at some time or other; they may do so regularly, or they may do so for short periods and then forget about it. In neither case is it harmful. Boys in particular are aware of their penises, obviously so since they stick out, and it is quite normal to handle them. Only if a child masturbates compulsively and furtively should you be concerned: there may be an underlying emotional cause for which you should seek help; otherwise you should not worry about it and not draw your child's attention to it. It is all part of his SEX EDUCATION which should be kept as natural as possible.

MEASLES
A VIRAL INFECTION spread by exhaled droplets. It is highly infectious from just before the beginning of the illness to about four days after the rash appears. The INCUBATION PERIOD is eight to 14 days. Measles is now an uncommon infection in the United States because of the high rate of measles IMMUNIZATION.

■ PREVENTION Measles should be prevented by immunization because the complications can be grave, and occasionally fatal. Immunization is usually given at about 15 months of age, in combination with MUMPS and RUBELLA vaccine, but measles can occur in the first year of life. If a baby is at high risk of catching measles, an injection of immunoglobulin within six days of exposure can prevent or modify measles. A measles vaccine booster injection given before entry to school is likely to be recommended for all children in the

United States by 1990. Measles can occur in a mild form even after immunization, but in such cases there are no serious complications.

Keeping suspects in quarantine is not particularly effective because the carrier is highly infectious before symptoms occur, and the disease spreads most rapidly at that time.

■ SYMPTOMS First, a very runny nose, red eyes (CONJUNCTIVITIS) and a dry COUGH. FEVER is mild before the rash develops, but then the child's temperature can rise dramatically.

The rash appears about four days after the onset of symptoms, starting behind the ears and rapidly spreading over the face and body. As the red areas of the rash merge, the skin has a blotchy appearance. The rash fades to a brownish color after a few days, and the skin becomes dry and scaly.

Koplik spots occur in the mouth in the early stages of measles, before the rash appears. Typical of measles, these are small, white spots that look like grains of sand and develop inside the cheeks, close to the molar teeth; they stand out against the red, inflamed membranes of the mouth.

■ ACTION If you suspect measles, get urgent medical advice. It is important to diagnose and report cases of measles to the health department so that measures can be taken to prevent a local epidemic.

The fever should be treated immediately with acetamenophen and a tepid bath. See also *FEBRILE CONVULSIONS*.

The child may feel ill enough to want to stay in bed, but this is not essential.

Bright light may hurt his eyes because of the associated conjunctivitis, so a shaded room can help; however, the room does not need to be in total darkness. Music or tape-recorded stories can help to relieve the boredom if the eyes are too painful to allow the child to read.

■ COMPLICATIONS, ranging from mild to severe, are common. They include PNEUMONIA, EAR INFECTIONS and ENCEPHALITIS. All complications tend to be more severe in undernourished and chronically ill children, so it is particularly important that such children are immunized against measles. However, even normal children are at risk from encephalitis which may be life threatening or cause serious brain damage. With few exceptions all children should be immunized against measles.

■ TREATMENT ANTIBIOTICS are not routinely used, but secondary BACTERIAL infection is common, and they may well be necessary at this later stage.

Children whose immunity is depressed from any cause should be given an immunoglobulin injection if they come in contact with a person who has measles. This helps to boost immunity and prevent the disease.

■ OUTLOOK Most children recover completely, but prevention is better than cure. Countries that have a low immunization rate still have a high incidence of infection.

MECONIUM

The sticky green-brown substance produced in the baby's bowel before birth. It is usually passed by the baby in his first stool after birth. If the unborn baby is distressed or asphyxiated before or during birth, he may pass meconium that stains the amniotic fluid and may be sucked into the lungs.

MEDICAL SPECIALISTS

There are many different types of medical specialist who have trained in particular branches or specialties of medicine. In a large hospital, you are likely to encounter, either as individuals or as departments, any of the following:

– Allergist: specialist in ALLERGY.

– Anesthetist/anesthesiologist: specialist in giving ANESTHETIC.

– Cardiologist: specialist in HEART-DISEASE.

– Cardiovascular surgeon: specialist in heart and blood vessel surgery.

– Child developmentalist: specialist in assessing delayed child development.

– Dermatologist: specialist in skin disorders.

– Endocrinologist: specialist in endocrine gland problems such as DIABETES, thyroid disease.

– Gastroenterologist: specialist in diseases of the stomach, intestines, liver and esophagus.

– Geneticist: specialist in how diseases are inherited.

– Gynecologist: specialist in diseases of the female reproductive organs.

– Hematologist: specialist in diseases of the blood including HEMOPHILIA and SICKLE-CELL ANEMIA.

– Immunologist: specialist in dealing with disorders of the IMMUNE system.

– Infectious diseases: specialist in dealing with INFECTIONS.

– Intensivist: specialist in INTENSIVE CARE for children and/or adults.

– Neonatologist: specialist in INTENSIVE CARE for new-born babies.

– Nephrologist: specialist in kidney diseases.

– Neurologist: specialist in diseases of the BRAIN and nervous system such as EPILEPSY.

– Neurosurgeon: specialist in BRAIN and spinal cord surgery.

– Obstetrician: specialist in caring for pregnant women and delivering babies.

– Oncologist: specialist in CANCER.

– Pediatrician: specialist in children's disease; may also have a sub-specialty, for example pediatric cardiology.

– Opthalmologist: eye surgeon; eye doctor.

– Orthopedist: specialist in bone and joint surgery.

– Otolaryngologist: ear, nose and throat surgeon.

– Plastic surgeon: specialist in cosmetic surgery.

– Psychiatrist: specialist in mental disorders.

– Radiologist: specialist in X-rays, CAT SCANS, ULTRASOUNDS and other imaging procedures.

– Rheumatologist: specialist in ARTHRITIS and other rheumatic diseases.

– Urologist: specialist in the medical and surgical treatment of kidney, urinary tract and male reproductive organ diseases.

MENARCHE
See *PUBERTY*.

MENINGITIS
Infection of the membranes covering the brain and spinal cord (meninges) by BACTERIA or VIRUSES.

▇ SYMPTOMS The infection can be preceded by a SORE THROAT. FEVER, HEADACHE and VOMITING and usually evolves within hours. Neck stiffness, CONVULSIONS, PARALYSIS and COMA may follow. Most cases of bacterial meningitis occur in children under age two but it can occur at any age.

▇ ACTION Get medical advice if you are worried about meningitis; it is a medical emergency and will require prompt treatment. The signs of meningitis are not always obvious at first, so if a sick child is not improving with treatment for any of the symptoms above, meningitis should be considered. If in doubt, take the child to the hospital emergency room.

▇ CAUSES Infection usually reaches the meninges through the blood, but bacteria can spread directly to the meninges from the sinuses or the ears. Bacterial meningitis may also arise as a complication of skull FRACTURE or of SPINA BIFIDA.

▇ INVESTIGATIONS LUMBAR PUNCTURE and BLOOD TESTS.

▇ TREATMENT Bacterial meningitis is treated with ANTIBIOTICS, mostly given intravenously or by intramuscular injection for one or two weeks depending on the bacteria involved and the severity of the infection. Some children may need INTENSIVE CARE support if the illness is severe. Fluids may be given intravenously and it may be necessary to monitor pulse rate, blood pressure and temperature frequently. In severe cases, assisted ventilation and monitoring of the pressure inside the head may be necessary. There is no specific treatment for viral meningitis, which is usually a milder illness than the bacterial type. IMMUNIZATION is available against *Hemophilus influenzae* b bacteria, the most common cause of bacterial meningitis in childhood. Tracing and treating contacts of some types of bacterial meningitis is important.

Bacterial meningitis may be complicated by pneumonia or septic ARTHRITIS.

▇ OUTLOOK Nearly all children suffering from viral meningitis make a complete recovery, but some with bacterial meningitis die or survive with disabilities such as hearing impairment, EPILEPSY, HYDROCEPHALUS or CEREBRAL PALSY. Before antibiotics were available, bacterial meningitis was almost always fatal. Today, less than one in 20 children with meningitis die. Research is going on to develop vaccines to prevent the other common types of bacterial meningitis. The success of the *Hemophilus influenzae* b conjugate vaccine suggests that this may be possible.

MENSTRUAL PROBLEMS
A girl starts to menstruate usually about two years after the growth spurt that marks the onset of PUBERTY. But this is variable.

It is important that girls (and boys) understand about menstruation. Girls should not be worried or embarrassed when they begin to have periods, or feel inadequate that their friends have started when they have not.

■ PROBLEMS If periods begin before the age of ten, or have not started by 16, your daughter should see your doctor to determine if there is a problem (see also *PUBERTY –* precocious and delayed).

The first few periods are often irregular both in timing and flow. This is normal and happens because these first cycles are not related to the production of an ovum (egg) by the ovary (ovulation): thus, although menstruating, the girl may not yet be fertile.

Many girls suffer some pain and cramping with their periods. The first few cycles may not be painful, but the problem can develop later and is difficult to pinpoint because the pain is often spasmodic. It may be associated with nausea.

It is thought that period pains may be due to hormonal imbalance, leading to high levels of a group of chemicals synthesized by the developing uterine lining. These chemicals, known as prostaglandins, are responsible for uterine contractions during labor. This may explain why period pains are cramp-like; and prostaglandins may also be responsible for contraction of the muscle of the intestine, with attendant nausea.

■ SIMPLE REMEDIES Heat applied to the lower abdomen from a heating pad, massage and simple painkillers (particularly aspirin and ibuprofen, which both inhibit prostaglandin action) are often helpful.

■ MEDICAL TREATMENT If the pain persists despite simple remedies, your daughter should get medical advice. Your doctor may prescribe further painkillers, or, occasionally, a low-dose contraceptive pill or progesterone-only pill to correct the hormonal imbalance.

Pre-menstrual tension is uncommon in adolescent girls. If your daughter suffers from irritability, DEPRESSION, HEADACHES, CONSTIPATION and a bloated feeling due to water retention, two to 12 days before each period begins, discuss it with your doctor.

■ ALTERNATIVE TREATMENTS Rest, reducing salt intake, and taking vitamin B6 may be helpful.

MENTAL HANDICAP

The social consequence of mental retardation. Children whose general intelligence lies within the lowest 3 percent in the population are considered to have some degree of mental retardation. The definitions used to classify 'mild', 'moderate' and 'severe' retardation are to some degree arbitrary and reflect society's growing ability to cope with the problem.

■ CAUSES A substantial proportion of 'mildly retarded' children go undetected. 'Moderately retarded' children and adults are simply identified as the least able of the population that functions independently within society. 'Severely retarded' persons are not capable of functioning independently. There may be no identifiable cause of their problem. However, more than two-thirds of the severely retarded children have identifiable disorders such as CHROMOSOMAL abnormalities. Other causes include malformation syndromes, INHERITED DISORDERS, INFECTION or damage by RUBELLA, ALCOHOL or other agents during the pregnancy, very severe BIRTH ASPHYXIA or serious illness or injury in childhood.

■ SYMPTOMS Mental handicap may be suspected from birth if a specific condition such as Down syndrome or MICROCEPHALY is present. Usually, delayed MOTOR DEVELOPMENT and, especially, LANGUAGE delay raise suspicions. Severe EPILEPSY in early childhood is likely to be associated with mental handicap, and a third of children with CEREBRAL PALSY turn out to be mentally retarded. Conversely, one in three severely mentally retarded children has epilepsy, and one in five has cerebral palsy. Psychiatric disorders such as ANXIETY, DEPRESSION and AUTISM are relatively common in retarded children, but may be difficult to manage because of the disordered or very limited communication abilities of these children, and because of the lack of appropriate facilities for assessment and treatment. Two-thirds of severely retarded children have a degree of visual impairment and one in six has an appreciable hearing loss.

■ ACTION If mental retardation is suspected, the child should be referred to a child development clinic the staff of which usually includes pediatric developmental specialists, pediatric neurologists and geneticists as well as social workers, nurses and educational psychologists.

■ INVESTIGATIONS may include chromosome tests; BLOOD and URINE TESTS for intra-uterine infection or biochemical problems, and EEG RECORDING. A CAT SCAN of the brain does not usually reveal a specific diagnosis, except when detailed physical examination suggests a particular disorder. Developmental,

psychological and educational testing may be done to assess the seriousness of the deficit and the degree of intellectual development that is possible.

■ TREATMENT For the very severely and multiply disabled retarded child with poorly controlled seizures, long-term institutional care may be required. This is difficult to find since such institutions are limited and often expensive and located at a distance from the family. Home care, with additional nursing and physiotherapy support may offer an affordable, more stimulating and loving environment. Some centers have respite care programs to offer parents a short-term break or 'holiday' from caring for their severely disabled child. Your doctor may be a good source of information about community support facilities.

Schooling for the mentally handicapped child: There have been considerable improvements in the schooling offered to mentally retarded children, some of whom were considered uneducable until the early 1970s. Recently, through federal legislation, there have been moves made to integrate retarded and disabled children into public school programs. Many pupils placed in special schools for the mentally retarded may benefit from the wider curriculum and range of social stimulation present in public school systems, provided special teachers are available.

GENETIC COUNSELLING is important for families. The recurrence risk of mental retardation is 10 percent unless a specific non-inheritable cause is found.

Treatment of visual or hearing problems, or epilepsy may lead to improvement. Physiotherapy can help motor development; speech therapy is useful for communication problems, and clinical psychologists and child psychiatrists may be able to help in the management of BEHAVIORAL or psychiatric disorders and, indeed, for distress suffered by their families.

Educational and health services for children with mental handicap are much better developed than those for adults. Access to adult sheltered workshops and supervised group homes is often limited. Alternatives such as adult institutional care is expensive, less stimulating and often hard to find. Community support for appropriate programs is growing but money to fund these efforts is often lacking. The issue of adult placement is often very stressful for families.

National societies concerned with the mentally handicapped publish useful literature and may offer practical support.

■ OUTLOOK Most mentally retarded children develop with time and teaching at their own rate, but often reach a plateau at puberty. Autistic children with mental retardation show particularly slow progress, whereas some children with language problems continue to improve into adult life. A few with severe seizure disorders deteriorate in adolescence despite all treatment.

MENTAL RETARDATION

See *MENTAL HANDICAP* and *LEARNING DISORDERS*.

MESENTERIC ADENITIS

Swelling of the lymph nodes in the abdomen, in response to INFECTION. Mesenteric adenitis may result from a local abdominal infection, or from a general VIRAL infection. It is thought

to be a cause of stomach ache in childhood. However, this is rarely certain as there is often no visible, external sign of the internal inflamed lymph nodes.

■ SYMPTOMS The features of this condition are vague. The stomach ache is mild or moderate, and there may be a slight FEVER. The child can move around without much discomfort, and does not look unduly ill. There are no specific diagnostic tests, but the white blood cell count may be increased as in any infection.

■ ACTION The child may gain some comfort from fluids, acetamenophen and bed rest. But if the pain persists, or the child cannot move about easily, or he looks sick, you should contact your doctor to be sure he does not have APPENDICITIS.

■ OUTLOOK Mesenteric adenitis is a vague condition that may recur. Always get medical advice, however, if you suspect that appendicitis may be the problem.

MICROCEPHALY

A child with an abnormally small head (and brain). This may be a ressessive INHERITED DISORDER; a non-genetically determined CONGENITAL ABNORMALITY (caused, for example, by infection of the fetus with *rubella*) or acquired after birth as, for instance, following profound BRAIN DAMAGE from trauma or cardiac arrest. Most microcephalic children are MENTALLY HANDICAPPED.

MIDDLE EAR INFECTION (*OTITIS MEDIA*)

An INFECTION of the middle ear by BACTERIA or VIRUSES that invade the middle ear from the nose and throat through the Eustachian tube. Commonest in young children, particularly those under five years. Some children seem especially vulnerable, including those with a CLEFT PALATE, Native Americans and possibly some children with allergies.

■ SYMPTOMS EARACHE, DEAFNESS; also more general symptoms (especially in infants) such as FEVER. If the eardrum perforates, a discharge of green or yellow mucus may be seen coming from the ear.

■ ACTION Always get medical advice if you suspect your child has an ear infection. See also *EARACHE.*

■ TREATMENT If the appearance of the eardrum suggests middle ear infection, your doctor will prescribe a seven to ten day course of ANTIBIOTICS. The course should be completed even if your child feels better in a day or two. Acetamenophen may help to relieve the pain in the first day or two. The doctor should check your child's ears at the end of the course of treatment to ensure that they have returned to normal.

Tonsillectomy does not decrease the frequency of middle ear infections.

■ OUTLOOK For infants and younger children, there is a slight risk of GLUE EAR with hearing impairment after an ear infection. If there is any doubt, his hearing should be checked one or two months afterwards. Children may have repeated bouts of middle ear infection.

MIGRAINE IN CHILDHOOD

Migraine is severe, recurring headaches, usually affecting only one side of the head at a time, often preceded by visual disturbances or aura (typically flashing lights), and accompanied by NAUSEA and VOMITING. The child may look pale and complain of nausea and STOMACH-ACHE. The aura is thought to be due to abnormal constriction of intracranial arteries, the headache to dilation of scalp blood vessels. Migraine often runs in families, and is commoner in older children.

■ CAUSES Unknown. Individuals may identify specific triggers, including stress and some foods (such as chocolate and cheese).

■ INVESTIGATIONS There is no specific test for migraine, and all children complaining of headache do *not* have migraine. Severe, recurrent or persistent headache in a child requires medical assessment and advice. It is important not to overlook migraine (some episodes may prove a nuisance for the child at school). Conversely it is important not to call every headache migraine, since headache complaints may be an appeal for attention or the sign of serious brain disease.

■ TREATMENT Give acetamenophen as soon as possible. Taking an analgesic (painkiller) early may prevent a full-blown attack in some children. During an attack the stomach may empty more slowly than usual: for this reason some doctors recommend metoclopramide, which speeds stomach emptying, to enhance painkiller effectiveness.

If the migraines are very severe and/or frequent, the doctor may prescribe vasoconstrictors such as ergotamine and caffeine. If taken at the very onset of symptoms, they may abort an attack. Due to their side-effects, these drugs are usually only used in older children and in adolescents.

■ SELF-HELP Encourage the child to lie down in a darkened room.

■ OUTLOOK Many children grow out of migraine.

MINIMAL BRAIN DAMAGE (MBD)

It is common for some developmental or behavioral difficulties in children to be ascribed to 'MBD' without evidence of actual brain damage. However, children who have suffered BIRTH ASPHYXIA and subsequently display neurological abnormalities, are more likely to have impaired language, co-ordination and attention in later years. Similarly, children who have suffered major HEAD INJURIES are likely to show memory difficulties, irritability and impulsiveness. It cannot be inferred, conversely, that children who sleep badly, make a slow start at school or have tantrums, have suffered brain damage.

Children with a relative language delay or disorder are better described as having a specific developmental language problem than having MBD. Children who are verbally fluent but immature, or incompetent at motor or perceptual-motor activities, are best described as having a specific MOTOR DEVELOPMENT problem – see CLUMSINESS. See also ASPERGER SYNDROME.

MOLES (NEVI)

All pigmented spots and patches are called moles. Most are harmless but they can be unsightly.

■ INCIDENCE 95 percent of people have some sort of pigmented mole.

■ TYPES OF MOLE Apart from the commonly occuring small, flat, brown moles, there are larger moles which may be covered with hair ('giant hairy nevi'). These are usually found on the body. 'Café-au-lait' spots, pale brown patches are found in association with neurofibromatosis, a rare condition. Malignant melanoma, a form of skin cancer, is very rare in children, but is capable of developing in any large pigmented mole.

■ ACTION Nearly all moles are harmless, but if you are worried about one get medical advice. If any mole is seen to be enlarging, bleeding, itching, or changing its appearance in any other way, then don't put off getting medical advice.

■ TREATMENT Large moles can be removed surgically: your doctor will advise about this. Occasionally a mole becomes infected, usually through being scratched. Simple ANTIBIOTIC treatment is the remedy. Itchy moles are not true moles but histiocytomas, benign, dark spots of unknown cause. No treatment is needed for most moles, but occasionally they are removed surgically if there is suspicion about their nature or the patient wants this for cosmetic reasons.

MONILIA
See CANDIDIASIS.

MORO REFLEX

An automatic response by a new-born baby to a sudden noise or movement. The baby throws out his arms and legs, and then brings them back together with slight shaking movements. The reflex usually disappears by the age of three months. Eliciting the reflex may distress the baby and cause him to cry out and be unsettled. The Moro reflex is used by doctors to assess neurological development.

MOTION SICKNESS

Much worse in some families than in others, and some cars provoke it more than others. Children often start to suffer from travel sickness around five or six years of age, and stop in their teens. Prevention is effective, using medications such as dimenhydrinate or antihistamines (sold over the counter: note dosage instructions for children carefully). Most antihistamines cause drowsiness, but children vary in their susceptibility to this.

■ SELF-HELP Avoid reading or close work while travelling. In public vehicles, sit near the front preferably with some fresh air and free from cigarette smoke. Don't give a child heavy or fatty meals before or during a journey. Make sure the child faces forward, and looks out of the window if in a car or train. For air travel, giving dimenydrinate a half hour before take-off may prevent air sickness.

MOTOR DEVELOPMENT

Most children follow a developmental sequence of sitting (five to 12 months), crawling (six to 14 months) and walking (nine to 19 months). This is generally regarded as normal motor development.

About one child in 20 does not crawl, but instead creeps on his tummy, rolls over and over or shuffles on his bottom. Such children may sit and walk a little later than average, but eventually have no motor or performance difficulties. Some children stand and walk as their first means of mobility.

Many specific patterns of motor development tend to run in families. Boys tend to be a little slower in their motor development than girls.

MOUTH ULCERS

Common at any age, painful, small, white, round ulcers may occur on the tongue, gums or anywhere in the mouth, and can cause fretfulness and real difficulty in eating. They are probably caused by a VIRUS, and may be associated with illnesses, or simply be associated with fatigue or psychological stress.

■ ACTION Medicated candies or gels used for teething in babies can be helpful, because of their local anesthetic content. Acid foods such as orange juice may sting. Bland foods may be better tolerated. Get medical advice if they last longer than a week or two, or recur frequently.

MULTIPLE PREGNANCY

A pregnancy with more than one baby. It is suspected if the womb seems large, or if more than one heartbeat is heard. It can be confirmed by ULTRASOUND SCAN.

Twins occur in about one in every 80 births. They may be produced from either one fertilized egg constituting monozygotic or identical twins; or from two separate fertilized eggs, forming dizygotic or non-identical twins. The latter is more likely when there is a family history of twins, or if the mother has taken a fertility drug.

Triplets occur naturally in about one in 900 pregnancies. However, they are becoming more common as a result of the use of fertility drugs and test-tube (*in vitro*) fertilization.

■ PRENATAL CARE of women with twins or triplets requires careful management, because complications such as ANEMIA and high BLOOD PRESSURE occur more frequently than in single pregnancies. In general, the mother will gain more weight and need more rest. Additionally, the individual babies may have problems of their own.

For example, one baby may not receive as good a blood supply from the placenta as the other, and may grow more slowly than his twin. The premature onset of labor is more common in multiple pregnancies: the average length of pregnancy for twins is 35 weeks.

■ LABOR AND DELIVERY In 70 percent of twin pregnancies, the first twin lies head down and is born normally. The doctor may then need to rupture the sac around the second twin to facilitate his delivery. The birth of the second twin usually follows ten to 15 minutes after the first birth. If the first twin lies head up in the womb, or there are other complications, delivery is likely to be by CESARIAN SECTION. Triplets are more frequently delivered by Cesarian section.

■ BREAST FEEDING more than one baby is difficult but can be successful. The mother must consume sufficient calories and fluids daily: this cannot be prescribed precisely other than to encourage the mother to eat and drink to her fill. It may be possible to breastfeed the babies together or separately, or to use a bottle alternating with breast feedings. The various options are best discussed with your doctor or pediatrician.

■ TWIN CLUBS have sprung up in many places, offering a valuable self-support group (equipment, know-how, friendship and gossip) for parents with multiple births. There is now a national organization for parents with twins.

MUMPS

A VIRAL INFECTION, spread by exhaled droplets. The sufferer is infectious during the week before he develops symptoms; and he remains infectious for about a week after onset. The INCUBATION PERIOD is 14-21 days. Mumps is now an uncommon infection in the United States because of the high rate of mumps IMMUNIZATION.

■ SYMPTOMS The illness begins with FEVER, feeling generally sick,

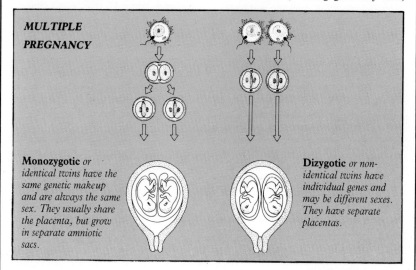

MULTIPLE PREGNANCY

Monozygotic *or identical twins have the same genetic makeup and are always the same sex. They usually share the placenta, but grow in separate amniotic sacs.*

Dizygotic *or non-identical twins have individual genes and may be different sexes. They have separate placentas.*

MUMPS

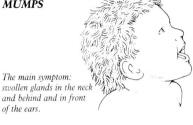

The main symptom: swollen glands in the neck and behind and in front of the ears.

HEADACHE and loss of APPETITE. Swelling of the salivary glands below and in front of the ear (parotid glands) and less commonly under the jaw (submanolibular glands) begins a day or two later and lasts for about a week. Eating is painful because it causes movement and stimulation of the inflamed glands. The cardinal sign of mumps is the disappearance of the 'angle of the jaw' because of firm swelling beneath the ear. This is *not* always seen; about one third of infections fail to produce an apparent swelling.

VOMITING and ABDOMINAL PAIN sometimes occur.

▨ ACTION The pain and fever can be treated with an analgesic, typically acetamenophen.

A bland, fluid diet is often necessary until the pain subsides. Certain foods and liquids, particularly those that are sour, stimulate secretion of saliva, and these should be avoided as they can cause intense pain.

The mouth should be kept clean with a regular mouthwash.

Complications include ENCE-PHALITIS, infection of the testes (orchitis) in boys and DEAFNESS. If symptoms such as drowsiness, pain in the testes in boys or any unexpected symptoms appear, get medical advice.

Keep the child out from school until the swelling has subsided (usually about seven days from the beginning of the illness).

IMMUNIZATION is available against mumps in combination with MEASLES and RUBELLA, and is given at about 15 months of age.

▨ OUTLOOK Mumps occasionally causes serious complications such as MENINGITIS or deafness. Inflammation of the testes can sometimes cause sterility, but this is very rare. Prevention is better than taking the risk. The mumps vaccine is effective and does not produce significant side-effects.

MUSCULAR DYSTROPHY

Progressive weakness due to degeneration of muscles. There are different types, all inherited. Duchenne and Becker's dystrophies are inherited on a recessive GENE at a known site on the X chromosome so only boys are affected, though girls can be carriers of the disease.

In limb-girdle dystrophy, a dominant gene is usually involved and one of the parents is affected.

The defect directly causing the condition is thought to be in the voluntary muscle cell membrane where the protein (dystrophin) is deficient or abnormal.

▨ SYMPTOMS The child may be late in walking and shows progressive weakness over a number of years. Muscles are slowly replaced by fibrous tissue and fat which may make them look bulky. Speech, bowel and bladder control are affected later. A quarter of affected boys are unable to walk by 18 months of age, delayed LANGUAGE DEVELOPMENT is common, ability to run, jump, rise from the floor or climb stairs is very limited at any stage of development.

▨ TREATMENT There is no cure, but mechanical aids and appliances, suitable seating, physiotherapy, hydrotherapy and suitable education contribute considerably to making it possible to manage the child at home. GENETIC COUNSELLING is required to make parents aware of the risks of the disease occurring in their future children.

National muscular dystrophy associations and local parent groups provide literature and support to the parents.

■ OUTLOOK The most common muscular dystrophy (Duchenne) progressively leads to loss of ability to walk at ten to 12 years of age, and death from respiratory failure or INFECTION in late adolescence or early adulthood.

The milder form tends to give slower deterioration and survival until middle age.

MYOCARDITIS

A rare but dangerous disease in which there is inflammation of the heart muscles, usually caused by a viral INFECTION. See *HEART-DISEASE*. The symptoms occur suddenly, and begin with acute breathlessness and general illness: there are signs of HEART FAILURE. Most children recover completely, although treatment is often continued for a number of years. Occasionally the damage to the heart muscle is permanent and long-term care by a heart specialist is required.

MYOPIA

See *SHORTSIGHTEDNESS*.

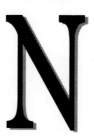

NAIL BITING

A tension habit common in children (and some adults). The child is often unaware that he is doing it. The habit is generally harmless, but some adults may find it unattractive. Measures aimed at stopping the habit – prompting the child to stop when you see him biting, applying unpleasant-tasting liquids to his nails or giving rewards for unbitten nails – usually fail unless the child himself wishes to stop.

NAUSEA

The inclination to vomit, often accompanied by churning of the stomach, sweating, pallor, excessive salivation and dizziness. Most commonly associated with GASTROENTERITIS or MOTION SICKNESS; can accompany many illnesses, for example EAR INFECTIONS.

■ ACTION Nausea as such is difficult to treat. Motion sickness is usually preventable with appropriate medication taken before travelling. Otherwise, don't give the child solid food and give him sips of clear fluids or ice cubes to suck.

NEBULIZING MASK

A device frequently used in the treatment of ASTHMA that transforms liquid medications into a fine mist, which is then breathed in through a mask. In this way, drugs such as bronchodilators can be directed to their site of action in the airways of the lung.

■ USES To treat severe attacks of asthma. This may take place in the hospital, or in the doctor's office, or occasionally at home (if the family have had full instructions on the use of the nebulizer). If the treatment fails to relieve the asthma within a specified period, then a potentially serious situation may be developing. Hence parents using nebulizers at home need to be carefully instructed when to seek medical consultation.

Nebulizers are also used to give regular doses at home of drugs that prevent asthma, such as sodium cromoglycate or beclomethasone, if the child is too young to use other sorts of inhalers effectively.

NECROTIZING ENTEROCOLITIS

A serious condition of new-born and specially of premature babies, in which there is a disintegration, or necrosis, of the intestinal wall. Depending on the severity of the episode, it may carry a variable risk of permanent damage to the bowel, and occasionally have fatal consequences.

■ CAUSE is not understood. It seems to occur when there has been both BACTERIAL INFECTION and poor blood supply to the baby's intestine

(as may occur as a complication of BIRTH ASPHYXIA or RESPIRATORY DISTRESS SYNDROME). The baby becomes very ill, his abdomen swells and feeding is no longer tolerated. He may pass blood in his stools.

■ TREATMENT consists of ANTIBIOTICS and resting the intestine; that is, giving the baby no food by mouth until the bowel heals. A small number of babies require surgery to remove affected segments of the bowel.

NEPHRITIS

A general term referring to inflammation or swelling of the glomeruli in the kidneys. A glomerulus is the loop of capillaries (or fine blood vessels) that functions as a cup-like filtration system in the kidney. In these microscopic structures water and waste products pass out of the blood to enter a system of fine tubes, in which some water and filtered chemicals are selectively reabsorbed. The term nephritis is often used as an abbreviation for the more specific disorder of glomerulonephritis. It tends to affect children of school age.

■ CAUSES Nephritis usually follows two to three weeks after a bacterial skin or throat INFECTION. The ANTIBODIES produced by the body to the BACTERIA cross-react with and attack the glomeruli causing them to swell.

■ SYMPTOMS The most striking feature in most cases is the passage of bloodstained or 'smokey' urine. This may be accompanied by vague lassitude or headache. Damage to the glomeruli prevents the normal filtering process of the kidney. Salt and water are retained by the body and proteins are lost through the urine, causing edema, most commonly seen as swelling around the eyes and of the feet, and high BLOOD PRESSURE.

■ ACTION The development of red or smokey urine or EDEMA must be reported to a doctor without delay.

■ TESTS A URINE TEST will confirm the presence of blood and protein. BLOOD TESTS may detect the antibodies that cause the nephritis. More important, they will show how the kidney is functioning.

■ TREATMENT Initial assessment usually requires admission to the hospital. The severity of nephritis is highly variable – some cases need no treatment, others need medicines to control the raised blood pressure. The amount of fluid your child drinks may need to be carefully balanced against the amount of urine he passes. In the most severe cases, the kidneys may temporarily stop functioning. Some form of dialysis (clearing the body of the waste products usually excreted in the urine) will then be required.

■ OUTLOOK Normally the kidneys recover spontaneously and completely. There may be blood in the urine for many weeks; this is not in itself a sign that the nephritis is worsening. Uncommonly the kidneys do not fully recover but progress to chronic RENAL FAILURE over a matter of years. Should this happen the child should be cared for by a pediatric nephrologist, and plans will be made for long-term dialysis and immunotherapy and, in some cases, kidney transplantation.

NEPHROBLASTOMA
See *WILM TUMOR*.

NEPHROTIC SYNDROME
The condition arises when the kidneys allow blood proteins to escape into the urine. The microscopic filtering units of the kidney (glomeruli) are largely responsible for excreting waste products from the blood and stabilizing the blood chemistry. The cause of nephrotic syndrome is unknown.

■ SYMPTOMS The main symptom is EDEMA or swelling or puffiness particularly of the face, and around the eyes and ankles. The child usually does not feel particularly sick. He may be somewhat drowsy (lethargic).

■ ACTION If your child develops edema you should get medical advice. Your doctor will do a URINE TEST for protein if he or she suspects nephrotic syndrome.

■ TREATMENT is with steroids. The swelling usually remains unchanged for the first week or two, but usually by six weeks there is a decrease in the protein loss in the urine, an increase in the volume of urine passed, and a steady dissolution of the swelling.

■ OUTLOOK Nephrotic syndrome may recur, but most children eventually grow out of it. A small minority of children continue to need long-term care, because of the ultimate risk of kidney failure.

NEW-BORN SCREENING TESTS
Blood samples for a variety of neonatal screening tests, including tests for neonatal HYPOTHYROIDISM and phenylketonuria, are performed on every baby around the third day after birth. Collection of a sample of blood is done by pricking the heel and allowing the blood to drip onto a specially prepared

card made of a heavy filter paper. In some states the screening test also checks for CYSTIC FIBROSIS. If you and your baby leave the hospital early, arrangements must be made to have this test done at your doctor's office, outpatient clinic or at home, when the baby is six or seven days old.

NICOTINE
See *SMOKING*.

NIGHT TERRORS
The sleeping child suddenly appears to be in a state of intense fear. Unlike NIGHTMARES, he does not wake up, and has no recollection of the event afterwards. Witnessing a child's terror can distress parents, but there is no need to wake him or discuss the event with him. They are not a cause for serious concern, and the child grows out of the problem by the early school years.

NIGHTMARES
Bad dreams that are sufficiently frightening to wake a child: nightmares can be recalled immediately. They are essentially no different from the bad dreams of adulthood. They are sometimes, but not always, related to a recent emotional upset. They are a common reason for night-waking in older children. Many children go through periods of frequent nightmares that then stop for a time. If your child wakes from a nightmare, calmly reassure him and help him to settle back to sleep, talking about something that will distract him from the fear. There is no need to discuss the content of the nightmare.

NITS
See *LICE*.

NOISY BREATHING
See *STRIDOR, ASTHMA, CROUP*.

'NORMAL' DEVELOPMENT
The development of 97 percent of children in growth, co-ordination, language and social behavior is considered to be 'normal'. The remaining 3 percent, considered to show FAILURE TO THRIVE or DEVELOPMENTAL DELAY, may require investigation or treatment, typically for motor, language, visual or hearing impairment. In many developed countries, babies and children under five years of age are checked for normal development as a part of well-child visits to their doctor or health center. Health professionals performing these checks-ups are trained to take into account family and other special circumstances, and to avoid causing parents unnecessary anxiety when a child falls below so-called 'normal' in some aspect of the testing process.

■ SIGNS OF ABNORMAL DEVELOPMENT Failure to: respond to sounds; to 'fix' the eyes on objects or to visually follow the movements of others during early infancy; to walk by 18 months; to use three-word phrases appropriately by the age of three years. All these require investigation.

Often enough, though, a child shows delayed development in one of these respects as part of an inherited pattern. For example, the baby who does not crawl, but moves from place to place by inching along on his belly or bottom or by purposeful rolling over and over, may well be late to walk, but usually turns out to be 'normal', especially if his father or mother followed the same pattern.

■ ACTION If your child shows one or

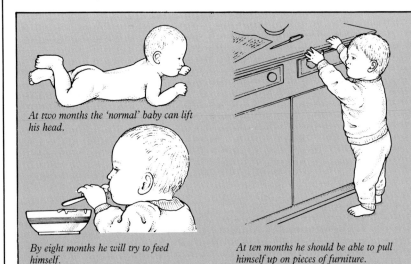

At two months the 'normal' baby can lift his head.

By eight months he will try to feed himself.

At ten months he should be able to pull himself up on pieces of furniture.

more of the signs described above, don't be alarmed, but get medical advice in any case. Be sure that your baby's vision and hearing are checked early in infancy and frequently thereafter, particularly if you think he may have trouble hearing or seeing.

■ TREATMENT   Physiotherapy, speech therapy or special teaching techniques can help to accelerate development.

■ SELF-HELP Spend time playing with your child. An excellent book, *Play With A Purpose* by Dorothy Einon (Pantheon, 1985), provides endless ideas for constructive activities and games. Variety of experience, sharing your child's interests, ensuring an adequate diet and conversation, within the limit of your child's understanding, all help. Children learn most from their parents' involvement and interest in them.

■ OUTLOOK depends on the cause

of the delay, if any. It may be possible to remedy visual and hearing defects. Motor (physical mobility) delay, language delay and SPEECH DISORDERS may well resolve if due to a lag in maturation or a family tendency. But see also *MOTOR DEVELOPMENT, SPEECH DISORDERS, DEVELOPMENTAL DELAY, MENTAL HANDICAP, CEREBRAL PALSY, LEARNING DISORDERS.*

NOSE, FOREIGN BODY IN
Children of two to three years of age may put a wide variety of objects into their nostrils, including beads, small toys, paper, and cloth. These may be less easily noticed than foreign bodies in the ears, because the space inside the nose is much larger.

■ SYMPTOMS The usual sign is a discharge from the nostril (from that side of the nose containing the object), which may become green, brown or foul smelling.

■ ACTION The object needs to be re-

NORMAL DEVELOPMENT

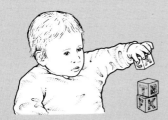

By twelve months he will be building towers of bricks.

moved by a doctor. In most cases the object can be simply removed with special tweezers. Rarely, in difficult cases, the child may be referred to an ear, nose and throat specialist.

NOSEBLEED

A frightening, but seldom serious problem.

■ CAUSES The bleeding usually comes from a small vein just inside the nostril, on the inner wall of the nose. Such veins can be broken by direct injury, typically falls or playground fights, or indirectly by a COMMON COLD. Generalized VIRAL infections, such as MEASLES, and any high temperature may also set off a nosebleed. Some children have exceptionally fragile veins in the nose and bleed without any obvious cause. The low humidity found in homes with hot air heating systems can increase the chance of a nosebleed. Very rare causes are those diseases that affect blood clotting, such as HEMOPHILIA or LEUKEMIA.

■ ACTION Almost all nosebleeds can be stopped by simply squeezing the child's nose between the thumb and finger, just below the bony part. Pressure should be just enough to stop the bleeding and keep the nose completely still, and should be continued for ten minutes, then released, and repeated if necessary. It helps if the child's head is held forward, so that the blood flow can be seen. If tilted back, blood runs down the child's throat, is swallowed, and may later cause vomiting and unnecessary distress. After the bleeding has stopped, the child should rest quietly, and avoid blowing his nose or sniffing.

There is no need to apply ice or to put any sort of plug into the child's nose.

■ GET MEDICAL ADVICE if the bleeding has not stopped after gentle pressure for 20 minutes, or if nosebleeds are recurring frequently.

■ TREATMENT Recurrent nosebleeds can be treated simply by sealing off (cauterizing) the vein, using either a silver nitrate stick, or an electrical form of cautery. This is usually done in a hospital clinic, but some doctors will do this in their office. If a nosebleed cannot be controlled with cauterization, your doctor may have to pack the side of the nose (nostril) that is bleeding with Vaseline gauze and leave this in place for a few days until healing occurs.

■ TESTS If, besides nosebleeds, there are other signs that the child could have a blood disorder, your doctor will arrange for BLOOD TESTS – but serious disorders accompanying nosebleeds are exceedingly rare.

■ OUTLOOK The amount of blood

lost is unimportant, although it may seem to be copious. Children who are likely to have nosebleeds can be taught how to deal with them, using the method described above.

NUTRITION

See also APPETITE, WEANING, VITA-MINS. The ideal diet for a child contains adequate protein for growth and repair of body tissues, plus sufficient carbohydrates and fats to provide energy for daily activities. Adequate quantities of all essential classes of foods should be provided to avoid specific nutritional deficiencies. There should be plenty of fiber and a liberal intake of fluids. A balanced diet in childhood promotes growth, the development of strong teeth, the prevention of obesity and the promotion of good eating habits and health as an adult.

In the first two years of life, most of a child's nutritional requirements are provided by milk, which is a well-balanced food containing carbohydrate, proteins and fats. In the first six months, this is best provided in the form of the baby's own mother's milk or infant formula. Thereafter, a transition is made to baby foods, and then to the normal household diet with homogenized or cow's milk as an important component. Skim milk is *not* recommended for young children.

Healthy nutrition is easier to define than to implement. The child's diet will reflect the household traditions and habits, later to be influenced by school peer pressures and media advertizing.

If you have questions or concerns about your child's diet or state of nutrition, speak to your doctor. He or she may feel that a discussion with a dietician would be helpful. Excellent books on healthy nutrition for children are available at many libraries and bookstores.

OBESITY

Obesity can be defined as excess weight in relation to height compared to the average child of the same age and height. There is no exact line between normal weight and obesity. Practially, the diagnosis is made by the appearance of the child rather than an arbitrary value of excess weight. (If the child thinks he is overweight but clearly is not, see ANOREXIA NERVOSA.)

■ CAUSES Obesity results from eating more than is necessary for that individual's needs; it is, however, hardly ever due to 'glandular problems' such as Cushing's disease – see ADRENAL DISORDERS. There may be a long-standing (sometimes family) habit of eating more food than is necessary for normal growth and activity.

▓ OUTCOME While severe childhood obesity may cause medical problems, mild obesity may not have serious consequences for future health. However, fat children may be teased and unpopular at school, less likely to be good at sport and more likely to be fat as adults. It is therefore worthwhile trying to get the child's weight back towards normal for both present and future well-being. Obesity carries definite health risks for adults including DIABETES, heart, chest and joint complaints.

▓ AVOIDING OBESITY While there is some evidence that fat babies grow to be fat children, a healthy, hungry baby who is plump should not be placed on a diet. However, as the baby becomes a toddler and pre-school child, if the propensity to fatness persists, you should try to instill good eating habits based upon three balanced meals per day and only small nutritious snacks. Eating high-calorie junk food such as French fried potatoes and soft drinks should be limited.

▓ ACTION 1 Mildly overweight, children often don't need to lose weight; it is enough to hold their weight steady while they grow. Concentrate on small changes in the diet to reduce calories and fat (perhaps replacing high-calorie snacks with fruit, but not cutting them out altogether), rather than trying to make drastic changes that will be hard to maintain. 2 A new pattern of exercise may help the child feel healthy and fit. However, this is only likely to succeed if it is fun, and supported by friends or family. Exercise as a prescription will fail. 3 If your child is definitely obese, get medical advice, and ask to be referred to a dietician. Don't leave this step until it is too late: once a pattern of fatness is well established, it is very difficult to reverse. And if it is a family feature, then it is a family responsibility to change eating habits.

OBSESSIONS

Many children between the ages of about six and nine years go through a phase of superstitious rituals, such as not stepping on pavement cracks, or dressing in a special way. These seem to help a child feel safe from bad luck in a world that is progressively seen as a dangerous place. These routines can be particularly irritating to parents in a hurry, but are otherwise usually without significance. Some older children become preoccupied in a similar way when anxious or under stress, for example during examinations. As the stress recedes, normal interests take the place of the obsession.

Usually the parents' best strategy is to ignore the obsession: it will fade as the child grows and becomes more confident. Distracting the child's attention or offering incentives may sometimes help.

▓ GET MEDICAL ADVICE 1 if an obsession seems to be dominating your child's life and seriously restricting his activities, 2 if he seems absolutely compelled to perform the ritual regardless of the situation and becomes distressed if prevented from doing so, or 3 if family life is being generally affected. Your doctor may refer you to a child psychiatrist. For most children, a few sessions discussing the problem can be helpful. Rarely, more intensive and longer treatment is required. See *AUTISTIC CHILD, FEARS.*

OPERATIONS
See *HOSPITAL, CHILD IN, ANESTHETICS.*

ORBITAL CELLULITIS
Occasionally CELLULITIS may involve the eyelids and the tissues surrounding the eye in its socket (orbit).

■ CAUSES BACTERIA.

■ SYMPTOMS The lids of one eye are swollen, red to violet in color and there is a discharge. The child is usually febrile and quite ill. Movement of the eye to look up, down or sideways may cause pain. Vision may be blurred. Do not confuse this with conjunctivitis. SINUSITIS may occasionally spread to cause cellulitis of the eye.

■ TREATMENT Take the child to your doctor or local hospital emergency room. Most cases respond well to ANTIBIOTICS given by intramuscular injection or intravenously. Your child may be referred to an opthalmologist (eye doctor) for assessment. Rarely, an operation may be needed to drain pus from the back of the eye.

■ OUTLOOK Early diagnosis and treatment usually ensure a full recovery. In severe cases, complications such as loss of vision in the eye or brain abscess may occur.

ORTHODONTICS
The branch of dentistry concerned with correcting irregular positions of the teeth, and the way the upper and lower teeth come together when biting. Treatment usually begins in late childhood when most of the baby teeth have been replaced by permanent ones: a successful result is more easily achieved during this period of development than if left until adolescence or later.

■ SYMPTOMS The teeth may seem to crowd the mouth because they are too large in proportion to the jaw. The upper teeth may protrude (buck teeth or overbite), or the lower teeth may do so (underbite).

■ TREATMENT Crowding of the teeth may simply be treated by removal of some premolar teeth (the teeth immediately behind the pointed canine teeth). The remaining teeth may then move into correct position by themselves, but usually an orthodontic appliance (a brace) is needed. It works simply by pressing teeth into the correct position and holding them there until they will stay in place by themselves. Some braces can improve the bite. The brace may be fixed or removable, and usually requires adjustment about once a month. It may have to be worn for between two or three years, and sometimes much longer, particularly if treatment is delayed. Once the child has become used to having the brace in his mouth, it causes no discomfort.

OSGOOD-SCHLATTERS DISEASE
A disease of the large bone of the lower leg (the tibia) in the region of the knee. The cause is unknown and the problem resolves by itself after a few months.

Symptoms include pain and swelling around the bone just below the knee. There is usually a LIMP. An X-ray confirms the diagnosis and treatment is rest for six to eight weeks. It is sometimes necessary to put the leg in a plaster cast to enforce adequate rest. There are no long-term complications.

OSTEOGENESIS IMPERFECTA

A rare INHERITED DISORDER. The child's bones are fragile (it is also called brittle bone disease), and fractures are common. The fractures heal normally, but some children suffer many fractures which cause severe deformities of the body and limbs.

OSTEOMYELITIS

A bone infection occurring most often in the ends of the long bones of the arm or leg. It may occur after a FRACTURE if the bone breaks through the skin (compound fracture).

■ SYMPTOMS The illness may start abruptly. The child may complain of severe pain in the bone; he may recently have had an infected sore on the skin. There is usually redness and swelling of the skin over the part of the bone that is infected. He is reluctant to move the painful limb.

Other symptoms include FEVER, HEADACHE, loss of appetite and generally feeling ill.

Sometimes the illness starts slowly with only slight pain or swelling as the first sign.

■ ACTION Pain or swelling over a

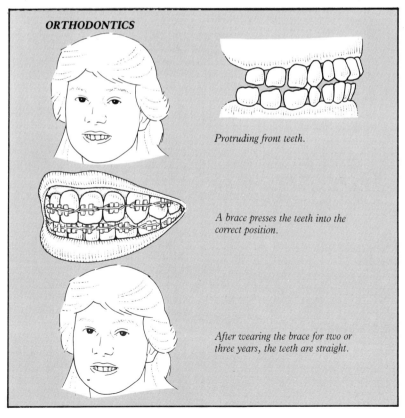

ORTHODONTICS

Protruding front teeth.

A brace presses the teeth into the correct position.

After wearing the brace for two or three years, the teeth are straight.

bone is always a clue. Take the child to a doctor without delay, especially if he seems sick.

■ TESTS include BLOOD TESTS and X-rays of the painful limb. A bone scan may show early signs of the infection. X-rays may not show definite signs of infection in the early stages.

■ TREATMENT The earlier treatment is started, the better the results. ANTIBIOTICS are needed in high doses, usually given into a vein for a few days until the child is better. To ensure all infection has been eradicated, antibiotics are usually given by mouth for about six weeks.
  The pain is treated with analgesics and bed rest.
  An operation is occasionally necessary to drain the infected fluid (pus) that collects within the bone.
  Once the pain disappears, physiotherapy prevents the muscles from becoming weak.

■ OUTLOOK is usually good if the treatment is started early. Occasionally, the infection causes complications of bone growth, and this must be checked for a number of years after the infection has cleared. This problem is most common if the infection occurs in infancy.

OTITIS
See *MIDDLE EAR INFECTION, EXTERNAL EAR INFECTION.*

OTITIS EXTERNA
See *EXTERNAL EAR INFECTION.*

OTITIS MEDIA
See *MIDDLE EAR INFECTION.*

OVERBREATHING
Breathing more deeply or rapidly than necessary, often through fear or anxiety. Medical term: hyperventilation. This results in excess carbon dioxide being released from the lungs. The body's chemical balance is disturbed, the blood becomes alkaline and nerves and muscles become excitable.

■ CAUSE Usually the result of anxiety, sometimes reflecting a more serious underlying psychological disturbance.

■ SYMPTOMS are dizziness, faintness, a feeling of 'pins and needles' in the hands and feet, and eventually spasm of muscles of the arms and legs.

■ ACTION 1 The symptoms are frightening, so reassure the child firmly and calmly. The first time this happens, the child should be seen by a doctor. Only when the diagnosis is sure should parents proceed to try to reverse the disturbance. 2 The imbalance may be reversed if the child breathes in and out of a paper bag, thereby re-breathing his own carbon dioxide.

■ TREATMENT Try to identify the underlying cause of anxiety and, if possible, relieve it. You may need medical advice for this. Careful assessment of the child's feelings and fears, including inquiry into the family and school backgrounds, may be necessary. Many children experience temporary anxieties during their school years, which pass in due course with no long-term consequences.

OVERDOSE
See *POISONING.*

OVERDUE BABY

Born later than the expected date of delivery (gestation to maturity normally lasts 40 weeks). Also called 'postmature'. The overdue baby often has wrinkled, flaky skin and long nails. He may pass MECONIUM while still in the womb. Postmaturity carries little risk for the baby until the pregnancy reaches 42 weeks. After that, the placenta may begin to fail, and the volume of water surrounding the baby (amniotic fluid) decreases. There is then also a risk of sudden unexplained death of the fetus in the womb, resulting in STILL BIRTH. Almost all obstetricians recommend induction of labor after 42 weeks of pregnancy.

OVERWEIGHT
See *OBESITY.*

PQ

PAIN

The experience of an unpleasant, potentially harmful stimulus. Specific nerve endings in the skin and other body surfaces respond to extreme and painful stimuli; and they are distinct from those that transmit normal sensations such as touch, temperature and stretching.

■ SYMPTOMS Perhaps the most intense, gnawing pain is caused by increased pressure within an enclosed space, for example a bone, ear or dental root. A whole range of lesser pains may be perceived as sharp, throbbing, colicky, burning or tight.

Pain has a protective function: if we didn't feel it, we would not naturally withdraw from danger. Pain also indicates disease. But pain of psychological origin can of course be just as unpleasant as physical pain and deserves equal attention.

Pain can be acutely and obviously localized in sensitive areas such as the mouth or the hands, but may be more difficult to pinpoint elsewhere. Localizing pain is a particular problem in the very young. Parents can do no more than respond to signs of severe trouble, such as irritability, pallor, vomiting or immobility.

■ ACTION The first, common-sense step for mild pain is to give the child acetamenophen in the pain-killing dose recommended by your doctor. People tend to under-use painkillers, unaware of their application in an extraordinarily wide range of conditions from HEADACHES to CUTS and BRUISES.

Clearly, intense, highly distressing pain requires medical advice.

■ TREATMENT A bewildering range of painkilling drugs is available today, but most pain in childhood is best treated by a simple painkiller (analgesic) such as acetamenophen or codeine. It is generally best to use a single-ingredient remedy because this means you are in control of the dosage. Aspirin should not be used in children – see *REYE SYNDROME*.

More powerful analgesics are given to children for specific conditions such as pain following surgery, malignant disease or juvenile ARTHRITIS, but should be given only under your doctor's supervision. Some of the powerful analgesics are addictive and are only used for short periods. Opiates (morphine/heroin/demerol) tend to cause respiratory depression in babies.

■ OUTLOOK Children are relatively tolerant of pain. A child will often be active soon after surgery or a bone fracture. This may be because pain causes less fear in some children, rather than because children are less sensitive to pain. Relaxation exercises or distraction can help a child to tolerate pain.

PAIN IN THE EYE

There are several causes. If it is mild and the eye is red and itchy, it may be due to CONJUNCTIVITIS.

Inflammation of the inside of the eye (as in uveitis) may produce a more severe pain, made worse by looking at light. Your child may also complain of blurred vision. There are a number of conditions associated with uveitis, such as RHEUMATOID ARTHRITIS.

If the pain is severe or prolonged, you should get medical advice without delay. Infections of the eyelids or globe of the eye itself (see *ORBITAL CELLULITIS*) can be dangerous and progress rapidly. Likewise if there is any chance of injury or a foreign body in the eye, urgent medical attention is required – if necessary at the emergency department of your local hospital.

PALPITATIONS

See *ARRHYTHMIAS*.

PARALYSIS

Causes in childhood include diseases of muscle, peripheral nerves, the nerve-to-muscle (neuromuscular) junction, nerve roots, the spinal cord (as, for example, in POLIOMYELITIS) or the brain; biochemical disorders (for example abnormal potassium levels); hormone disorders (see *ADRENAL DISORDERS*) and poisons (see *POISONING*). See also *BRAIN TUMORS, TETANUS*.

■ ACTION Paralysis is always a reason to get urgent medical advice.

■ INVESTIGATIONS depend on the suggested cause and site, and include: muscle biopsy; nerve conduction studies; tests of the neuromuscular junction; an X-ray of the spinal cord (myelogram); brain scan (see *CAT SCAN*) and BLOOD TESTS.

■ TREATMENT depends on the cause, severity, site and duration. It may mean INTENSIVE CARE with respiratory support if breathing is affected; or it may mean rest of affected parts, drug treatment, surgery, physiotherapy or hydrotherapy.

■ OUTLOOK Some muscle diseases, such as MUSCULAR DYSTROPHY, lead to deterioration and death in adolescence. Neuromuscular disease may respond to long-term drug treatment. Spinal paralysis may respond to spinal surgery, but this is rarely indicated. Brain surgery may help acute paralysis (for example after trauma or BRAIN TUMOR), but not chronic paralysis (for example with CEREBRAL PALSY).

PARASITES

Organisms that live off others (the term parasites is often used in contexts outside of medicine and biology). Parasitic organisms may be microscopic, as in the case of MALARIA, or much larger, such as WORMS, which may infest the bowel. Parasites may enter the body in many ways: the child's hands, food or drink may be contaminated; in other cases the parasite may pass through the skin, as happens with mosquito-born malaria.

PARONYCHIA

An INFECTION of a finger-nail (also called a whitlow). It is usually caused by BACTERIA, but occasionally a VIRAL or FUNGAL infection can occur. The organisms enter the fold of skin around the nail through a break in the cuticle.

▓ SYMPTOMS A painful, red swelling begins suddenly; eventually pus is discharged if the swelling is not lanced by a doctor. Occasionally a more long-term infection is caused by habitual chewing or picking at the cuticles.

▓ ACTION If the infection is superficial, cleaning and soaking in an antiseptic solution can cure it. If there is swelling, and the finger is throbbing, see your doctor. There is no danger of losing the affected finger nail.
A fungal infection will require an antifungal cream or tablets. The viral infection, herpes whitlow, resolves with time and rarely needs

specific antiviral treatment.
A chronic infection results in continuing redness and swelling of the skin, with occasional discharge of pus. This usually requires antibiotic treatment.

▓ OUTLOOK is good if the infection is treated adequately.

PATENT DUCTUS ARTERIOSUS
See *CONGENITAL HEART-DISEASE.*

PEAK FLOW METER
An instrument to measure airflow out of the lungs, chiefly used in the management of ASTHMA, both in the diagnosis and the monitoring of progress during or between attacks.
Children with severe asthma may be given a peak flow meter to use at home. This is a useful method of following the progress of the condition between consultations with your doctor.

PEAK FLOW METER

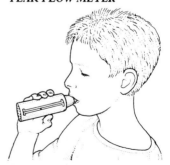

A peak flow meter is easy enough for a two-year-old to use: he simply has to exhale into it.

PECTUS EXCAVATUM (FUNNEL CHEST)
A relatively rare deformity in which there is a deep hollow in the middle of the chest.

■ CAUSE Unknown. It sometimes runs in families.

■ SYMPTOMS The deformity does not impair physical health: the problem (if there is one) is parental concern and, occasionally, a psychological one for the child. He may suffer from poor self-image, embarrassment and refusal to take part in sports, especially swimming.

■ TREATMENT A consultation by a chest surgeon may be helpful. Operations are rarely recommended because the risks usually outweigh the benefits.

PEPTIC ULCER

An ulcer caused by inflammation of the lining of the upper intestine (the mucosa), due to excess acid production within the stomach. It is uncommon in childhood. The ulcer usually develops in the stomach or duodenum. Such ulcers can arise acutely, or over time. BACTERIAL INFECTION may be a cause. There may be a family history of ulcers.

■ SYMPTOMS Acute: VOMITING blood (hematemesis) after severe infection or trauma, or when using high doses of aspirin (not recommended in children – see *REYE SYNDROME*). Chronic: vomiting and recurrent ABDOMINAL PAIN in the upper half of the abdomen. Black stools containing blood (melena) may sometimes be present. Secondary PYLORIC STENOSIS associated with vomiting may develop.

Severe, acute abdominal pain caused by a perforation of the ulcer into the abdominal cavity and causing PERITONITIS is rare.

■ INVESTIGATIONS BLOOD TEST to identify ANEMIA. Gastroscopy –

(examination of the stomach with a tube under ANESTHETIC). A barium X-ray of the stomach and upper intestine may identify the ulceration.

■ MANAGEMENT BLOOD TRANSFUSION may be required; antacids and ulcer-soothing drugs, some of which have side-effects, will be necessary for several weeks. Small, frequent meals may help and aggravating foods should be avoided. Surgery may be required for perforation with peritonitis, pyloric stenosis or severe, persistent symptoms.

■ OUTLOOK Drugs will help to heal the inflamed mucosa. Surgery is not often required, but may be necessary for children with chronic, upsetting symptoms, or major complications.

PERIODONTAL DISEASE
See *GINGIVITIS*.

PERITONITIS

This occurs when the membrane covering the intestine and the inner surface of the abdomen becomes inflamed, as in APPENDICITIS or following a leak or perforation of some part of the intestine. Peritonitis may progress rapidly, leading to SHOCK and life-threatening INFECTION. It is a medical emergency.

■ SYMPTOMS The signs of impending peritonitis are usually clear. The child is pale, very sick and feverish, and unwilling to sit up or eat. Depending on the underlying cause, there may have been preceding VOMITING, DIARRHEA or CONSTIPATION. There is severe ABDOMINAL PAIN, which may start in one area and spread as the situation gets worse. The wall of the abdomen is held tense and is tender to touch; the child cannot tolerate any pressure placed on the abdomen. Internal pressure is also painful, and the doctor may need to check for this by examining with a finger inside the rectum. If untreated, the condition will worsen, the pulse rate will go up and the child will become distressed or, worse, listless and shocked.

▨ ACTION This is an emergency. Take your child to the nearest hospital emergency room. See *SHOCK*.

▨ TREATMENT See SHOCK.

PERTUSSIS
See *WHOOPING COUGH*.

PETIT MAL SEIZURE
A form of EPILEPSY in which the child briefly displays a distant or glazed look, with minor movements of the eyelids and mouth. There is no jerking or loss of posture as in GRAND MAL SEIZURE. Many such episodes may occur daily.

▨ CAUSE Abnormal electrical discharge in the brain.

▨ SYMPTOMS Eyes glaze or roll up; some facial movements; pallor; episodes last a few seconds only. Occasionally, this type of seizure is continuous (petit mal status epilepticus) giving rise to a false impression of mental deterioration/retardation. Most sufferers respond well to anti-epileptic drugs.

▨ OUTLOOK If the condition is not diagnosed and treated, learning problems may result. However, most inattentiveness in school is due to simple lack of concentration (or day dreaming), not to petit mal epilepsy. Most children grow out of petit mal by mid-adolescence. In the majority of cases, the condition is innocuous. Occasionally, petit mal is followed by other forms of seizures in later childhood and young adulthood.

▨ TESTS The clinical diagnosis can be confirmed by an EEG, which characteristically shows a three-per-second spike and slow wave pattern.

PHARYNGITIS
See *SORE THROAT.*

PHENYLKETONURIA (PKU)
An inherited disease of metabolism. The child is unable to process a substance – phenylalanine – digested from protein in the diet. Approximately one in 15,000 babies are affected.

▨ SYMPTOMS An untreated child will become MENTALLY HANDI-CAPPED, with signs of DEVELOPMENTAL DELAY by four months. Such children often have blond hair, blue eyes, a funny musty smell, ECZEMA and poor head growth (MICROCEPHALY). One third will have convulsions and many will become HYPERACTIVE and difficult to manage socially.

▨ TESTS All children are screened shortly after birth. Several drops of blood are placed on a card which is sent to the laboratory for analysis of the phenylalanine level. This test is not valid if the blood was taken before the baby was fed. If your baby is discharged within 24 hours of delivery, the test is usually done three to seven days later as an outpatient. If this test is positive, further BLOOD TESTS must be performed to confirm the diagnosis.

▨ TREATMENT The aim is to prevent BRAIN DAMAGE in susceptible children. Dietary treatment should begin as soon as the diagnosis has been made. Milk substitutes from which phenylalanine has been largely removed are used in the early months, and parents must follow a special diet once the child is on baby foods. Natural foods in which the phenylalanine content is known are gradually added. Blood levels of phenylalanine must be monitored frequently. 'Overtreatment' or too low levels are associated with lethargy, anorexia, anemia, rash and diarrhea. Undertreatment or too high levels are associated with brain damage.

The highly controlled diet essential in infancy and childhood is often stressful for the child and family. Dietary control may be relaxed in adolescence, and many adults with the condition will manage a normal diet.

Mothers who suffer from phenylketonuria must return to a strict diet before conception and throughout pregnancy, otherwise the baby may be at risk from microcephaly and CONGENITAL HEART-DISEASE.

PHIMOSIS

A tightening of the foreskin around the tip of the penis. Passing urine will cause 'ballooning' of the foreskin, and the urine stream will be poor, possibly reduced to a dribble. A tight phimosis is an indication for CIRCUMCISION.

Phimosis may be present from birth, but is more commonly caused by recurrent BALANITIS. Pulling back the foreskin with too much force may also cause a phimosis. Retraction of the foreskin should not normally be attempted before the age of one year.

PHOBIAS

A phobia might be described as a fear that has grown out of all proportion. The child is frightened not only of some object, but also pictures of the object, stories about the object or a place where the object might have been.

Developing fear is an essential part of growing up safely. Sometimes a real and reasonable fear (say of dogs once the child has been chased by a snapping dog) develops into a phobia. Some phobias are easier to understand than others, for example fear of the dark. Some, on the other hand, are totally imaginary and may never be explicitly defined by the child. Most fade away as the child's confidence and knowledge of the world increase.

■ACTION Don't ridicule your child's fear (and don't let other children tease him). Hold his hand firmly while walking calmly past the house with the dog, and talk about looking brave. If he is terrified, calm him down while trying not to rush away. Next time, approach more cautiously; try to deal with the feared situation or object, rather than avoiding it; but don't inadvertently cause your child great or repeated distress in your wish for him to be brave.

Get medical advice if the child's panic is worsening, if the number of phobias increases, or if they don't diminish after a few months.

Phobias in older children are rarer and less easily resolved without help. Isolated phobias of spiders are common and normally not much of a problem; but if the phobia interferes with your child's enjoyment of life and social activities, get medical advice. A consultation with a clinical psychologist or child psychiatrist will probably be suggested.

PHOTOTHERAPY

Treatment by ultraviolet light of a

new-born baby with JAUNDICE.

The principle of the therapy is the bleaching effect that light has on bilirubin, the yellow waste product of hemoglobin breakdown – hemoglobin that is released from red blood cells that are destroyed for a variety of reasons. The bilirubin in the tissues below the skin is chemically transformed by the ultraviolet light into colorless and harmless derivatives.

Blue or white light is directed at the baby through the transparent cover of his incubator or crib. The baby is left naked in order to expose the maximum area of skin to the light. His eyes are covered for protection from the brightness of the light.

The baby may need extra feedings because phototherapy causes water to evaporate from the skin at an excessive rate. For healthy full-term babies, phototherapy will only be needed for two to three days. For the premature baby and the baby with BLOOD GROUP INCOMPATIBILITY, longer periods of phototherapy may be necessary. Side-effects are usually trivial – the baby may have a slight skin rash and loose stools.

PICA
See *ANEMIA*.

PIGEON TOES (INTOEING)
The child's toes are turned inwards. Sometimes one of the bones of the lower leg (the tibia) is involved.

Intoeing actually helps to prevent a small child from falling backwards, so that intoeing is normal in children up to three years of age. It can also occur as part of a CLUB FOOT or with some abnormalities of the nerves and muscles of the foot, as in CEREBRAL PALSY.

■ SYMPTOMS Pigeon toes may make a child trip over his feet, so that he appears clumsy or accident-prone. It is most noticeable when he

starts to walk and when he walks about without shoes.

■ ACTION In most cases the problem is mild, and resolves on its own.

■ TREATMENT Surgery is rarely needed and is only justified if the deformity is severe in an older child.

■ OUTLOOK Intoeing almost always improves without treatment.

PINK EYE
See *CONJUNCTIVITIS*.

PINWORMS (ENTEROBIASIS)
Pinworms are the most common bowel PARASITES in children in the United States. They are not likely to cause symptoms other than an itchy bottom at night, when the adult worms emerge to lay eggs at the anal opening. The worms may be visible as white threads.

■ TREATMENT consists of medication such as pyrantel pamoate or mebendazole if the child is over two years. It is usually advisable to treat the whole family. Unfortunately, recurrences are frequent.

PITYRIASIS ROSEA
A skin rash of unknown cause, consisting of oval patches on the trunk that persist for about six weeks, then disappear.

■ SYMPTOMS A 'herald patch' is the first sign: a small red patch of skin about one inch (2 cm) in diameter, somewhere on the child's chest, back or stomach. A few days later, numerous oval patches, smaller than the herald patch, cover the upper body. The usual distribution of the rash is such that it would be completely covered if the child wore a short-sleeved, turtle-neck sweater.

The rash is often distributed on the back in a pattern that resembles a Christmas tree. The lesions are red, with a faint scaly surface. They do not usually itch, but cause great anxiety to parents. The child is not ill, but may have had a mild sore throat during the weeks before the appearance of the rash.

■ ACTION There is no need to isolate the child. It is wise to get medical advice in order to be sure of the diagnosis.

■ TREATMENT No specific treatment is needed, unless the rash is very irritating, when a mild soothing cream may be prescribed.

■ OUTLOOK *Pityriasis rosea* is not a serious condition, and will completely disappear in two or three months. After the rash has gone, there may be areas of increased and decreased skin pigmentation, particularly in black patients. These clear up with time. There are no long-term effects, nor is there a connection with other skin problems. (It is *not* related to PSORIASIS or ECZEMA.)

PKU
See *PHENYLKETONURIA.*

PLAY THERAPY
At one level, this consists of psychological treatment using play to help a young child express and resolve emotional problems. This would normally require regular individual sessions with a specially trained therapist.

At another level, play therapy may be utilized in the hospital to distract and occupy the small child. This is now recognized as an important and constructive part of the hospital's work with sick children. See *CHILD PSY-CHOTHERAPY.*

PLEURISY
An inflammation of the outer lining of the lungs, or the inner lining of the chest wall. Although fairly common in adults, it is rare in children.

■ CAUSES Any INFECTION of the lungs, such as PNEUMONIA or TUBERCULOSIS, can result in pleurisy.

■ SYMPTOMS In addition to the symptoms of the underlying infection or disease, pleurisy causes pain with each breath, which may be felt in the chest, the abdomen or the shoulder. The pain is sharp and severe; it prevents the child from breathing deeply.

■ ACTION Pleurisy is unlikely to be the first sign of illness in a child: if a child has these symptoms, he should be seen by a doctor for physical examination and tests such as a chest X-ray.

■ TREATMENT and OUTLOOK See the various underlying diseases – PNEUMONIA, TUBERCULOSIS.

PLUGGED EARS
See *WAX IN EARS, EARS, FOREIGN BODIES IN, WATER IN EARS, EXTERNAL EAR INFECTION.*

PNEUMONIA
An INFECTION of part or all of the lungs.

■ CAUSES A wide range of BACTERIA or VIRUSES.

■ SYMPTOMS The child will usually have a COUGH and a FEVER. Very young babies may only display rapid breathing, and appear generally ill.

Older children may have no chest signs, but have high fever and delirium; other children (with other types of pneumonia) may experience pain, or may cough up phlegm, often colored green or yellow. The child may be BREATHLESS.

■ ACTION Children with pneumonia are often seriously ill and need to be hospitalized. In milder forms pneumonia may be treated at home. However, pneumonia always requires medical advice and care: don't hesitate to call a doctor if your child has symptoms and signs of pneumonia.

■ INVESTIGATIONS X-rays of the chest may be performed to confirm the diagnosis and reveal the extent and type of pneumonia. BLOOD TESTS and tests of the sputum (phlegm) may help to determine the type of infection actually causing the pneumonia.

■ TREATMENT ANTIBIOTICS are prescribed for the many types of pneumonia due to BACTERIA. They are usually given by mouth. If the child is too ill, they may be given by intramuscular injection or intravenous drip. Antiviral agents are available to treat some viral pneumonias but are only used in severe cases. If the bacterial or viral pneumonia is severe, the child may be given oxygen through a mask or in a tent; in extreme cases the child may need life support on a ventilator (a tube inserted into the wind pipe and attached to a machine that 'breathes' for the child).

■ PHYSIOTHERAPY In some bacterial pneumonias, chest physiotherapy may help to encourage coughing, to move mucus or phlegm to the upper airways from which it can be coughed up and spat out, and to improve breathing. The physiotherapist may teach parents how to perform the treatment.

■ OUTLOOK following pneumonia is good for almost all children. Unless there is an underlying cause (such as CYSTIC FIBROSIS), continuing problems are rare. Occasionally, damage to the lung leads to BRONCHIECTASIS and recurrent infections.

POISON IVY (POISON SUMAC, POISON OAK RASHES)

In the United States, skin contact with the resin from poison ivy, poison sumac or poison oak is the most common cause of direct contact allergic rashes.

■ CAUSE These plants all contain a resin to which most people are highly allergic. Poison ivy grows as a shrub or vine in woods, vacant lots and wilderness areas throughout the Unites States except in the southwest. Poison sumac is found mainly east of the Mississippi River and grows as a shrub or tree, never as a vine. Poison oak is most common on the West Coast and grows as a shrub. Each has a distinctive leaf pattern – see illustration.

Most rashes occur in summer but the resin can stick to clothing and garden tools so exposure to the resin may occur year-round. A history of direct contact with the plant is common, but indirect exposure to contaminated clothing or animal fur may confuse the diagnosis. Smoke from fires burning scrub containing these plants can carry the resin and cause a rash on exposed skin, and severe swelling of the lining of the air passages.

■ SYMPTOMS The rash is the same

for all three plants. One to three days after skin contact with the resin, the area is red, itchy and has blisters and small bumps. The area may be linear, spotty or may involve large areas depending upon where the resin contact occurred.

■ ACTION Try to avoid poison ivy, poison sumac or poison oak by knowing what these plants look like and where they are found.

If exposed, minimize the effect by washing the skin thoroughly as quickly as possible, preferably within five to ten minutes. Contaminated clothing and tools must also be washed. For mild reactions, calamine lotion is helpful, as are cold compresses. Oral antihistamines such as chlorpheniramine may give some relief to the itch. All moderate or severe rashes should be seen by your doctor.

POISONING

Medicines are the most common poisons taken by children, followed by household chemicals, seeds and plants. Eighty percent of serious accidental poisoning occurs in children under five years of age, usually when the family is under stress. Many poisonings can be prevented by locking medicines away, using child-proof medicine containers and by keeping household cleaners and garden supplies up out of reach.

■ IMMEDIATE ACTION If unconscious, see *EMERGENCY RESUSCITATION.*

Phone your local poison control center (usually listed in the front pages of the telephone book) or emergency room for immediate advice.

Medicines: Your poison center may recommend inducing vomiting

POISON IVY

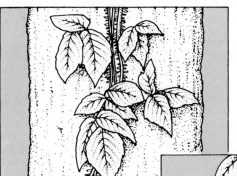

Poison ivy

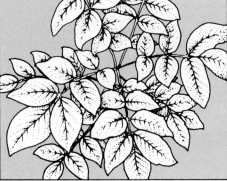

Poison sumac

with syrup of ipecac before going to the hospital emergency room. Look for the empty container, and take it with the child to hospital.

Household and garden chemicals: Take the child to hospital, with the container from which the substance was taken. If there is likely to be a substantial delay, give milk and water or whatever is recommended by the poison center. Don't make the child vomit – it could cause corrosive damage to the esophagus (feeding tube) and the throat.

What to expect at the hospital: The toxicity of the poison will be assessed. In some cases, vomiting will be induced by syrup of ipecac to expel any unabsorbed poison from the stomach. Or a tube may be passed through the nose or mouth into the stomach through which the stomach contents will be washed out. For certain poisons, antidotes are given to neutralize their effect. Some children will be detained overnight in the hospital for observation.

Your local poison control center can supply you with information about poison-proofing your home.

POLIOMYELITIS (POLIO)

An INFECTION caused by the polio VIRUS, of which there are three types. The disease is spread by infected stools (fecal-oral route) or possibly by exhaled droplets. The INCUBATION PERIOD is from three to 14 days, and children are most infectious from a week before to a week after the symptoms appear.

▣ PREVENTION IMMUNIZATION is essential, and ought to be routine.

▣ SYMPTOMS Most polio virus infections are asymptomatic. HEADACHE, FEVER and loss of APPETITE occur first.

These symptoms are usually mild and no serious illness result. However, in some cases severe muscle pains and stiffness occur.

In some children, PARALYSIS follows. This can involve the muscles of the arms and legs, or the muscles involved in breathing and swallowing. Paralysis is more common in older children and adolescents; in children who have had an operation or any intramuscular injection during the incubation period; and in children who have been involved in strenuous physical activity just before the onset of symptoms.

ENCEPHALITIS is a rare but grave complication.

▣ TESTS The virus can be found in throat swabs and stool specimens. BLOOD TESTS can also confirm the diagnosis.

▣ ACTION Because the symptoms are similar to those of COMMON COLD or INFLUENZA, the diagnosis may not be obvious early in the illness. If your child has any suspicious symptoms and for some reason has not been immunized, always mention this to your doctor.

▣ TREATMENT depends on the symptoms. Even if there is no paralysis, rest is essential to prevent and limit paralysis if it should develop. If paralysis occurs, admission to the hospital is essential. Splints and physiotherapy will prevent stiffening of joints.

If the muscles of breathing or swallowing are paralyzed, the child could well be put on a ventilator machine to help with breathing.

Since a child with polio continues to be infectious for a week or more after the illness has started, everyone looking after the child should be immunized and use careful hand-washing after each contact with him.

■ OUTLOOK depends on the severity of the infection, but any paralysis that occurs, usually continues to improve for about a year after the illness. However, permanent paralysis is a possibility. Prevention is better than any treatment. The polio vaccines are very effective and safe.

PORPHYRIA

The porphyrias are a group of uncommon diseases caused by inherited deficiencies of enzymes necessary for the production of heme, an essential component of hemoglobin, the oxygen carrier in red blood cells. The incidence is as low as one in 30,000 in the general population.

■ SYMPTOMS There are many types of inherited porphyria, each with its own set of symptoms. In the types where there is over-production of porphyrins in the blood stream (for example, congenital erythropoitic porphyria), the child develops striking photosensitivity of the skin. Exposure to sunlight may result in blistering, scarring and in severe cases damage to fingers and toes. Excess facial and body hair and skin pigmentation may also occur.

In acute intermittent porphyria, skin sensitivity is rarely a symptom, but patients may suffer sudden ABDOMINAL PAIN and neurological or psychiatric disturbance. Fortunately this condition and the acquired, non-inherited, form of the disease rarely occur in childhood. POISONING with lead and hexachlorobenzine can also produce the condition.

■ ACTION Avoiding sunlight is essential for the photo-sensitive child. In severe cases, the child may need to wear protective clothing and a specially constructed glass helmet which absorbs ultraviolet rays. The home may need special windows with ultraviolet-absorbent glass, and the child's movements may need to be restricted. Children with a family history of the acute form should avoid certain drugs such as barbiturates, sulfonamides and alcohol.

■ TREATMENT Disturbances in body fluids may occur in severe attacks. Water restriction and intravenous extra salt and glucose given under careful supervision in the hospital may dramatically improve the patient's condition. Long-term management requires careful control of infections and avoidance of alcohol and certain drugs. A diet high in carbohydrates, adequate in protein and low in fat is beneficial. Excessive exposure to sunlight should be avoided. A dermatologist may recommend special prescription creams to protect against ultraviolet and near ultraviolet radiation. A medical alert necklace or bracelet should be worn.

■ OUTLOOK With sound preventive measures and prompt treatment, most forms of porphyria can be controlled sufficiently for the child to live a useful and happy life.

POSTNASAL DRIP

The flow of mucus from the nose down the back of the throat. This is the usual cause of COUGH when a child has a COMMON COLD, HAY FEVER or ALLERGIC RHINITIS. The cough is usually described as 'tickly'. It should not be suppressed as it keeps the mucus out of the child's lungs. If possible the cause should be treated.

PREMATURITY

Born before 37 weeks of pregnancy. The full term of pregnancy is 40 weeks.

▨ CAUSES In the majority of cases, labor begins prematurely for no apparent cause. A baby may, however, have to be delivered prematurely because of maternal or fetal problems. Hypertension developing in the mother during pregnancy is the most common reason.

▨ PROBLEMS The more premature the baby, that is, the shorter the duration of the pregnancy, the more immature the baby's normal physiology. Thus premature babies have poorly developed sucking and swallowing mechanisms. They tend to spit up feedings more easily, and are therefore at risk of inhaling milk into the lungs.

Most premature babies become JAUNDICED, and are susceptible to HYPOTHERMIA, INFECTION and RESPIRATORY DISTRESS SYNDROME. They often develop ANEMIA when they are two to three months old.

▨ TREATMENT Some premature babies (those born around 36 weeks of gestation; not those born after very short pregnancies) can be nursed by their mothers. However, feedings may need to be given through a narrow tube passed through one nostril into the stomach. (If tube feedings are needed then special nursing help will be required, which may be available only in the special care nursery.) The feedings may be either breast milk that has been expressed by the mother or a donor (if the hospital funs a human milk bank), or a commercially prepared milk (formula). Because such babies have small stomachs, they need to be given tube feedings in small amounts at frequent intervals. Babies born after shorter gestation with very low birth weight will need INTENSIVE CARE.

Premature babies of less than 35 weeks' gestation, together with most babies of less than 4+ lb (2,000 gm), require at least close observation with special attention to temperature control and feeding.

However, sick babies and those below 30 weeks' gestation and less than 1 lb (500 gm), will often need additional or intensive care. This may require one nurse to be assigned at each work shift to observe and care for an individual baby. Additionally, fluids and nutrients may need to be given intravenously, ANTIBIOTICS may be required for infections, other drugs may be indicated to stimulate breathing or support heart function, and frequently a period of artificial ventilation is called for. The care of such babies requires a highly complex form of treatment; it is very technical. But you should ensure that, as parents, your central role in being with your baby is not overlooked.

▨ OUTLOOK For other than the smallest and sickest premature infants, the outlook is generally good. The majority of such babies live and grow up to be normal children. But each baby's problems are highly individual, and you should ask the doctors to discuss with you what they believe the outlook is for your child.

PRENATAL DIAGNOSIS

There continue to be rapid advances in the field of prenatal diagnosis, with the identification of more disorders of the fetus long before birth. The various prenatal tests can diagnose certain CONGENITAL or INHERITED DISORDERS, and assess the maturity of the fetus.

■ ULTRASOUND SCAN is used:
– To assess the size and rate of growth and, towards the end of pregnancy, the maturity of the fetus at the time of expected delivery.
– To confirm MULTIPLE PREGNANCY.
– To assess the position of the fetus and placenta if AMNIOCENTESIS (see below) is under consideration.

■ BLOOD TESTS The mother's blood can be tested to show whether the fetus has certain congenital abnormalities.

■ AMNIOCENTESIS involves taking a sample of the amniotic fluid surrounding the fetus. The fluid can be tested to discover whether the fetus has certain congenital or inherited diseases. The test is rarely performed before 12-14 weeks, but it can be used late in pregnancy if there is a risk of premature birth to assess whether the fetal lungs are mature enough for the baby to breathe effectively outside the uterus.

An ultrasound scan (see above) is usually performed beforehand to confirm the position of the placenta and to determine whether more than one fetus is present. An area on the mother's lower abdomen is anaesthetized and a needle is inserted into the amniotic sac to withdraw a small amount of amniotic fluid. This contains cells from the fetus that can be examined for CHROMOSOMAL ABNORMALITIES (such as DOWN SYNDROME). This test is offered to older women in whom the risk of a Down syndrome child is greater than average. Chemical tests can also be performed on the amniotic fluid and the cells within it to identify a variety of rare fetal, genetically-determined abnormalities.

The procedure involves essentially no risk to the mother and only slight discomfort. However, if an amniocentesis is carried out early in pregnancy, there is approaching a 1 percent chance of it being followed by an abortion. When performed late in pregnancy to assess maturity of the fetus, the risks of still birth are very small.

■ CHORIONIC BIOPSY is a fairly new procedure whereby a needle is inserted through the abdominal wall or via the vagina into the uterus. A few cells from the developing placenta are removed and tested for specific genetic and chromosomal abnormalities. The advantage of this test is that it can be done earlier in the pregnancy than amniocentesis (see above); it may, however, carry a greater risk of causing an abortion. The risk to the mother is slight. Although uncomfortable, the procedure is not painful.

■ FETOSCOPY is a procedure used to examine the external appearance of the fetus, and also take blood samples to test for certain inherited abnormalities. A needle containing a device to inspect the fetus is inserted into the uterus. The risk of abortion following this procedure is about 4 percent, so fetoscopy is only used when information cannot be obtained in any other way.

■ PSYCHOLOGICAL CONSIDERATIONS are important. Before embarking on these tests, make sure that you understand the procedure, the risks to the fetus and what specific information will be gained from performing the test. You may be under a great deal of stress waiting for the results, and support from your doctor or GENETIC COUNSELLOR and partner may be helpful. You and your partner may want to discuss in advance what your approach will be if the tests reveal a serious abnormality.

PROLAPSE, RECTAL
See *RECTAL PROLAPSE*.

PROTRUDING EARS ('LOP' EARS)
Children's ears sometimes stick out to a degree that leads to embarrassment and ridicule. A simple cosmetic operation can be performed, usually in the early school years, to correct the anomaly. A narrow strip of cartilage is removed from the ear to allow the ear to flatten.

However, many parents (and children) choose to live with the problem, perhaps encouraging the child to wear his hair long.

PSORIASIS
A relatively common skin condition of unknown cause, characterized by raised red patches that tend to come and go. There are several different types: the commonest in children consists of many small round patches (about the size of a finger-nail or less); less common is scalp psoriasis, in which thick scales form on the scalp beneath the hair; and generalized psoriasis, which is very rare, affecting the entire skin.

Overall, about 1 percent of the population have psoriasis at some time in their lives. It may run in families, and is less common in children than in adults.

■ SYMPTOMS The red patches of psoriasis are due to areas of skin with a rich blood supply growing faster than normal skin. The main symp-toms are the reddened appearance of the skin, and its scaliness. Occasionally there may be itching and, if cracks occur, pain.

■ ACTION Children who develop any new rash should be seen by the family doctor or pediatrician. The diagnosis of psoriasis depends on the appearance and distribution of the rash, together with a consideration of how it initially developed. Referral to a specialist may be needed for confirmation of the diagnosis and, in severe cases, for special treatment.

■ TREATMENT There is as yet no total cure. In many cases the rash fades on its own, sometimes permanently.

Many different types of creams and ointments are used. These include: steroid ointments, used under instructions from a doctor mainly for the most angry patches, but restricted to courses of short duration, and not used on the face; tar preparations, which tend to be rather messy, may be prescribed as bandages, a thick paste, or liquid to put in the bath. Coal tar preparations may be recommended to be used in conjunction with ultraviolet light therapy.

Scalp psoriasis is treated with an ointment containing salicylic acid to soften the thick scales, followed by frequent washing with a coal tar based shampoo.

Make sure you have clear instructions from your doctor before using any of these treatments.

■ LONG-TERM MANAGEMENT Chronic psoriasis, which is rare in children, comes and goes. Treatment helps to speed up the clearing of individual lesions, but there is no way of preventing recurrence.

■ OUTLOOK An individual acute bout of psoriasis commonly clears in six to 12 weeks. Relapsing and chronic psoriasis may, rarely, be a lifelong condition. It is sometimes complicated by a form of arthritis.

PSYCHOSIS

A mental condition in which there is alteration and disintegration in the way a child is able to think; as a result, there is a change in the way he behaves. The child seems to be in a different world; he is withdrawn; he acts strangely. He loses (or seems to lose) the skills and abilities he previously had. There are many different types of psychosis; their causation is unclear; no doubt the abnormality is in the brain. AUTISM and SCHIZOPHRENIA are two serious mental illnesses in which a child may be described as being psychotic; they usually have a gradual onset. A child may also develop a psychosis as a sudden and brief reaction to a severe physical illness or a great stress. In these cases, there is usually complete recovery.

PUBERTY

A time not only of sexual development, marking the end of childhood and the beginning of adolescence, but also of change in physical appearance and of changing emotional outlook. The stages of puberty occur in a set order, but there is wide variation among individuals as to when they occur. Girls usually begin and end puberty earlier than boys.

■ STAGES OF PUBERTY – GIRLS
The first sign of puberty is usually the growth spurt. This begins around ten years, and most girls have reached their final adult height by 15. Breast development and the appearance of pubic hair can start as early as ten years, with underarm hair a little later. Menstruation begins, on average, between 12 and 13 years of age.

■ STAGES OF PUBERTY – BOYS
The first signs, around 12 to 13 years, are enlargement of the testes and growth of pubic hair. The growth spurt also begins around this time. The penis starts to lengthen and erections become more common than in childhood. Ejaculations, starting as early as age 12 years, at first contain no sperm. Underarm, body and facial hair then appear and the voice begins to deepen.

■ PROBLEMS OF PUBERTY
Delayed or precocious puberty: get medical advice if your daughter begins her periods before the age of ten, or has not started by the age of 16; if your son is much shorter than his classmates (because his growth spurt is delayed), or if he shows no signs of puberty by 14.

Although delayed puberty may be perfectly normal, it warrants further investigation because it can be a sign of pituitary disease or of TURNER SYNDROME in girls. It may be a sign of ANOREXIA NERVOSA, and it sometimes occurs in girls who engage in intensive sports such as gymnastics. The tendency sometimes runs in families.

Precocious puberty is much commoner in girls than in boys. It may be normal, but usually warrants investigation: causes include ovarian, testicular and ADRENAL problems. There are rare cases of BRAIN TUMORS causing precocious puberty in boys.

Breast development in boys at puberty is commoner than many parents realize. One or both breasts may be involved. This is not 'abnormal', and soon resolves naturally, but nonetheless report it to your family doctor, who should be able to offer reassurance.

PULLED ELBOW
See *DISLOCATION OF A JOINT.*

PULMONARY STENOSIS
See *CONGENITAL HEART-DISEASE.*

PYELITIS, PYELONEPHRITIS
See *URINARY TRACT INFEC-TION.*

PYLORIC STENOSIS
The pylorus is the exit passage of the stomach: the pyloric sphincter is a ring of muscle which closes off the stomach until the stomach contents have been liquefied and are ready to pass out into the intestine. In some babies (usually boys) between three and eight weeks of age, the ring of muscle grows too fast, becomes very tight (stenosed), and cannot open up properly.

▓ SYMPTOMS Because of the build-up of pressure in the stomach after a feeding, milk that cannot pass into the intestine is vomited. As the condition progresses, the vomiting becomes more frequent and more forceful – projectile vomiting is characteristic (the milk will project one or two feet out of the mouth, often out of the baby's crib and on to the floor). The baby does not absorb enough fluid from the intestine because of the blockage, and may become DEHYDRATED.

▓ TREATMENT The doctor can usually make the diagnosis by examining the baby during a feeding and feeling the enlarged pyloric muscle through the abdominal wall. In that case, hospital admission will be recommended for an operation.

▓ OUTLOOK The wound usually heals up well and the baby is able to feed normally soon afterwards.

QUARANTINE
See *INCUBATION PERIOD.*

QUINSY
See *TONSILLITIS.*

R

RABIES

Rabies VIRUS is endemic in some parts of North America. Skunks, bats, foxes, raccoons and woodchucks are the most commonly infected wild animals. Rabies also occurs in unimmunized domestic dogs and cats. The virus is present in the saliva of the infected animal and is transmitted by bites or licking of open wounds, the eye or mouth. The INCUBATION PERIOD is usually nine days to more than one year, but averages two months. In rabies-endemic areas children must be taught *not* to touch or pet wild animals. All contact with strange animals, including household pets should be avoided. Household pets should be immunized. Animal immunization programs are the major weapon in preventing rabies spread.

■ ACTION If a child is bitten by a suspect animal, clean the wound with soap and water. Take the child to the hospital emergency department.

A suspect dog or cat that has bitten a human should be captured, confined and observed by a veterinarian for ten days. If the animal displays no symptoms of rabies in that time, it is unlikely to be infected. In some municipalities the police may help you locate and contain the suspect animal. Since clinical signs of rabies in a wild animal are hard to interpret, a suspect wild animal should be killed at once, and the brain examined for rabies.

■ TREATMENT In high-risk cases, both human rabies immunoglobulin and rabies vaccine are given. One half of the rabies immunoglobulin is injected into the wound, the rest is injected intravenously. Five doses of rabies vaccine are given by injection one each on days 1, 3, 7, 14 and 28. This can prevent the disease from developing. Early treatment and immunization after a bite from a suspect animal are crucial.

■ OUTLOOK Once symptoms appear, the infection is almost invariably fatal. Among other problems, the virus causes muscle spasms, which prevent drinking and swallowing, and paralyze the muscles used in breathing.

RASH

A very vague term applied to almost any skin irritation or eruption.

Doctors diagnose rashes mainly by recognizing their appearance and distribution on the body, a skill which most parents are unlikely to possess. However, certain rashes do have a highly characteristic appearance and can be easily recognized by parents. CHICKEN POX, once seen, is unmistakable, as is URTICARIA.

■ ACTION Unless you are certain that you recognize the rash, and also that your child is not ill in any other way, you should get medical advice for any unexplained skin rash. If the child is unwell, this is essential.

One rash, for example, requires urgent action: the purpura rash of MENINGITIS. If a child becomes ill, feverish, and develops a faint rash of tiny dark red spots, which may become larger, meningococcal meningitis is a possible cause (see *MENINGITIS*). Take the child to a doctor immediately.

For further information see specific entries – *DIAPER RASH, ECZEMA, URTICARIA, DERMATITIS, MEASLES, CHICKENPOX, RUBELLA.*

RECOVERY POSITION
See *page 234.*

RECTAL PROLAPSE
A rare condition in the United States that may occur with MALNUTRITION and occasionally in CYSTIC FIBROSIS, and very rarely with bowel PARASITES. Pressure in the rectum causes a protrusion of bowel from the anus.

■ SYMPTOMS The protruding bowel looks red and moist. Parents are likely to be alerted to the problem if the prolapse causes discomfort when passing stools.

■ IMMEDIATE ACTION An icepack made from crushed ice placed in a small plastic bag will reduce soreness, while getting medical advice. If due to malnutrition or cystic fibrosis, these conditions need to be treated or rectal relapse may recur. If parasites are suspected, your doctor may ask for a stool specimen. Parasite infestations can be eliminated by appropriate medication.

RECURRENT ABDOMINAL PAIN
Some children have bouts of abdominal pain that seem to recur again and

again. Sometimes there is an apparent pattern of events that lead to the onset of the pain – perhaps at the beginning of the school year or just before exams. Usually, however, there is no such obvious pattern. Parents sometimes worry that each episode is APPENDICITIS. There may be associated NAUSEA and pallor, but the abdomen is not particularly tender and there are no signs of PERITONITIS.

■ CAUSE There seems to be a link in some cases with STRESS, although there may not be any obvious signs of ANXIETY. Discussing the pattern of episodes may help the child and family understand that the pain functions as a stress signal and is not a sign of a serious abdominal problem. Muscles in the bowel may well be contracting in response to tension. In other cases, recurrent abdominal pain may sometimes by due to increased gas being produced in the intestines.

■ ACTION If the episodes seem stress-related and if the family can recognize the pattern, there will be less anxiety and efforts can be made to cope with any underlying problems. The individual bout of pain may be helped by acetamenophen, and rest and reassurance, and it invariably disappears within a couple of days. A visit and discussion with your doctor may be helpful and reassuring.

For children with no obvious stress-inducing factors, a trial of increasing fluids and fiber in the diet may be helpful. Many children outgrow their recurrent abdominal pain episodes, although some may have an irritable colon as adults.

See also *PUBERTY* for recurrent lower abdominal pain before and during periods; also pain at ovulation time.

RECOVERY POSITION

A vital, basic element of first-aid. Putting an unconscious child (who is breathing and who has a heartbeat) in this position ensures that the airway to the lungs is kept open, that the tongue cannot fall back into the throat (so obstructing it) and that vomitus can drain easily from the mouth. However, don't attempt to move a child with neck or back injuries into the recovery (or any other) position without professional help. In this case, the patient should be lying flat on his back and the airway should be kept open in this position.

RECOVERY POSITION

1 *Open airway: see EMERGENCY RESUSCITATION.*
2 *Place the child's arm by his side, then lift his near buttock and place the hand underneath, fingers straight. Grasp the*

far leg behind the knee and cross it over the near leg; move the far arm across the chest as shown in **3**.
3 *Support the child's head as shown, and with the other hand get a grip on his clothing in the vicinity of the far hip. Pull the child's whole body towards you, supporting him while temporarily on his side against your chest.*

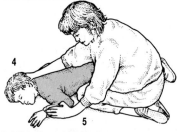

4 *Adjust head once more as shown, jaw forward, to ensure airway is still open. Still support the body against your knees.*
5 *Bend arm as shown.*

6 *Bend knee.*
7 *Pull other arm from under the child. Leave it as shown.*
8 *No more than half the chest should be left in contact with the ground. Finally check that the casualty's resting position is stable – one purpose of the recovery position is to prevent him from rolling.*

RENAL FAILURE

The point at which health deteriorates as a result of chemical inbalance in the body produced by poor kidney function. It may occur rapidly, or gradually over a number of years. Rare in children.

▨ SYMPTOMS The child feels ill, has a poor appetite and passes less urine than normal. He may also become ANEMIC, develop RICKETS and have high BLOOD PRESSURE. Growth is affected if kidney failure progresses slowly over many months or years.

▨ MANAGEMENT A child with kidney failure will be given a special diet low in protein (but high in other energy sources) and low in salt and phosphorus. His fluid intake will be regulated as excess fluid cannot be filtered out by the kidneys. Drugs may be necessary to treat the high blood pressure. He may require blood transfusions for anemia.

Eventually kidney failure will require dialysis to keep the chemistry of the body in equilibrium. Most children would then be placed on a waiting list for a suitable donor for kidney transplantation.

▨ DIALYSIS A means of carrying out the filtering work of the kidneys. There are two methods – hemodialysis and peritoneal dialysis. In hemodialysis, blood is led from an artery

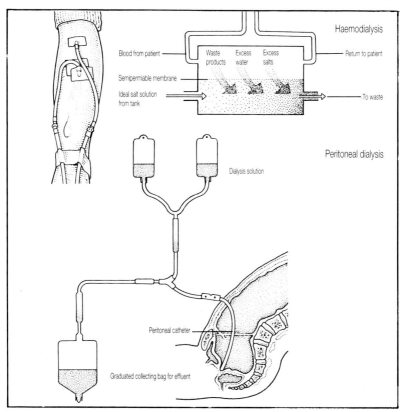

Haemodialysis

Blood from patient

Waste products | Excess water | Excess salts

Return to patient

Semipermiable membrane

Ideal salt solution from tank

To waste

Peritoneal dialysis

Dialysis solution

Peritoneal catheter

Graduated collecting bag for effluent

in the arm via a piece of fine tubing to the kidney machine where the waste products are removed; the filtered blood is then directed back through another tube to a vein in the arm. This treatment is usually needed for a period of several hours two to three times a week. In peritoneal dialysis, a tube is inserted into the abdomen and a special fluid allowed to run in. The fluid flows over the peritoneum, the lining that covers the bowels and major abdominal organs. The waste products in the blood cross the peritoneal membrane into the fluid, which is then allowed to slowly drain out of the abdomen. This cycling of the fluid is repeated until the chemical balance of the body is improved. It can be performed overnight or during the day when the dialysis system is arranged so as to allow the child to be up and moving about.

■ KIDNEY TRANSPLANT Replacement of a non- or very poorly functioning kidney by a healthy one. The healthy kidney may be donated by a living person (usually related to the child) or may come from someone who has recently died. The diseased and the donated kidneys are carefully matched for tissue type to minimize the risk of rejection. Steroids and drugs that suppress the immune system are also given to help prevent rejection.

In recent years the success of renal transplantation has been dramatic. About three-quarters of transplants are completely successful, and are being undertaken at progressively younger ages (vital for those babies born with untreatable damaged or malformed kidneys).

RESPIRATORY DISTRESS SYNDROME (RDS)

A breathing difficulty of PREMATURE babies caused by lack of surfactant, a chemical that coats the lung surface, preventing collapse of the small airways of the lungs. Surfactant does not appear in the fetal lungs until around 28 weeks of pregnancy, and RDS affects 70 to 80 percent of babies born at, or before, this time. (See also *PREMATURITY*.) The incidence and severity of RDS decreases with maturity at birth, so that only 10 percent of babies born around 34 weeks of pregnancy will develop RDS. It is very rare in full-term babies.

■ CAUSES Prematurity is the major cause. Put another way, immaturity of the lungs is a component of the general immaturity that characterizes the premature baby. However, RDS may occur in full-term babies who suffer BIRTH ASPHYXIA or HYPOTHERMIA, although in many such cases the picture does not simply result from surfactant deficiency.

■ SIGNS Within the first hours following birth, the baby will have breathing difficulties: he will breathe rapidly, his chest will be drawn in and he will make grunting noises while breathing in and out. However, these signs can occur in conditions other than surfactant deficiency such as MECONIUM aspiration, PNEUMONIA or CONGENITAL HEART-DISEASE. A chest X-ray helps to determine the reason a particular baby is experiencing distress with his breathing.

■ TREATMENT is aimed at keeping the premature baby alive and well until he starts to make his own surfactant. This often begins 48 to 72 hours after birth. Recently surfactant extracted from calf's lungs and artificially manufactured surfactant have proven effective in treating

RDS when they are instilled under pressure into the baby's airways.

Babies with RDS receive INTENSIVE CARE. The oxygen level in their blood is measured at regular intervals by BLOOD TESTS or by the continuous use of a skin monitor, or of an umbilical catheter (a small tube inserted in the artery of the UMBILICUS). If the level drops, oxygen is given either by enriching the air of the INCUBATOR or by ventilation. The latter involves placing a tube through the baby's nose or mouth into the trachea (the upper air passage). The tube is then connected to a ventilator (breathing machine), that takes over the work of breathing. Over the following days, most babies recover sufficiently to breathe without the ventilator. The smallest and sickest babies may, however, require weeks of assisted ventilation. During the course of intensive care, all body systems receive support: regulation of the body's temperature; PHOTOTHERAPY for jaundice; fluid regulation; feeding by tube into the stomach; and many other details of care including stimulation and maximal contact of the baby with his parents.

▧ COMPLICATIONS may arise with ventilation. These include lung collapse, leakage of air from the lung into the chest cavity (pneumothorax), PNEUMONIA and chronic oxygen dependency. Very high concentrations of oxygen can damage the retina of the eye, but this can usually be prevented by monitoring the blood's oxygen level. Some babies with severe RDS need long-term ventilation.

▧ OUTLOOK Babies whose lungs are not damaged will grow to be healthy, and even those with the most severe lung damage usually recover from breathing difficulties by the time they are 12 to 18 months old.

REYE SYNDROME

Severe VOMITING, FEVER, confusion and CONVULSIONS following a VIRAL INFECTION such as INFLUENZA and CHICKEN POX or other viral illness. This is a rare condition. In some cases it has been shown to be related to a child taking aspirin. For this reason, never give aspirin or medication containing aspirin to a child or adolescent. Use acetamenophen instead for pain and fever. The number of cases of Reye syndrome in the United States has fallen with the decrease in the use of aspirin by children but cases still occur.

▧ ACTION If Reye syndrome is suspected, the child must be urgently admitted to the hospital for treatment.

▧ INVESTIGATIONS Blood glucose is usually low. Other BLOOD TESTS will also be needed to confirm the diagnosis.

▧ TREATMENT Correction of fluid imbalance. Treatment of convulsions and raised pressure in the brain. Artificial ventilation, management of liver failure and correction of clotting problems will be the priorities. Patients are severely ill and should be managed in an intensive care unit.

▧ OUTLOOK may be fatal, but full recovery is possible. After five to seven days, rapid improvement in liver and brain function is usually seen in surviving patients.

RH INCOMPATIBILITY

Destruction of a new-born baby's red blood cells (erythrocytes) that occurs when the baby is Rh positive and the mother Rh negative. The technical term for the condition is *Erythroblastosis fetalis*.

Most people have the Rh ANTIGEN on the surface of their red blood cells: they are Rh positive. Those who don't have this antigen are Rh negative. During pregnancy some fetal red blood cells cross the placenta. If the mother is Rh negative, exposure to the antigen results in sensitization and the production of anti-Rh ANTIBODIES. If it is a first pregnancy, the effects may be insignificant. However, in subsequent pregnancies, if the fetus is Rh positive, the mother's immune response is more vigorous. Her antibodies cross the placenta, and destroy the fetal red blood cells. If severe, this will result in fetal anemia and EDEMA; and after the baby is born, severe jaundice that results from the release of hemoglobin and its break-down product, bilirubin, from the destroyed red blood cells. Jaundice does not occur in the uterus because the placenta filters the bilirubin from the fetal blood.

■ PREVENTION AND TREAT-MENT If the mother has not developed any Rh antibodies, then the destruction of the baby's red blood cells can be prevented. The mother is given a substance called Rhogam immediately after birth that destroys the Rh positive cells in her blood (the fetal cells that would otherwise sensitize the mother's immune system, and that cross into the mother's circulation in large numbers at the time of delivery), and hence prevents the development of antibodies that would cause problems in the next pregnancy. All mothers who are Rh negative should be given Rhogam after delivery. If the mother has already developed antibodies, then the baby may be deliberately delivered prematurely

to avoid excessive destruction of his red blood cells.

This same process can also occur when the fetus' blood type is A, B or AB and the mother is type O (A-O, B-O and AB-O incompatibility), or when the fetus is type A and the mother type B, or vice versa (A-B and B-A incompatibilities). These incompatibilities are much less common than Rh incompatibility and are less apt to cause serious difficulties.

RHEUMATIC FEVER
A disease common in developed countries. Its occurrence in the United States has decreased for several decades, but recent outbreaks in some parts indicate that it is still a problem. It is caused by the same *Streptococcus* BACTERIUM that causes SCARLET FEVER, bacterial TONSILLITIS and SORE THROAT. It occurs mainly in schoolchildren and causes ARTHRITIS, FEVER, abnormal movements (CHOREA) and/or inflammation of the heart. It can have the unwelcome long-term effect of HEART-DISEASE by damaging the heart valves.

■ TREATMENT is aimed at quieting the inflammation with corticosteroids and aspirin. This is usually done in hospital with careful monitoring of the blood salicylate (aspirin) levels. Bedrest is recommended for three weeks if there is no heart involvement, and longer if there is.

The long-term outlook depends upon the severity of the heart involvement.

If a child has had an episode of rheumatic fever, he should be given the ANTIBIOTIC penicillin regularly for several years in order to prevent a recurrence, which can further damage the heart. If he has heart problems as a result of the illness, he will always need the protection of antibiotics when having a tooth out, and indeed if undergoing any other operation, in order to prevent further heart complications.

RHEUMATOID ARTHRITIS
See *JUVENILE RHEUMATOID ARTHRITIS.*

RICKETS
A curable disease of bone, due to a disturbance in the way calcium is deposited in bone. This is a process requiring vitamin D, which is formed in the skin when the skin is exposed to sunlight. This is now a rare problem in the United States: all milk is fortified with vitamin D.

■ SYMPTOMS Bone pain, BOW LEGS, weakness and possibly other signs of VITAMIN DEFICIENCIES.

■ TREATMENT Vitamin D is taken for several months. An excess of vitamin D can be harmful so give only as directed by your doctor.

ROSEOLA INFANTUM
A relatively common INFECTION caused by human herpes VIRUS type 6 which affects children between six months and two years of age. The INCUBATION PERIOD is about ten days.

■ SYMPTOMS There is a sudden onset of high FEVER; FEBRILE CONVULSIONS can occur. This lasts for three to five days and the temperature then returns to normal, whereupon a fine, pink rash spreads rapidly over the body within a few hours.

■ ACTION The fever is the only real problem, and this should be treated with tepid baths and acetamenophen. Some parents mistake the infection for measles. In the case of *Roseola*, the temperature returns to normal when the rash appears and the child looks and feels much better, whereas with measles the fever continues after the rash appears.

■ OUTLOOK The child always recovers fully.

ROUNDWORM
See *FUNGI AND FUNGAL INFECTIONS.*

RUBELLA
A VIRAL INFECTION, also known as German measles. This infection is now uncommon in the United States because of the high rate of IMMUNIZATION in childhood.

The INCUBATION PERIOD is 14-21 days. A child can pass on the infection during the week before he becomes ill, and remains infectious for up to five days after the rash has appeared.

■ SYMPTOMS The illness starts with a rash consisting of fine pink spots on the face and trunk that gradually merge and last three to five days. The lymph glands at the back of the scalp and behind the ears usually enlarge. They are seldom painful, but are easily felt. There may be slight FEVER, a runny nose, CONJUNCTIVITIS and a general feeling of being unwell.

In young children, the symptoms are often so mild that the diagnosis is never made. Other viral infections can give a similar picture, so the diagnosis is often difficult to make with certainty.

In adolescents and adults, the symptoms tend to be more severe and can be followed by pain and swelling of the joints, which usually lasts for a week or two.

■ ACTION There is no specific treatment, but the fever should be treated with an analgesic such as acetamenophen and a tepid bath if necessary.

If the joint pains are severe, aspirin will help but it should not be used in children because of the risk of REYE SYNDROME.

The child with *Rubella* should avoid contact with pregnant women who are not immune to *Rubella*, since infection of the fetus in early pregnancy can cause CONGENITAL RUBELLA SYNDROME. Children who have been recently immunized against *Rubella* cannot transmit it.

■ PREVENTION Immunization is offered as part of MEASLES, MUMPS and *Rubella* immunization, given at about 15 months of age. This vaccine is very effective in preventing *Rubella*. Its widespread use has resulted in a major decline of cases of *Rubella* in the United States, and an almost complete disappearance of the congenital *Rubella* syndrome. Prior to getting pregnant, all women should have a BLOOD TEST to determine whether they are immune to *Rubella*. If they are not, they should be given the *Rubella* vaccine.

■ OUTLOOK The joint symptoms do not cause permanent disability. Long-term complications are rare, although ENCEPHALITIS has been recorded in association with *Rubella*.

RUPTURE
See *HERNIAS*.

S

SALT IN THE DIET
Salt intake is a health issue for adults, largely because of its apparent association with high BLOOD PRESSURE. However, for healthy children, salt should be considered a normal and essential dietary ingredient. Salt loss and dehydration may occur in hot weather, or through excessive sweating, vomiting or diarrhea leading to weakness and lethargy.

However, in light of current views on the long-term relationship between excessive salt intake and adult health, it is prudent to discourage children from regularly adding salt to all their food.

SCABIES
An itchy skin eruption due to infestation with the mite *Sarcoptes scabei*.

■ CAUSE The tiny mite, hardly visible to the naked eye, is transmitted by close personal contact with an affected person. It then burrows into the new host's skin. Once installed, the female lays eggs, leaving a track, or burrow, in the skin, which may be visible as a white tortuous thread-like line. The invasion causes an allergic reaction, resulting in red raised itchy swellings.

■ SYMPTOMS Itching, worse at night, and thickening of the skin as a result of constant scratching. Common sites for the lesions are between the fingers, the inside of wrists, the elbows, the genital area and the arms and feet generally. Close contacts (typically of mothers and babies) need to be examined and treated. Secondary INFECTION of the infected site may cause IMPETIGO.

■ ACTION Effective treatment is easily obtained at the drugstore. Your doctor should be consulted if you suspect scabies infection in your baby.

■ TREATMENT Infected children over the age of two years should bathe, dry, and then apply lotions or creams containing lindane or crotamiton over the entire body below the head. Because scabies can affect the head, scalp and neck in young children, treatement of the entire body is required. The medication should be removed by bathing after eight to 12 hours for lindane, or 24 hours for crotamiton. For children less than two years, lindane should be used cautiously. Sulfur ointments applied for three consecutive nights are an alternative. Permethrin is also effective. Each member of the household – parents and children – should be treated at the same time. Wash all clothing and bedding used by the child (or other affected family members) in a washer using hot water and a hot drying cycle. Clothing that cannot be laundered should be removed and stored away from people for several days to a week.

■ OUTLOOK Correct treatment as described should eliminate the scabies infection; however, itching can persist for up to a week. Scabies can return of course, even after treatment, if contact with an affected person recurs.

SCALDS
See *BURNS*.

SCAR
A mark on any part of the body, internal or external, where repair of an injury has occurred.

■ CAUSE Scar tissue is the growth of firm, fibrous material which joins together separated tissue, typically after a cut. The scientific term for the fibrous material is collagen, and it is also found in ligaments and tendons. Any injury or cut can lead to scar formation, but the more ragged the cut, the more extensive the scar. An infected or dirty cut will produce more scar tissue than a clean one, while a widely gaping wound on the skin will produce a bigger scar than a tightly closed wound. Cuts in the skin are thus stitched to give as slender a scar as possible.

Burns to the skin also cause scarring over wide areas where scar tissue entirely replaces the lost skin. For this reason, skin grafts are applied to areas of full thickness burn, and special dressings used to reduce scar formation.

A keloid is a scar on the skin which has become very prominent, and may need special treatment by a plastic surgeon. Keloid scars occur more commonly in dark-skinned people than in whites.

■ ACTION To minimize scarring, cuts should be cleaned to remove all dirt and grit (see *CUTS AND GRAZES*). If the skin edges are separated, they should be brought together either by special band-aids or by sutures (stitches). Stitching is usually performed by a doctor or in the emergency department of a hospital.

■ TREATMENT If a scar is unsightly, it may be possible to improve it by plastic surgery: your doctor can advise.

■ OUTLOOK Scars tend to fade with time, and to become smaller. They are usually red at first, but gradually turn white, usually within a year. Permanent scars on the face can be well hidden by special masking creams. Ask your doctor about them.

SCHIZOPHRENIA

A rare illness of adolescents (and adults), almost unknown in younger age groups.

■ CAUSES Onset is often gradual and intermittent. The adolescent loses interest in school work and withdraws from friends, seems to lose touch with reality, and may become preoccupied with unusual ideas. You may notice mood swings that exceed what you would expect for his age. Sometimes the illness appears suddenly (typically at an obviously stressful time) with HALLUCINATIONS and inexplicable behavior. See *PSYCHOSIS*.

■ ACTION Your doctor will recog-

nize the possibility of schizophrenia, and refer your child to a child psychiatrist.

■ TREATMENT Hospital admission may be recommended and treatment with major tranquillizer drugs (chlorpromazine is the commonest, but there are many). Psychotherapy may also be used. The family will need advice to cope with what is often a relapsing illness. Most adolescents recover sufficiently to return to a normal school and friendships after treatment. However, the long-term outlook is variable and, in some cases, gloomy.

SCHOOL ATTENDANCE PROBLEMS OR SCHOOL PHOBIA

Attending school for the first time, or changing school, is an ordeal for some children. For the nervous child, it may require special preparation: stress the enjoyable parts of school life; emphasize that you will be looking forward to his return each day.

Reluctance to go to school may be expressed directly or take the form of 'symptoms' such as headaches, feeling sick or having a stomach ache just before it is time to leave for school. These are symptoms the child is no doubt experiencing, but which disappear once it is clear that he can stay off school. Sometimes what starts as a genuine physical illness may seem to linger on – see *ANXIETY, STRESS SYMPTOMS*. This may indicate that something is worrying your child at school; it can also be due to changes or worries at home: Is someone ill? Are there other FAMILY PROBLEMS?

■ ACTION Talk to your child and his teacher; deal with anything in the school routine that your child identifies as worrying.

If the worry is about you or something at home, try to ease his anxieties; but remain consistent and firm (but not unkind) in presenting school attendance as the norm.

Problems may re-surface after a holiday break or an illness; the routine of going to school needs to be re-established as quickly as possible.

If reluctance to attend school is accompanied by major distress or continues for more than a week or two, investigate, with his teacher, whether there are specific difficulties at school such as LEARNING DISORDERS, bullying in the school playground or teasing in class.

If the problem continues, talk to your doctor, who may suggest seeing a pediatrician, clinical psychologist or a child psychiatrist.

SCHOOL MEDICAL INFORMATION

Many schools ask parents to complete a questionnaire concerning their child's health at school registration. Some districts have strict immunization requirements and parents must show proof that the child is up-to-date with his shots at the time of registration. If your child has a serious medical problem such as heart-disease, epilepsy, cystic fibrosis or bad asthma, review with your doctor what is medically important to tell the school about your child's condition. The school will want to know about activity restrictions, medications, special diets and what to do in an emergency and who to call. Your doctor or clinic may have pamphlets about the disease, which may help you explain the problems to your child's teacher and/or principal.

SCOLIOSIS

Abnormal curvature of any part of the spine. It can be caused by any problem with the bones of the spine (the vertebrae), or the muscles designed to support the spine equally on either side. But sometimes no cause is found.

Scoliosis is most common in childhood. Doctors usually monitor children with scoliosis for several years as the curve may or may not worsen with time. It may become more severe during periods of rapid growth, and stop progressing when growth ceases.

■ SYMPTOMS Deformity is usually the only symptom in childhood. The condition can however cause pain at a later stage because of long-standing structural strain. Scoliosis can occur in young children, but it usually appears for the first time at ten to 12 years. Sometimes it is discovered during a routine physical examination.

■ ACTION If you think that your child may have scoliosis, get medical advice. Your doctor may suggest that the child see an orthopedic surgeon. This does not necessarily mean that the child will need an operation.

Scoliosis in the lower part of the spine is usually not particularly severe, but may be more problematic if it affects the spine in the region of the chest.

■ TESTS X-rays will reveal the degree of scoliosis, and may help to detect the cause. They are also essential, at regular intervals, to monitor progress.

■ TREATMENT depends on many factors:

If the scoliosis is mild, no active treatment may be necessary. Examinations and X-rays done every six to 12 months indicate whether there is any change that requires treatment.

A brace may be fitted to keep the spine as straight as possible.

Sometimes an operation is suggested. Various types are available, but the common aim is to stabilize the spine in the best possible position and prevent further curvature of the spine.

▇ OUTLOOK depends on the cause and on the treatment.

SCURVY

Caused by a deficiency of vitamin C in the diet. This is very rare in developed countries. Vitamin C is present in most fruit and vegetables, including potatoes, but is partly destroyed by cooking. Symptoms include bleeding gums and slow healing of skin after cuts and bruises. See *VITAMINS*.

SEAT BELTS

Research has clearly shown that seat belts and proper infant/child car seats save lives and minimize injuries in an automobile accident.

For babies, birth to nine months The rear-facing baby car seat is a toughly constructed, padded, semi-reclining seat, held in place by an adult seat belt. Use of these seats is required by law in all states. They can be used as a reclining seat outside the car. Other

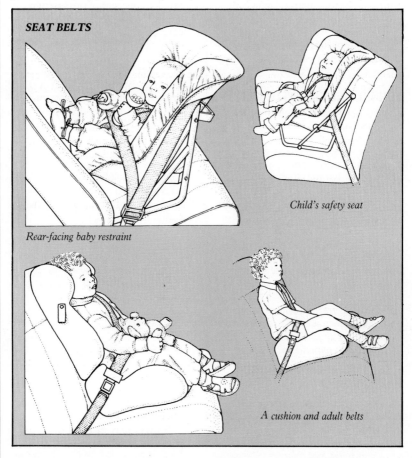

SEAT BELTS

Rear-facing baby restraint

Child's safety seat

A cushion and adult belts

variants of the car seat for babies are currently being evaluated and introduced to the market. Ensure that you select a model that bears the seal of approval by the American Academy of Pediatrics, 'Make Every Ride a Safe Ride', and install it correctly. Some hospitals have loan systems for baby car seats allowing you to rent one at minimal cost. Ask your doctor.

For young children, six months to four years As soon as a child can sit up he can, in principle, use a child's safety seat. These usually have two shoulder and two hip straps and also a strap between the legs, giving a comprehensive support. Follow fitting instructions carefully.

Older children, four years onwards, can use adult seat belts in the back seat, with booster seats until the seat belts fit correctly. A correctly fitting belt puts pressure on one shoulder and over both hips; the belt should not ride up on to the abdomen. If children use an adult seat belt without a booster seat, the belt could compress the abdomen on impact, and damage the liver and spleen.

Child safety harness also needs a booster seat. Child/adult adjustable seat belt not as satisfactory – and still needs a booster seat.

All passengers in front and back seats should wear a form of restraint or seat belt at all times. This is required by law in most states.

SEPARATION ANXIETY

The normal reaction of babies and young children when separated from parents or other persons with whom they are familiar. Before about seven months, babies allow themselves readily to be held and cuddled by strangers. They then become gradually unsure of anyone new or unfamiliar, and will cry and protest if picked up by them.

As mobility increases, the toddler shows separation anxiety by playing close to their parents or friends if in a strange place, or protesting vigorously if left at a new babysitter's or day care. He has not yet understood that you are going to return. It is natural for him to be angry with you if he has to be left unexpectedly with strangers for a few hours; but short periods of separation will not damage him. Most infants and toddlers adjust quite quickly to a new babysitter or day care provided the care is consistent, loving and stimulating. Parents may upset the development of this new caregiver relationship by overstressing the problem, lingering too long when dropping the child off and always being available to 'rescue' the child if he becomes 'too upset'. For those children not in day care, well-judged, regular opportunities in the first few years to spend periods of time away from parents are beneficial for most children. Some preschool children adapt more readily to separation than others: it is a matter of temperament, development, parental anxiety, skill and luck.

However, by three years, most children cope with strange places and strange people for short periods, given some encouragement.

All children regress in their behavior – go back to behaving younger than their age – if upset by new situations such as the arrival of a new sibling, starting at a new day care or babysitter's or being admitted to the hospital. This should resolve in a short time with firm loving support for the child.

If separation anxiety is a major problem for your toddler or preschooler, discuss this with your doctor.

SEX EDUCATION

A subject that worries most parents. But in order to grow up safely, your child will need to know facts about his body, the names used for sexual parts of it and how these relate to sexual feelings and relationships.

He needs this knowledge in the same way he needs to know about roads and traffic for his own safety. In both cases, what he needs to know changes as he grows. There will be many opportunities to explain the facts in increasing detail as he grows up.

■ A PARENT'S ROLE Facts which *you* give your child have the advantage of being communicated in words which you choose, and of being accompanied by your beliefs and attitudes. This will not be true of playground conversations. If you have talked openly with your child he will be more comfortable coming back to you to discuss what he learns from sex education and family living classes at school, as well as from playground talk.

Studies of children and adolescents have shown that they prefer sex education from their family, provided the information is accurate and relatively complete for their age. Since more than 30 percent of 9th-graders are sexually active, do *not* wait too long.

There is no evidence that if parents have explained sexual reproduction and feelings to their child, he is more likely to experiment than others who know nothing. If anything, a child who has accurate information will be *less* at risk of pregnancy, sexually transmitted disease or even SEXUAL ABUSE. He is less likely to be sexually active by 'accident'.

Of course, you will tailor what you say to your child's level of development; he will not understand or remember what is beyond him. There are books that help to explain all aspects of the body's working.

These can also give the parent a useful idea of the language and ideas a child can understand at different ages. When (or before) your child reaches puberty, he may also appreciate an up-to-date book to read for himself. Your library or local bookstore have a good selection. The books are no substitute for explaining your own views, but can make it easier. You may also find help in dealing with these topics from your local school or community health center. See *SEXUALITY, PUBERTY, MASTURBATION, PERIOD PROBLEMS.*

SEXUAL ABUSE

In the United States, this term includes the legal offences of incest, unlawful sexual intercourse and indecent assault, together with other forms of inappropriate sexual activities between adults and children, including the practices of fondling and flashing and the involvement of children in producing pornography.

■ INCIDENCE Surveys of adults have shown that between 10 and 25 percent were sexually abused to some degree during their childhoods. Sexual abuse is actually diagnosed in less than one child per 1,000 each year. Abusers are far more likely to be family members or close family contacts than strangers.

■ SYMPTOMS and signs that might suggest the possibility of sexual abuse include: inappropriate flirtatious behavior (for the age of the child); infection of the sexual organs with organisms normally sexually transmitted, such as gonorrhea and chlamydia; unexplained abdominal pain; sudden unexplained changes in behavior; unexplained problems at school and truancy; depression or withdrawal; 'clingy' behavior in young children; low self-esteem and feelings of worthlessness in older children; bedwetting or soiling if accompanied by other symptoms; attempted suicide or self-injury.

■ OTHER SIGNS Any evidence of injury in a child, which cannot be explained, should lead to questioning about physical or sexual abuse.

■ ACTION If any adult suspects that sexual abuse may be happening, he or she should seek help from a doctor, or a social worker. *Above all, tell someone.* Sexual abuse that is kept a secret continues to occur and to harm the child.

■ INVESTIGATION Once an allegation of sexual abuse is made, public health professionals will interview the child and others involved, and will decide what is best for the child's safety. This might involve admitting the child to the hospital for a while. However, if the person alleged to be responsible for the abuse is not in the family home, investigations will be carried out without removing the child from home. The police will be involved if there are grounds for suspecting that a criminal offense has been committed. Medical examination of a sexually abused child should take place in a pleasant room (usually not available in a police station) by doctors specially trained in child care and in legal (forensic) medicine.

■ OUTLOOK The sad truth, borne out by long-term studies, is that sexual abuse in childhood causes long-term emotional problems. It is possible that more active counselling at the time of the abuse may help to lessen this. As the taboo on speaking about sexual abuse is lifted, more

adults may be able to seek professional help in dealing with their psychological problems caused by childhood sexual abuse; and help with the psychological problems that result in their inclination to abuse children.

■ PREVENTION Increasing emphasis is placed on educating children to say "No" to behavior that feels uncomfortable or wrong. Many schools have programs, starting in the elementary grades to teach this approach.

■ FURTHER READING *No More Secrets for Me* by Oralee Wachter (published by Penguin) is a sensitive study. Your library should have several helpful books on the subject. If you have discussed sexuality with your child from a young age, he may feel more comfortable coming to you if there is a problem in this area.

SEXUALITY
See *PUBERTY, MASTURBATION.*

SHINGLES
See *CHICKEN POX.*

SHOCK
As a medical term this denotes the effects of the circulation system failing to deliver blood and oxygen to all parts of the body effectively. It occurs after: severe blood loss; excessive fluid loss, as in prolonged VOMITING or severe BURNS; overwhelming INFECTION, some insect stings; and some forms of HEART-DISEASE.

■ SYMPTOMS A child with shock is pale, cold, sweaty and anxious, with a fast pulse and possibly rapid breathing. He may also complain of thirst, feel sick or lapse into unconsciousness.

■ IMMEDIATE ACTION Call an ambulance, or ask someone else to do so; place the child flat on his back; stop any bleeding with firm pressure; and, if necessary, start EMERGENCY RESUSCITATION without delay. If it seems likely that the child will need an ANESTHETIC in hospital, withhold drinks and food.

■ TREATMENT in hospital: Oxygen, intravenous fluid and/or blood will be given, along with appropriate drugs. The cause of shock will be treated.

SHORT STATURE

There are many causes of a child being significantly short in height, including congenital short stature. This is the most common cause. Short stature runs in some families. Rarer causes include:

– Deficiency of various hormones, but typically those produced by the thyroid, adrenal and pituitary glands.
– Chromosomal abnormalities such as TURNER SYNDROME.
– Chronic illness such as severe HEART, kidney (see *RENAL FAILURE*) or liver disease.
– Disorders of bone development such as ACHONDROPLASIA.
– Steroid treatment for diseases such as JUVENILE RHEUMATOID ARTHRITIS.

■ SYMPTOMS will depend on the cause of the problem. See the separate entries mentioned above. If there is a problem it may well be recognized during a routine physical examination.

■ ACTION If you think that your child is significantly shorter than all the other children you know of a similar age, get medical advice. Your doctor will examine your child and accurately measure his height. This is then entered on a percentile chart, which gives the average height and weight for every age and for both sexes.

The doctor will want to know the exact height of both parents, and to get some idea of whether there are many short people in the family.

If there is no obvious medical problem, and if the members of the family are short (in particular the parents) the doctor may decide simply to watch your child's growth to see if it increases at the normal rate. Charts are available (based on the parents' height and the child's current height), which will predict the height that the child is likely to reach as an adult.

If there is any possibility of a medical problem, tests may be necessary, performed either by your doctor or by a pediatric endocrinologist.

■ TESTS include X-rays of the bones to discover the child's 'bone age'. This shows how the bones are maturing and can help with diagnosis; BLOOD TESTS to measure hormone levels and to detect CHROMOSOMAL abnormalities; investigations for kidney or liver problems, and also for MALABSORPTION.

■ TREATMENT depends on the cause – see the separate entries mentioned above.

If your child has a hormonal problem, treatment is usually available to replace hormones that are lacking.

Until recently, there has been no effective treatment for children who are 'normal' but short, and for those with chromosomal or genetic abnormalities such as Turner syndrome or achondroplasia. There is experimental evidence that daily injections with growth hormone can increase the height to the normal range, but there are also convincing arguments against increasing a child's height for purely cosmetic and psychological reasons. The treatment is not routinely available and is expensive. Furthermore, an excess of growth hormone may increase the possibility of developing diabetes.

■ OUTLOOK Many short children will eventually reach an adult height that is within the normal range. For those who do not, developing a positive self-image is essential.

The pros and cons of intervening with growth hormone must be carefully assessed for each case.

SHORTSIGHTEDNESS (MYOPIA)
When the eye sees distant objects as blurred and near objects clearly. This may be due to the globe of the eye being 'longer' than it ought to be or the lens or cornea bending the rays of light too much.

You may suspect your child is shortsighted if he sits close to the T.V., holds books close to his eyes, or complains of not being able to see the blackboard at school. The problem can be corrected by EYE GLASSES, which are fitted after an EYE TEST.

Because vision changes with age, regular eye tests are important.

SHYNESS
This can be worrying or infuriating, and it rarely responds to reprimand or coaxing. Often best ignored unless it interferes with new activities, or making friends; or suddenly worsens and becomes incapacitating. In these cases, talk to your child's teacher or your doctor. See also FEARS, PHOBIAS.

SIBLING RIVALRY
It is a rare child who would not like to be the permanent center of parental attention; learning to share anything, from affection to toys, takes time. Sharing is hardest when one child is ill or upset or feels at a disadvantage. The very existence of a brother or sister can constitute a direct threat and a very apparent need to compete for attention. Often enough, children squabble most and press their demands hardest when parents are busiest. So runs the vicious circle of sibling rivalry.

There is little you can do, apart from scrupulously paying equal attention to each of your children; if you have a favorite, keep that information to yourself.

When a new baby is due, prepare your child or children by talking about it well ahead of time. Explain the changes in routine that will be necessary. Make sure you or your partner always has some time exclusively for the other child or children, ideally when the other parent is busy with the new baby. Don't use special names for the baby that you used to give the older child, and don't always put the baby first. Don't belittle the child whose behavior regresses when the newcomer arrives. Being jealous of a new baby may make a child aggressive or unkind (sometimes interspersed with being very loving). Remember that a child cannot properly understand that a baby is unable to look after himself. It often takes many months for the child's ill feelings toward his new brother or sister to disappear.

The relationships between siblings over time show a wide range of patterns: don't expect your own children to relate in the same way as you did with your brothers and sisters. Sometimes bitter fighting early on may be replaced with closeness, but the reverse is also true.

When the going gets rough, remind

yourself, and the jealous child, that jealousy, like any other emotion, is something he must learn to handle.

Make sure that visitors dont forget the elder child when coming to see a new baby: if there is a gift for the baby, there should be one for him too – and he should be greeted first.

SINUSITIS

INFECTION in the sinuses; rare in children.

■ SYMPTOMS Pain and swelling over one of the sinuses, usually following a cold. Children with sinusitis may become feverish and quite ill. Pain, redness and swelling around the eye may be due to infection in the maxillary or ethmoid sinuses (and of the eyelids and globe of the eye itself – periorbital cellulitis).

■ ACTION Mild symptoms can be treated with decongestant nose drops (for example, ephedrine 0.25 percent), and acetamenophen.

■ GET MEDICAL ADVICE if the pain is severe, there is local tenderness or FEVER. If the eyelid becomes red and swollen, your child should be seen by your doctor.

■ TESTS An X-ray of the sinuses may be performed to confirm the diagnosis.

■ TREATMENT An ANTIBIOTIC will be prescribed, together with decongestant nose drops. If this does not bring about a cure, your child will be referred to an ear, nose and throat specialist. A needle may be inserted into the sinus to remove the infected fluid, and antibiotics given by injection intravenously.

■ LONG-TERM MANAGEMENT

SINUSITIS

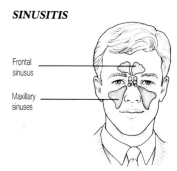

Frontal
sinusus

Maxillary
sinuses

Main symptoms: pain, redness and swelling.

Sinusitis is not usually a persistent problem of childhood, but milder symptoms caused by ALLERGIC RHINITIS may re-occur.

SIX-WEEK CHECK
See *'NORMAL DEVELOPMENT'*.

SLEEP PROBLEMS
The amount of sleep needed varies enormously from child to child, and from age to age. In the pre-school years, many children have difficulty in falling asleep, and may wake habitually during the night. In older children problems may include SLEEP-WALKING, NIGHTMARES, NIGHT TERRORS or talking in their sleep.

■ CAUSES Difficulties in falling asleep and night-waking may arise in a child accustomed to having contact with you at the time of going to sleep. Disruption in routine or illness may start sleep problems in a young child who has previously been sleeping through the night.

However, there is a range of normal night-time behavior. Many normal children and parents value the bedtime routines or rituals. And in most instances the 'problem' is the inconvenience caused to parents.

■ ACTION Try to establish a bedtime routine. Be consistent about the pattern and duration of the routine – the story, drink, and so on. It will normally follow as a matter of course over the years that the duration and degree of contact will progressively decline. If your child cries on waking and does not fall asleep again, try to settle him with a minimum of contact, and avoid a complete repetition of the bedtime rituals. If you cannot resolve the problem, ask your doctor for advice. He or she may suggest consulting a clinical psychologist.

Adults should perhaps recall or recognize that for some children (and adults), particularly those with a nervous disposition or colorful imagination, night-time and falling asleep can be worrisome. Such children need consistent sympathetic support and not 'treatment'.

■ OUTLOOK Difficulties in falling asleep and night-waking rarely persist into the school years; but the cumulative effect of broken sleep can take its toll on the parents' capability and psychological health.

SLEEP-WALKING
Some children are prone to sleep-walking: it may happen particularly at times of stress. There is no need to wake them, just gently return them to bed. Sleep-walking children almost always avoid potential hazards in the house, but with younger children it may be a wise precaution and give you peace of mind to ensure you are woken: attach something to the child's bedroom door that will make a noise if he opens it to leave the room.

SMALL-FOR-DATES BABY
Babies of a LOWER BIRTH WEIGHT than would normally be expected for the length of pregnancy. The size of a baby depends on many factors. There is the size, health and age of the mother – mothers in their teens or over 35 years of age tend to have smaller babies. If the mother smokes, drinks, takes drugs or is severely undernourished during pregnancy, the baby is likely to be small (cigarette smoking is the most serious and avoidable factor in causing poor growth of the fetus). Babies of a MULTIPLE PREGNANCY tend to be small. CONGENITAL ABNORMALITIES and CONGENITAL INFECTION also affect the growth of the fetus, and hence the baby's birth weight.

Most small-for-dates babies have no major problems after birth and will usually 'catch up' in weight and height by the end of their first year. If a fetus has had a prolonged period of poor growth in pregnancy, then he is likely to remain relatively small in later life.

New-born small-for-dates babies are more likely to suffer from HYPOGLYCEMIA and HYPOTHERMIA. The smaller the baby, the more serious the risks of other complications. Thus even a full-term baby who weighs under 4+ lb (2,000 gm) at birth will need close observation, if not admission to a special care nursery.

SMOKING
Out of every 100 men in most developed countries, 25 will die prematurely of tobacco-related diseases, mainly cancer and heart-disease. Women who smoke are also at increased risk. Nicotine, the active drug in tobacco, is extremely addictive, causing intense craving in regular users if stopped. It is also a powerful tranquillizer. The act of sucking on a cigarette is in itself extremely soothing. The self-conscious adolescent, who does not yet know what to do with his hands in company, can find lighting and smoking a ciga-

rette an ideal way to keep his hands busy.

These powerful inducements to smoke don't even include the obvious pleasure of doing something of which adults disapprove, and of being part of a group that demonstrates its independence by smoking in secret.

Studies have shown that in some countries about one third of 14-year-olds smoke every day. Many of these will continue to smoke in adult life, when they will greatly increase their risk of cancer, heart attacks, artery disease, strokes, and, for women, the risk of a premature baby as well as a diseased one.

■ ACTION Children attach more importance to the immediate effects of smoking – cost, smell on breath, staining of fingers, damage to fitness for sports – than to the threat of future disease. So it seems that parents explaining the dangers should emphasize these immediate draw-backs – although of course the long-term health hazards must be stated too.

Above all, remember that your child is probably smoking to copy another child. Tackling the problem from this angle is easier said than done, but removing or diverting (even temporarily) the peer group pressure to smoke can be the most effective maneuver of any.

Children also mimic adult behavior, so if you smoke, try to stop. Many local branches of the Lung Association and the Heart Foundation sponser programs to stop smoking. Some are directed at adolescents. Prevention is always easier than trying to overcome the addiction.

SMOKING DURING PREGNANCY

This affects the growth of the fetus, causing LOW BIRTH WEIGHT, short length and, to a lesser degree, small head size. As it is not known how many cigarettes a day affect an individual baby, smoking in pregnancy should be avoided altogether.

SMOKING, PASSIVE

Research has shown that passive smoking (living or working in an environment in which people smoke) is detrimental to the health of babies, children and adults. Infants and children who live in a home where people smoke have more respiratory symptoms, more prolonged colds and are more likely to need hospital care than those who live in a smoke-free environment. Exposure to smoke can be particularly serious for children with CYSTIC FIBROSIS and some children with ASTHMA and chest diseases.

SNAKE BITES AND VENOM DISEASES

Of the more than 3,500 known species of snakes, only 200 are poisonous to man. Venomous species common to North America include rattlesnakes, water moccasins and copperheads. In the United States about 7,000 snake bites occur each year but less than 20 are fatal. Most are due to rattlesnakes, coral snakes and water moccasins.

■ SYMPTOMS Some snake bites cause a local reaction with local pain and swelling, bruising of the skin and oozing of fluid in blisters. Some bites are inconspicuous with no local reaction. Snake bites also cause generalized reactions. The venom from some snakes is a powerful anticoagulant and causes generalized bleeding, organ failure and death. The venom from other snakes contains neurotoxins or poisons to the nervous system with paralysis.

■ ACTION Immediately get a qualified first-aider to apply a tourniquet a few inches from the wound in an effort to further slow down the absorption of the venom. Immobilize the limb. Take the child immediately to the local hospital emergency department. The doctor will need a description of the snake to try to assess the type of poison in the venom. The wound will be locally cleaned, and the venom sucked out by syringe or pump from the fang sites. To be effective this must be done within two hours of the bite. Topical antibiotics may be applied and tetanus immunization given if this is not up to date. Specific snake venom antisera are given as indicated.

■ OUTCOME Most children survive a snake bite but a small number of bites are fatal despite therapy. Teaching children about poisonous snakes in your area and how to avoid bites is important for prevention.

SOILING (ENCOPRESIS)

An uncommon problem ranging from soiling underpants to frank defecation, day or night, in places and at times that are socially inappropriate. See also *CONSTIPATION, DIARRHEA, TOILET TRAINING.*

Some children just don't learn bowel control by the time they go to school. Children who are exceptionally constipated have difficulty in learning bowel control – the child may hang on' and avoid passing a stool if this has been painful in the past; some children resist attempts to regulate bowel action, to use the potty or toilet, particularly if their parents place a high premium on success – they may 'hang on' deliberately, and may soil their pants or pass stools at another time and elsewhere as a result.

Soiling usually indicates an emotional problem, particularly in a child who has previously adjusted to using the toilet. A minority of children who soil themselves may smear their feces on the floor or walls, indicating by such antisocial acts that there is a more serious underlying emotional disturbance.

Soiling is embarrassing and upsetting for children, even if they don't show it. Parents naturally become distressed, which can make it harder to resolve the issue. Treat any episodes of soiling as calmly as possible. Punishing the child will not help him to learn bowel control.

Get medical advice if your child is over three years old and soils persistently, soils and seems constipated, appears to be in pain on passing stools, starts soiling regularly after being toilet trained, or soils and smears his feces. Your family doctor or pediatrician may treat any medical problem. If, after medical investigation and the treatment of any associated constipation, the problem persists, help from a clinical psychologist or child psychiatrist may be suggested. Treatment will usually involve toilet training, which may include rewarding your child for passing stools on the toilet, while paying as little attention as possible to any episodes of soiling. The problem may take a few months and, rarely, years to resolve completely. Meanwhile, your child may be upset by teasing or comments at school or the nursery. To ameliorate this aspect of the problem, discuss with your child's teachers how you are handling the situation, and the best way of dealing with incidents at school.

SOLVENT ABUSE

Vapors are given off by a range of products used in the home, including adhesives, dry cleaning fluid, aerosol sprays and typing correction fluid. If actively inhaled these vapors lead to intoxication. In recent years many adolescents have experimented with these substances, mostly on an occasional or sporadic basis.

Damage as a result of solvent abuse is rare but can be serious or life threatening. The major risk is from accidents while intoxicated – inhaling vomit, falling in front of cars or from high buildings. However, rapid intoxication can alter the rhythm of the heart, and result in sudden death.

If you recognize that your child is abusing solvents, you should address the problem directly. Discuss the problem with him: if in doubt about how to proceed, ask your doctor for help.

SPEECH DISORDERS

By two years of age, most children will have started to talk. The child who talks early and well usually performs well in later learning difficulties. By the age of three, all but three or four in 100 children will be able to utter three-word phrases spontaneously and with meaning (not echoing what has been said to him).

The most common speech disorder is STAMMERING, common under the age of five when language is being acquired most rapidly. It usually resolves by seven years of age.

Physiological, psychological and environmental factors are all causes of stammering. It is twice as common in boys as in girls; and more than twice as common in children from large families. Identical twins tend to echo each other's speech problems.

Speech disorders can also result from structural abnormalities of the lips, teeth, roof of the mouth (palate), tongue, throat or voice box (larynx); or they can simply be due to difficulty in forming speech sounds or sequences of speech sounds. One in seven children entering school is described as having partially unintelligible speech.

■ SYMPTOMS Poor understanding of speech, HYPERACTIVITY, frustration, delayed or unclear speech. Other signs of problems in speech development that should be investigated include no words by 18 months of age, no intelligible speech to family members by 2+ years or to strangers by three years, no two-word phrases by two years, no simple sentences by three years or word endings consistently dropped after age five. If you are concerned about your child's speech discuss this with your family doctor.

■ INVESTIGATIONS Assessment by a speech therapist or speech pathologist and a clinical psychologist. Medical examination may show a local cause for articulation difficulties such as a disorder of the larynx or palate. Children with more severe language disorders may require a CHROMOSOME test, an EEG or a psychiatric assessment for, typically, elective mutism (deliberately staying silent for psychological reasons) or AUTISM. Hearing tests are essential, although only two children per 1,000 have a sufficiently severe hearing loss to cause major delay in acquiring language.

■ TREATMENT Children with speech or language disorders will benefit from speech therapy and a language-based teaching programme with plenty of adult contact. The public school system must provide free special education to all children with handicaps including speech and language.

■ SELF-MANAGEMENT When you talk to the child, make sure you

have his attention. Talk clearly and simply about the child's current interests and activities. Listen carefully to his speech. Be supportive and not punitive.

■ OUTLOOK Most children are intelligible by seven years and only one in 40 will remain difficult to understand. But while it is usual for speech difficulties to resolve, the child may well have spelling difficulties later. Severely restricted language development at five years carries a poor prospect for educational success, and many such children are classed as MENTALLY HANDICAPPED, AUTISTIC or both.

SPINA BIFIDA

The commonest major CONGENITAL ABNORMALITY of the nervous system, affecting typically one per 1,000 births. The baby is born with a defect in the spine or a cystic swelling over part of the spine (neck or back). This contains fluid and usually some nerve tissue – derived from malformed spinal cord and nerve roots.

■ CAUSE The neural tube, which forms the baby's spinal cord, closes between three and four weeks after conception. If this fails to occur, spina bifida results. Many such affected fetuses abort spontaneously. Spina bifida occulta results from partial closure of the spinal bony arch. This is quite commonly found on X-rays of children who have normal skin over the spine and is usually of no significance to the child's health.

■ COMPLICATIONS Spina bifida is often associated with HYDROCEPHALUS. In severe cases, there may also be abnormal angulation (kyphosis) or curvature (scoliosis) of the spine and abnormalities of BOWEL and bladder function. Disability depends on the site and degree to which the spinal cord has been damaged. Most children have partial or complete paralysis of the legs.

■ TREATMENT Immediately after birth, care is required to prevent INFECTION of the spinal cord and to treat infection if it occurs. Surgery may be performed to close the defect. Head size needs to be monitored to detect development of hydrocephalus. A shunt operation (a plastic tube placed in the brain to drain off excess fluid) is carried out if this occurs. Thereafter the individual patient's problems require a long-term management plan. Mildly affected children can often walk independently. Moderately affected children walk with aids and appliances, but severely affected children are chair bound. Bowel and bladder disorder require careful long-term medical and surgical care. Loss of sensation in the feet requires well-fitting footwear and good foot care. Loss of sensation higher in the legs carries additional risks such as painless fractures.

Care of the child with spina bifida extends to all aspects of his physical and emotional well being, to his schooling and employment, and to the needs of the whole family. The treatment plan is complex and requires the expertise of a team of many persons in a variety of professions.

■ PREVENTION Screening tests of the mother's blood to detect this abnormality in early pregnancy should be performed. A test of the amniotic fluid that surrounds the baby in the mother's uterus (amniocentesis – see *PRENATAL DIAGNOSIS*) and ULTRASOUND testing can contribute to prenatal identification of spina bifida. GENETIC COUNSELLING should be provided for subsequent pregnancies.

SPITTING UP

Babies often bring up a little milk at the end of a feeding. The milk will appear partially digested. Spitting up, as opposed to VOMITING is, by definition, more of a nuisance than a threat to health.

■ ACTION It may help to burp the baby in the middle of each feed as well as at the end.

SPLINTERS

Common-sense treatment – removing the foreign body with tweezers as gently as possible – is the answer unless it is embedded deeply, in which case get medical advice. Don't probe the area. Clean the affected area with soap and water first. Sterilize the tweezers first by passing the tips through a flame. Squeezing the flesh around the splinter can make the end of the splinter rise clear enough of the skin surface to give an adequate grip for the tweezers.

STAMMERING

Most children will stammer or stutter occasionally (as indeed do adults) under stressful circumstances. If stammering is persistent, get medical advice. Your doctor may suggest seeking the help of a speech therapist. See *SPEECH DISORDERS*.

STEALING

A child's sense of right and wrong develops over a period of years, not only through intellectual development but also through following the example set by others. The toddler or pre-school child who takes something often has no idea of what ownership means and indeed makes no distinction between taking and borrowing.

While this is clearly not true of older children, parents do need to think carefully about the context of theft. If faced with the knowledge that a child has, say, been shoplifting, ask yourself whether other children have been influential. A child will steal in order to imitate; to rise to a 'dare'; or because he is forced to do so, socially. He may also steal because he wants an object as compensation for something missing in his life. If the child is stealing from home, family relationships may well be implicated. Jealousy of a brother or sister may be the cause, as can the simple need to attract attention. Children need attention in order to thrive; sometimes the need can be desperate. Remember also that stealing and shoplifting may be related to a 'need' for money to buy drugs. Beware if the stealing is also associated with a change in behavior.

■ ACTION Your action will depend upon the age of the child and the factors mentioned above. Base any sanctions on the following common-sense principles:

First, the child should not benefit from the theft: don't let it become an attention-getting device. Rescuing an older child from a shoplifting charge may not be in his best interest if he then does not understand the consequences of the crime.

Second, the reasons why he stole should be openly discussed.

Third, try to explain *why* he should not steal – you may need to cover this again and again.

If a child steals persistently, discuss the problem with your doctor, who may suggest further help from a child psychiatrist or psychologist.

He or she will help you explore the reasons behind the child's behavior, which may be difficult for the family to tackle alone, especially if the problem is long-standing. Do *not* ignore this problem as it may be a sign of more serious underlying difficulties.

See also *LIES AND FIBS*.

STICKY EYE
See *CONJUNCTIVITIS*.

STILL BIRTH
The delivery of a dead baby after 28 weeks of pregnancy.

▨ CAUSES are mostly unclear; contributory factors include maternal DIABETES and high BLOOD PRESSURE, and CONGENITAL ABNORMALITIES of the fetus.

If your baby is still born you may be asked to give permission for a post-mortem examination (autopsy) in order to try to identify the cause of the death.

▨ MOURNING The parental distress following a still birth may be as great as that following the death of a child or an adult: feelings of shock and disbelief may follow, accompanied by intensive bouts of tearfulness; feelings of guilt, despair and anger are common. It may take a year for emotions to settle back to normal, but distress may resurface from time to time, especially around the anniversary of the loss.

Psychological studies have suggested, and many parents have found, that seeing and holding their dead baby helps, even though this may seem very stressful at the time. Taking photographs and being involved with the funeral arrangements may also be important to the parents. The doctors and nurses caring for parents normally provide opportunities for discussion about the baby's death, the results of the autopsy and also, if necessary, GENETIC COUNSELLING. A follow-up visit to the hospital is usually suggested several months after a still birth.

▨ REGISTRATION AND FUNERAL ARRANGEMENTS All still births have to be registered. Registration of a baby's first name is now also possible. The hospital staff will help with the necessary paper work. Funeral arrangements are made privately as they are for any death.

▨ NEXT PREGNANCY It is wise to allow time to mourn the death of your baby before conceiving again; you need sufficient rehabilitation to be able to cope with the anxieties of the next pregnancy and delivery. This may take some time – possibly over a year.

STILL'S DISEASE
See *JUVENILE RHEUMATOID ARTHRITIS*.

STINGS
See *BITES AND STINGS*.

STOMACH-ACHE
See *ABDOMINAL PAIN*.

STRAINS AND SPRAINS
Apply the RICE principle: R is for rest – it helps to stop bleeding, internal and external. I is for ice – apply ice cubes in a plastic bag or a bag of frozen peas; but take care that excessive cold does not burn the skin. C is for compression – firm bandaging will prevent further

bleeding into the tissues. E is for elevation – raising the affected part lets fluid drain away and reduces swelling. See also *FOOT INJURIES, BRUISING, PAIN.*

STRAINS AND SPRAINS

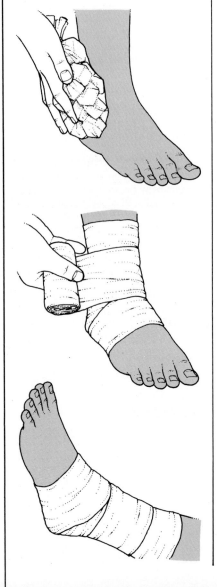

STRAWBERRY HEMANGIOMA
See *BIRTHMARKS.*

STRESS SYMPTOMS
Although children do not usually complain about stress in the same way as adults, they may well experience it in a variety of situations: when struggling at school, when experiencing failure in friendship, when frightened, if there are FAMILY PROBLEMS, illness or a threatened loss or BEREAVEMENT. The child cannot express his feelings; instead the stress is felt as a physical symptom: see *RECURRENT ABDOMINAL PAIN, HEADACHE, NIGHTMARES, ANXIETY, BEDWETTING, VOMITING,* having a PAIN anywhere. All are common ways of experiencing stress, and should not be ignored if they persist or keep returning.

■ ACTION Check with your doctor to be sure there is nothing physically wrong. Think about what could be distressing your child. He may or may not be able to tell you himself, but others (his teacher?) may have ideas. You may know yourself that there are family or other worries but may not have realized that your child has picked up the tension. Reassure the child, but remember the best remedy is to sort out the problem – whether the child's or your own. Your doctor can help.

STRIDOR
The name given to the noise that occurs while breathing in (inspiratory stridor) or breathing out (expiratory stridor).

■ CAUSES The commonest form in the new-born period is congenital laryngeal stridor. This is thought to result from a relative softness of the cartilage of the larynx ('voice box'). In older infants and children, stridor is often synonymous with CROUP or viral LARYNGITIS. Other rare causes include the inhalation of a solid object sticking at the level of the vocal cords.

■ SYMPTOMS There may be none other than the stridor. Additional features will depend on the cause of the stridor.

■ ACTION Stridor present from birth is not dangerous, but medical attention may be needed if the child contracts a respiratory infection. Stridor occurring for the first time should be taken seriously. This could be common viral laryngitis; or life threatening EPIGLOTTITIS; or the child could have inhaled something into the larynx or the wind pipe, in which case turn the child upside down and slap his back, and *summon urgent medical help.*

■ TREATMENT depends on the cause: *very* occasionally surgery may be necessary to relieve obstruction due to malformation of the larynx.

■ OUTLOOK Congenital laryngeal stridor improves as the child grows, and has usually disappeared by the age of one year, nearly always by two years.

STYE
An infection in the base of the eyelash that causes a small, painful boil on the eyelid.

Most styes need no treatment. Bathing the eye with cotton balls moistened with clean warm water may speed the healing process.

If your child repeatedly has styes, it is worth discussing the problem with your doctor, who may prescribe an ANTIBIOTIC ointment.

SUDDEN INFANT DEATH SYNDROME (SIDS)
See *COT DEATH.*

SUFFOCATION
An external obstruction to breathing cuased by such things as a soft pillow lying over an infant's face, or a plastic bag pulled over a baby's or a child's head, preventing air from reaching the lungs.

■ IMMEDIATE ACTION Remove the cause of suffocation. If the child is not breathing, see *EMERGENCY RESUSCITATION.*

■ PREVENTION Keep plastic bags out of reach; don't give a baby a pillow, and provide a mattress and crib of approved standards. Don't leave infants on waterbeds, especially face down.

SUGAR INTOLERANCE
Impaired absorption of sugar leading to watery DIARRHEA, flatulence (gas), COLICKY ABDOMINAL PAIN and sore skin around the anus and buttocks. The child may suffer from FAILURE TO THRIVE due to MALABSORPTION. An uncommon condition. See also *LACTOSE INTOLERANCE* and *GALACTOSEMIA.*

■ ACTION If your child has profuse watery DIARRHEA either after the introduction of sugar to the diet usually in the first few days of life, or after GASTROENTERITIS, report it to your doctor. A visit to the hospital may be needed for investigations.

■ MANAGEMENT depends on the type of sugar involved and whether the condition is primary (from birth) or secondary (acquired later in infancy or childhood). Specific sugar(s), usually lactose, are excluded and if the symptoms improve or disappear are introduced some weeks later as a challenge (see *LAC-TOSE INTOLERANCE*). Children with primary deficiency will require long-term feeding with specially prepared milks to exclude the appropriate sugars. The primary forms are inherited and further siblings have a one in four chance of developing the problem. There is no inherited pattern in the secondary form.

▆ OUTLOOK Primary types will persist through life and require continued dietary adjustment. The secondary form lasts for a period of months.

SUNBURN

Sunburn is essentially no different to any other sort of burn to the skin surface; it can cause problems varying from slight redness to very serious burns.

▆ SYMPTOMS The first sign is redness, and in mild cases this may be the only sign. Soreness develops after a few hours, and may be followed by BLISTERING. If the blisters break, fluid weeps from the raw surface of the skin. As the burn heals, ITCHING can be severe, and skin peels away in flakes.

▆ CAUSE Ultraviolet rays of medium wavelength are the 'burning' element of sunlight. These are not visible as light, and can pass through thin summer clothing or through hazy cloud cover. The burning effect is greatest between 11 am and 3 pm, when the sun is at its highest, and worst on beaches or in snow, because rays are reflected off the surface.

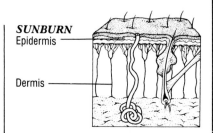

SUNBURN
Epidermis
Dermis

The changes which occur in sunburn take place in the dermis, the lower layer of skin. Here, the natural pigment melanin is produced in response to stimulus by ultra violet rays from the sun.

▆ ACTION Prevention is the best approach: whenever sunburn is likely, keep your child covered up with clothing and a sun-hat. Sunscreen creams are helpful; choose one with a high sun-blocking factor, say ten or 15, especially if your child has fair skin.

▆ TREATMENT If a child does get sunburned, soothe the pain, and limit the damage by cooling him off in a tepid bath or shower. The pain may be relieved by acetamenophen and the inflammation can be reduced by applying a 0.5 percent or 1 percent hydrocortisone cream, available at the drugstore. An antihistamine (or the old-fashioned remedy, calamine lotion) may help the itching. Try to keep blisters intact, but if they break, protect the skin with a clean dressing and an antiseptic cream.

▆ OUTLOOK Even severe sunburn leaves no permanent scars but HEAT-STROKE is a potential risk.

SUNSTROKE
See *HEAT EXHAUSTION*.

SWIMMER'S EAR
See *EXTERNAL EAR INFECTION*.

T

TANTRUMS

Most children have outbursts of kicking, yelling and foot stamping from as early as one year; they may continue up to three or four years. View them as angry responses to frustration – resulting from the child's own limitations, or because desires or a growing wish for autonomy are thwarted. Tantrums diminish as the child's skills, tolerance of frustration and ability to express himself increase.

Watch out for common situations when tantrums occur. Some are unavoidable, but some may be deflected by distracting the child's attention. Giving in to the demands of the child can be tempting, particularly in public; but such appeasement will only encourage the behavior over time and should be avoided. Since the child is fired by the anger of the moment, losing your temper or punishing him will not stop the tantrum, or reduce the likelihood of future outbursts. The best response is to ignore the tantrum as far as possible, calmly prevent the child from hurting himself or others, or breaking things, and reassure him when the episode is over. Praise your child in situations where he shows evidence of controlling a possible tantrum. See also *AGGRESSION, BREATH-HOLDING ATTACKS, HEAD BANGING.*

TAPEWORM

A PARASITE of the bowel, much less common than other intestinal infestations. The adult worm is made up of a 'head' portion which adheres to the bowel, and a tape-like 'body' consisting of flat segments that contain eggs. Individual segments break off and are passed in bowel movements. Each segment can be up to , in (6 mm) in size.

■ TREATMENT Medication such as niclosamide or praziquantel are both effective, but the latter is more expensive.

TEAR DUCT, BLOCKED

The tear duct is the tube that drains tears from the eye into the back of the nose; tears are necessary to keep the eye clean and moist. About 2 per cent of babies are born with some degree of obstruction of the duct.

■ SYMPTOMS The eye will be watery. If the tear sac becomes IN-FECTED, the eyelids may stick together (especially after sleeping) with yellow pus.

■ TREATMENT Keep the eyes clean. If they are sticky, wash with warm water using cotton balls. If there is infection, your doctor may prescribe ANTIBIOTIC drops or ointment. Your doctor may show you how to massage the tear duct. In some cases frequent daily tear duct massage may help open the blockage. If the baby still has problems after six months of age, a simple operation will relieve the blockage.

TEETH, DEVELOPMENT OF
See *TEETHING*.

TEETHING
A baby's first set of teeth starts to erupt, or break through the gums, at about five months. The two lower front teeth are usually first to appear, and are followed shortly afterwards by the two upper front teeth. The baby teeth are usually all present by the time a baby is three years old. The permanent teeth start to erupt at around five to six years, and this continues until the wisdom teeth come through in late teens or early twenties.

■ SYMPTOMS Your baby will appear irritable, will cry and will probably refuse feedings because of the soreness of his gums. Teething is not a cause for high fever or a rash.

■ TREATMENT Chewing appears to give some relief, hence the use of the traditional teething ring. A cool, wet, clean cloth to chew on often appeals to the baby. Application of a teething gel containing a local anesthetic may also give some relief. Consult your dentist, doctor or pharmacist about suitable preparations.

■ ACTION Clean the new teeth with a soft baby-size toothbrush using a fluoride toothpaste. Babies can try cleaning their own teeth when able to hold a spoon, but tooth brushing should be supervised until he is at least six years old. Some babies find chewing on a toothbrush soothing. Find out from your doctor whether the water in your area contains enough fluoride to protect your child's teeth. If it does not, ask your doctor about a fluoride supplement. Regular dental check-ups from the age of two or three years are recommended.

TEMPERATURE
See *FEVER*.

TETANUS
A rare disease caused by tetanus BACTERIA, which lie dormant in soil and can INFECT cuts and abrasions. Tetanus is also found in the mouths of many animals, whose bites can transmit the disease. It is, however, rare in most developed countries because of IMMUNIZATION. The INCUBATION PERIOD is between four and 21 days.

■ PREVENTION Immunization effectively prevents this lethal disease: its importance cannot be overemphasized.

■ SYMPTOMS Muscle pain and stiffness, caused by the tetanus toxin affecting nerves and causing muscle spasm.
   The spasms grow in frequency and cause severe pain; the jaw tends to be particularly affected, hence the term 'lock-jaw', the common name for the disease.

■ ACTION If you suspect tetanus, rush the child to the hospital immediately.

■ TREATMENT Tetanus antiserum and ANTIBIOTICS can lessen the severity of the disease. Hospital treatment, including sedation, will help the spasms, but these may severely affect breathing.

■ OUTLOOK is poor, despite modern improvements in treatment. Prevention by immunization

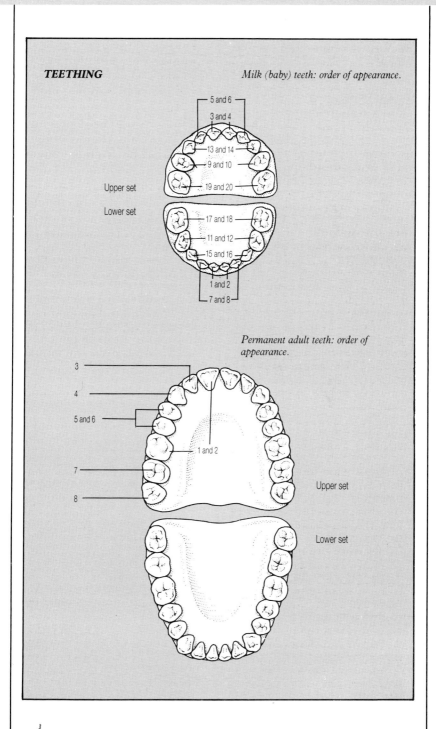

TEETHING

Milk (baby) teeth: order of appearance.

5 and 6
3 and 4
13 and 14
9 and 10
Upper set
19 and 20
Lower set
17 and 18
11 and 12
15 and 16
1 and 2
7 and 8

Permanent adult teeth: order of appearance.

3
4
5 and 6
1 and 2
7
8
Upper set
Lower set

is an essential protection for your child.

THALASSEMIA

A form of ANEMIA caused by abnormal hemoglobin formed in the body in place of the normal one. Hemoglobin (see *ANEMIA*) is the blood's oxygen carrier. In thalassemia the red blood cells become fragile and tend to break down. It is an INHERITED DISORDER. If both parents carry the GENE for the disease, they themselves are mildly affected, but there is a one in four chance of it occurring in a severe form in their children.

■ SYMPTOMS appear between six months and one year of age. There is pallor, listlessness and poor feeding. The spleen is always enlarged, as it tries to produce extra red blood cells. In older children growth is retarded. Children and adults with the milder form of the disease usually have no symptoms, except perhaps slight anemia.

■ TESTS BLOOD TESTS confirm the diagnosis.

■ ACTION INFECTIONS should be treated rapidly. If there is a family history of thalassemia, GENETIC COUNSELLING should be considered. Contact sports should be avoided: the enlarged spleen may rupture, causing severe bleeding.

■ TREATMENT of the severe form relies on BLOOD TRANSFUSIONS to counteract the acute anemia. The problem with transfusions is accumulation of large amounts of iron in the body; drugs may have to be used to get rid of this.

Recently, bone marrow transplants have been used to re-establish manufacture of normal hemoglobin.

Sometimes the spleen needs to be removed: it can grow so large that it presses upon and displaces other abdominal organs.

■ OUTCOME The severest form of the disease is fatal, but the recent development of bone marrow transplant treatment gives hope. Patients with milder thalassemia usually do not have any serious problems.

THE DYING CHILD

No amount of rationalization can relieve a parent's sense of shock and injustice when faced with the prospect of a dying child. Although each family is unique and the ability of family members to cope is often unpredictable, it is possible for even this tragic experience to enhance rather than destroy their integrity and emotional well-being.

There can be no absolute rules to guide anyone through the ordeal; the following suggestions are based simply on the observations and experiences of others who have suffered similarly, or who have been closely involved.

■ COMMUNICATION After parents have been told that their child's illness will have a fatal outcome they will have to deal not only with their own shock and disbelief but also, in the ensuing days and weeks, with meeting many different people: relatives, friends, health professionals, members of the clergy, in addition to the child. Expressions of anger or a retreat into silent grief may be natural but will help nobody, and may disturb the child's precious final days.

Parents should ask health professionals to explain all the facts clearly. It is often useful to write down questions before meeting with senior doctors and nurses as it is easy to forget what to ask during such stressful moments. Don't be afraid to ask the same questions again and again.

It may be helpful to meet with parents who have been through a similar ordeal or whose child had the same condition. Ask the nurse or your doctor if this is possible. Treat the child in as routine a way as possible: children are concerned with living normally, and if artificial celebrations are created – an early Christmas or birthday celebration – they may become upset.

Many clergymen will be a source of great comfort at this time and parents should not be reluctant to involve them, even if previous contact with them has been minimal.

Friends of the family may be uncertain how to cope and parents may need to encourage them to visit the child, or sometimes to discourage them if their interest and concern becomes too intrusive.

Above all, don't be afraid to talk to the child and to provide as much reassurance and honesty as you can.

■ THE PROCESS OF DYING Although death frightens most people, the physical process of dying should be, and can be, dignified and pain-free. Don't be afraid:
– to arrange for the child to die in a particular place – at home or in a favorite room in the hospital. Talk to the nurses about making the surroundings as warm and homely as possible;
– to include (or occasionally to exclude) relatives and friends in the visiting schedule;
– to discuss arrangements for pain relief repeatedly with the doctors and nurses;
– to talk to the child and to comfort him physically. The decision about what to tell the child will vary with the illness and other circumstances.

If you are in doubt about what to say, discuss this with the child's doctor; remember that lying to the child may make him lose trust in you.
– to be with the child after death.

■ BEREAVEMENT Although the pain of grief is intense, have no doubt that time is a great healer and that the mourning process will bring a sense of perspective and emotional stability, usually after a period of about nine months.

Many parents experience guilt: they may blame themselves in some way for the child's illness or, quite commonly, at feeling a sense of relief when the child finally dies, especially after a long illness.

It is important for parents to talk about their feelings with each other, with their other children and with close friends, their doctor or their clergymen. Be sensitive to the different pace and expression of grieving in different family members. Be patient.

Depression may well disturb patterns of eating and sleeping. Social contacts may be avoided. These are not harmful initially but may be if prolonged. Problems at work may follow, and if one parent finds it exceptionally difficult to cope with grief when the other does not marriage problems may arise. Be aware that this is a potentially destructive situation, and could well need help from a professional.

THROAT, INHALED OBJECT IN
See STRIDOR.

THUMB SUCKING
Many children find thumb or finger sucking comforting, usually when they are tired, bored or tense. A few continue to comfort themselves in this way into their early teens. It is not harmful and is best ignored: children stop

themselves when they are ready to do so. Thumb sucking does not cause protrusion of the upper front teeth. See also *COMFORT HABITS*.

TICS

Jerky, repetitive, habitual movements or sequences of movements. Very common in middle childhood; tics of the eyes, face or head are commonest of all.

■ CAUSES Poorly understood, but usually reflect underlying psychological stresses, the origins and nature of which will mostly be unknown to the child and family alike.

■ ACTION Most tics are best ignored, though this is difficult when they are annoying or worrying for the parent, and embarrassing for the child. Reassure him that tics nearly always disappear on their own over time. Ensure that the child's teachers avoid unnecessary public comment about the movements.

■ TREATMENT Get medical advice if the number or form of tics is increasing, if your child is being teased about them at school, or if he seems to be developing elaborate rituals and routines around them. Very rarely, it can be difficult to differentiate tics from the early symptoms of serious neurological disease. Depending upon your doctor's findings, he may suggest seeing a psychologist, neurologist or child psychiatrist. BEHAVIORAL TREATMENT can be effective as can working with the child and family to reduce stress. See also GILLES DE LA TOURETTE SYNDROME.

TOEING IN

See *PIGEON TOES*.

TOILET TRAINING

A child can only become toilet trained when he has reached a particular stage of development. It remains uncertain, however, what constitutes the exact components of development. This stage of development is not usually reached until 18 months of age (at the earliest). Most children learn bowel control first, followed by bladder control by day, then by night. There is great variation among children in how and when they gain such control; girls usually learn earlier than boys. Parents often feel strongly about toilet training but if started too early it is likely to fail, and to cause conflict and worry in the future. Avoid making toilet training a big issue. When the child begins to show he is aware that he is about to pass urine or move his bowels, sit him on the potty, without tension or fuss. Choose times when there is a reasonable chance of success, such as after meals. Praise success, stay relaxed and don't get upset about accidents. When he makes progress, reduce the use of diapers. Take advantage of sunny summer days to allow your child to be without a diaper in the backyard or park, or on the beach. See also *BEDWETTING (ENURESIS), SOILING, WETTING*.

TONGUE, APPEARANCE OF

Examining the tongue is not a very useful means of assessing illness. Normal children may have a 'coated' tongue at any time, but it is more commonly seen when the child has a FEVER, and/or is DEHYDRATED. A bright red or strawberry tongue may be seen in SCARLET FEVER and Kawasaki disease.

A 'geographical' tongue which looks like a pink-and-white map is not due to disease, and may be a CONGENITAL variant of normal. It causes no problems and is not a sign of illness. White plaques on the tongue and inside of the mouth that are sore, are usually a sign of CANDIDIASIS, and can be treated with antifungal drops. MOUTH ULCERS can also occur on the tongue, as well as the sides of the mouth. Sometimes these are due to HERPES virus and sometimes to unknown causes.

TONGUE-TIE
A small skin fold on the under-side of the tongue occasionally preventing full movement of the tongue's tip.

▧ SYMPTOMS Usually none.

▧ TREATMENT Surgery is rarely needed because the small skin fold stretches with time. Release of the fold is only done if there is a marked SPEECH DISORDER.

TONSILLITIS
INFECTION of the tonsils, usually by BACTERIA (such as *Streptococcus*); but may be part of a VIRAL infection of the respiratory tract, as in INFECTIOUS MONONUCLEOSIS. The condition varies widely in its severity.

▧ SYMPTOMS A very sore throat, FEVER, general malaise, sore neck (from the swollen glands that accompany the tonsillitis); in younger children there may be accompanying VOMITING, STOMACH-ACHE, general irritability or lassitude.

A severe complication of tonsillitis, quinsy, involves an abscess forming behind the tonsils. This requires hospital treatment without delay.

▧ ACTION 1 Give acetamenophen to lower the temperature and relieve the pain. 2 Encourage the child to drink a lot of fluids.

▧ GET MEDICAL ADVICE if you think your child has a bacterial tonsillitis. You may look inside the mouth and see bright red tonsils with whitish patches on them: this is typical of tonsillitis. It is often difficult even for the doctor to decide whether a child has a bacterial tonsillitis, or a viral throat infection, or pharyngitis (as in the earliest phase of many COMMON COLDS) simply by looking at the throat.

Note: the size of the tonsils is not a guide to whether or not they are infected – many children normally have large tonsils.

▧ TESTS The doctor will take a swab from the tonsils to determine whether the infection is bacterial.

▧ TREATMENT Penicillin is almost always effective against *Streptococcus*, the major bacterium causing tonsillitis. Erythromycin can be given if a child is known to be allergic to penicillin (a rare problem).

Tonsillectomy, the removal of the tonsils, is an operation performed infrequently today compared with a generation ago. It will be advised only if a child is losing considerable time from school, due to repeated attacks of bacterial tonsillitis, which are not controlled by antibiotic treatment; or if there are signs of chronic (persistent) infection of the tonsils. Chronic infection is rarely an indication for performing a tonsillectomy.

Since there are no specific antiviral agents to treat viral pharyngitis or tonsillitis, symptomatic treatment with fluids and acetamenophen is recommended.

▧ OUTLOOK Tonsillitis, both bacterial and viral, normally clears up without trouble, but may recur several times a year. As children grow, their tonsils become smaller; tonsillitis may, however, still be troublesome in teenagers and adults.

TOOTHACHE

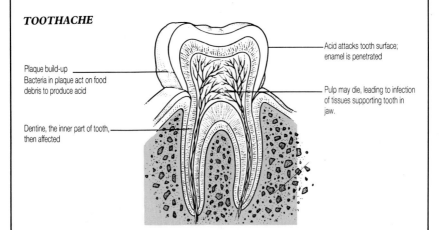

Acid attacks tooth surface; enamel is penetrated

Plaque build-up
Bacteria in plaque act on food debris to produce acid

Pulp may die, leading to infection of tissues supporting tooth in jaw.

Dentine, the inner part of tooth, then affected

TOOTHACHE

Extremely distressing pain in the teeth or jaws, which becomes worse while eating, but which may be present in between meals.

■ CAUSES In children toothache is commonly caused by tooth decay (*caries*). Poor tooth brushing results in the accumulation of a bacteria-containing substance called plaque, which clings to the teeth. The bacteria act on food debris and produce acids that attack the tooth surface. This eventually results in penetration of the tooth enamel, so that in due course the inner part of the tooth (the dentine) becomes affected, causing pain. If untreated, the pulp, which is the living part of the tooth, may die and lead to infection of the tissues which support the tooth in the jaw. This is usually the cause of more continuous toothache.

■ TREATMENT Pain on eating or drinking is usually a sign of dental decay, and will require early treatment by your dentist. If it persists after eating, the pain may be relieved by using a simple painkiller such as acetamenophen. More ad-

vanced decay, resulting in full-blown toothache, will almost certainly require an urgent visit to the dentist. Often, the only way of stopping the pain is to pull the tooth out.

■ ACTION See *TEETHING*, and talk to your dentist about preventive measures. Regular and thorough toothbrushing with a fluoride toothpaste, and the use of fluoride supplements where the local water supply does not contain sufficient fluoride, will help. So will the regular use of dental floss. Regular dental checkups are important to detect and treat cavities early.

TORSION OF THE TESTICLE

Twisting of the testicle. This can occur at any age. *Immediate action* is necessary: torsion cuts off the blood supply to the testicle, and treatment must be carried out within hours if the testicle is to be saved.

■ SYMPTOMS are severe pain in the testicle, groin and/or lower abdomen. The testicle will be swollen and tender. If torsion is suspected, get medical advice at once.

TREATMENT is by operation to reverse the twist and secure the testicle in its proper position. If the testicle is irretrievably damaged, it may be removed. The testicle on the other side may be stitched into position, to prevent it from twisting.

TOXOCARIASIS

Caused by ingestion of the eggs of the dog or cat roundworm, found in dirt contaminated by the animals' feces. If the eggs are ingested by the child, the parasites settle in different tissues of the body causing inflammation.

SYMPTOMS FEVER, ANEMIA, FAILURE TO THRIVE associated with COUGH and wheeze. Rarely, CONVULSIONS and generalized weakness may develop. Symptoms depend upon the number of eggs ingested and the degree of allergic response to them. Most people who are lightly infected have no symptoms. An enlarged liver and spleen or inflammation of the back of the eye (retina) may be detected. The child may show signs of failing vision. A history of eating soil (pica) is common.

PREVENTION Hygiene; appropriate, regular worming of cats and dogs, proper disposal of cat and dog feces.

INVESTIGATIONS BLOOD TESTS (including ANTIBODY tests); possibly a liver biopsy; chest X-ray.

TREATMENT Appropriate medication; attempting to eliminate the parasites; steroids such as prednisone may be used to treat troublesome symptoms. Prevention of further pica.

OUTLOOK Blindness may result if the effects on the eyes are allowed to advance. Rarely, the condition can be lethal if an exceptionally large number of eggs are eaten. However, most cases respond gradually (over six to 12 months), but well to treatment. Recovery is good if the child does not ingest more eggs.

TOXOPLASMOSIS

Toxoplasma gondii is a PARASITE that thrives within body cells. This parasite commonly infects dogs and cats. Humans are infected by accidentally eating the eggs. The eggs are found wherever dogs and cats defecate, such as in parks, backyards and sand boxes. Toxoplasmosis cannot be transmitted from person to person, except during pregnancy, from mother to fetus (congenital toxoplasmosis). This causes different symptoms than those of ordinary toxoplasmosis.

SYMPTOMS OF CONGENITAL TOXOPLASMOSIS A severe infection early in pregnancy can result in natural (spontaneous) abortion or still birth. Infections later in pregnancy may lead to the baby being born with signs of the disease. These may be mild or severe, and may in turn cause:
– Inflammation of the eyes, which can lead to BLINDNESS.
– Brain damage with MENINGITIS, ENCEPHALITIS or HYDROCEPHALUS. This may be obvious at birth, or give rise to CONVULSIONS or MENTAL HANDICAP which occur and are detected later.
– Inflammation of the liver, spleen and lymph glands can result in enlargement of these organs. JAUNDICE, ANEMIA and a bleeding tendency can occur.
– A red, blotchy rash.

SYMPTOMS OF INFECTION ACQUIRED AFTER BIRTH This

usually occurs after three years of age. The symptoms may be so mild as to pass unnoticed, or there may be signs of a more severe infection. Enlargement of the lymph glands is common, particularly those in the neck. There may be muscle pain. Symptoms may be similar to INFECTIOUS MONONUCLEOSIS or INFLUENZA.

■ TESTS BLOOD TESTS can confirm the diagnosis.

■ TREATMENT In severe cases, a combination of ANTIBIOTICS. Treatment of convulsions and hydrocephalus is described under those entries.

TRACHEO-ESOPHAGEAL FISTULA

A CONGENITAL ABNORMALITY where the trachea (wind pipe) and esophagus (food tube) fail to separate completely during development. The esophagus is usually incomplete (esophageal atresia), and there is an open connection between the trachea and the esophagus (fistula).

■ INCIDENCE Very rare: three babies in every 10,000.

■ SYMPTOMS From birth the baby is unable to swallow his saliva, and drools frothy mucus. Any attempt at feeding results in choking and distress.

In about 2 percent of those children, the fistula between the esophagus and the trachea allows food to spill over into the lungs. This causes recurrent attacks of PNEUMONIA.

■ ACTION *Immediate* specialist care is required. Doctors are trained to recognize and test for this condition at birth.

■ TREATMENT After diagnostic

tests and stabilization have occurred, surgery is required to separate the trachea and esophagus.

■ OUTLOOK Babies born at full term, and without other abnormalities or complications, have a better than 90 percent chance of survival, with an expectation of a healthy, normal life thereafter. If a baby is premature or has a very extensive abnormality, then his chance of survival is smaller.

TRANQUILLIZERS
See *POISONING.*

TUBERCULOSIS (TB)
An INFECTIOUS disease, common world-wide, but now relatively rare in developed countries. A tubercle, a microscopic mass of tissue, was one of the characteristic findings of the disease noted by early pathologists when examining victims' lungs.

■ CAUSE The BACTERIUM known as *Mycobacterium tuberculosis*, which is transmitted from person to person by inhalation of infected droplets. Ingestion of infected cow's milk is not a cause in North America, since all cattle are tested for tuberculosis, killed if positive and all milk is pasteurized.

■ PREVENTION In most parts of the United States and Canada, the risk of tuberculosis is so low that routine tuberculin skin testing and vaccination are *not* recommended. Testing is suggested for higher-risk children including native Indians and Inuits, those from high TB-prevalent neighbourhoods and those from countries where TB is common.

The use of TB vaccine, BCG, is controversial. It is not routinely used in North America.

■ ACQUIRING IMMUNITY The child, unknown to anyone, catches the infection and develops a 'primary complex' in the lungs. There are no symptoms, although its occurrence may later show on a chest X-ray, or when the child is shown on testing to be skin test positive. This first stage of the disease, in itself essentially harmless, gives immunity. However, the infection can spread through the body, causing such infections as tuberculous PNEUMONIA, MENINGITIS or bone, joint or skin infection which while uncommon in industrialized countries, can be serious and even life threatening.

■ SYMPTOMS of active tuberculosis include (early) loss of energy and appetite; (later) cough, sputum, weight loss and nocturnal sweating.

■ TREATMENT is by ANTIBIOTICS specific to tuberculosis. The patient usually has to take the drugs for several months.

■ OUTLOOK depends on the type of infection: for tuberculosis of the lungs and glands, treatment should be completely effective; tuberculous MENINGITIS is a grave disease, carrying a risk of permanent disabilities.

TUMOR OF THE EYE
An abnormal mass of tissue in the eye. The only significant tumor or cancer of the eye in childhood is retinoblastoma. It is very rare, can affect one or both eyes, and usually develops before the age of three years. The predisposition to this cancer may run in families.

■ SYMPTOMS The child may develop STRABISMUS; or when light is shone into the pupil, the reflection may appear white rather than red (as is usual). Untreated, sight will deteriorate and the eye will become inflamed.

An eye doctor will examine the inside of both eyes, usually under a general anesthetic, to determine the tumor's size and position.

■ TREATMENT Small tumors may be burnt out by a laser beam or treated with radiotherapy (X-ray). Sometimes, in order to save the child's life, it may be necessary to remove the affected eye.

■ OUTLOOK About 90 percent of children with retinoblastoma are cured. The radiotherapy may cause CATARACTS, which can be removed at a later date. If the child's eye needs removal, an artificial one can be fitted. Providing the vision is good in the other eye, he will be able to lead a normal life.

TURNER SYNDROME
A rare abnormality in girls where there is only one sex CHROMOSOME (an X) per body cell, instead of the normal two. Affected girls are of short stature and stocky, and some may be of slightly lower intelligence than might be expected from the family background. Hearing problems may also occur. Sometimes the diagnosis is not suspected until PUBERTY, when the girl's breasts fail to develop and her pubic hair growth is only slight. Periods do not start and she will be infertile. She can otherwise lead a normal life. If you have one child with Turner syndrome there is no added risk of further children suffering the same abnormality.

TWINS
See *MULTIPLE PREGNANCY.*

TYPHOID FEVER
A grave, INFECTIOUS illness now un-

common except in undeveloped countries, caused by the BACTERIUM *Salmonella typhi*.

■ CAUSE The infection spreads through poor hygiene, particularly by contaminated food or water. Uncooked food such as ice-cream, fruit, or unpasteurized milk products can carry the infection.

■ SYMPTOMS Gradual onset of fever, headache, loss of appetite, lethargy, abdominal pain and a pink rash (rose spots). The liver and spleen are enlarged. Complications may include OSTEOMYELITIS, MENINGITIS and septic ARTHRITIS.

■ ACTION Prevention is essential: avoid likely sources of infection, and have your child IMMUNIZED if visiting an area with a high infection rate. In high-risk areas, water should be boiled and uncooked foods avoided. Small children should be given only boiled or well-cooked food and drink, or bottled or canned drinks.

Immunization against typhoid enhances resistance to infection but the degree of protection is limited. It is recommended for all children at risk who are over one year. Babies under a year should be protected by strict application of the precautions listed above. Since the vaccine is not 100 percent effective, food and water precautions are essential when travelling in high-risk areas.

Consult your travel agent or your doctor for advice about whether you need immunization for travel to a particular country.

■ GET MEDICAL ADVICE if your child becomes ill in any way during or after a visit to a tropical or undeveloped country. Typhoid fever is diagnosed by BLOOD TESTS, and treatment with antibiotics is effective.

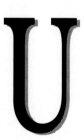

ULCERATIVE COLITIS

An uncommon inflammation and ulceration of the large bowel (colon and rectum) and sometimes the small bowel lining (mucosa). The cause is unknown. It occurs mainly in school-age children, but very rarely during infancy.

■ SYMPTOMS DIARRHEA, mucus and blood in the stools, loss of APPETITE and weight, ANEMIA, generally feeling ill and FEVER. VOMITING (occasionally), MOUTH ULCERS, joint pains, anal irritation, poor growth, eye inflammation, skin RASHES (particularly red swellings over the shins).

Rarely, acute ABDOMINAL SWELLING and distension of the bowel (toxic megacolon) may lead to perforation of the bowel and PERITONITIS.

■ INVESTIGATIONS Abdominal X-ray to determine the presence of characteristic gas shadows. BLOOD TEST for anemia and evidence of inflammation. A barium ENEMA to show the extent of bowel inflammation.

A pediatric gastroenterologist will need to examine the bowel and rectal passage, and possibly to take specimens of the lining of the bowel (biopsy). This process, called colonoscopy, is an examination of the large intestine using a flexible tube with a special light, that permits visualization of its lining to determine the extent of the disease.

■ TREATMENT A balanced, palatable, nutritious diet is recommended. Fatigue should be avoided and rest recommended but participation in school, social and athletic activities should be supported to the extent possible. Anti-inflammatory drugs such as steroids given by mouth and in enemas. BLOOD TRANSFUSION is occasionally necessary. Intravenous fluids may be necessary at times. Surgical colectomy (large bowel removal) and permanent ileostomy (creating a bowel opening on to skin of abdomen) may be necessary if the colitis does not respond to medical treatment. 'Pull through' procedures in which the distal part of the small bowel is brought down to the rectum, thus eliminating the need for a permanent ileostomy can be done in some patients.

■ OUTLOOK Medical treatment only may be required. Surgical treatment will be necessary for perforation or for severe or chronic symptoms with evidence of compli-cations. Many children accept, and are very much better with, an ileostomy if it is necessary. A 'pull through' procedure may be a more acceptable alternative. CANCER in very long-standing colitis is a risk in adulthood, so regular check-ups are advised. After the first ten years of illness the incidence of cancer rises by 20 percent per decade.

ULTRASOUND SCAN
A diagnostic technique employing high-frequency sound waves that are transmitted into the body. On reaching the organs, they bounce back and are picked up on a receiver, which converts them into pictures on a screen. Each organ, or part of an organ, has a characteristic appearance, so abnormalities in size or structure can be detected. The scan cannot reveal anything about the function of the organs, however, nor can all organs be clearly seen. The organs most readily examined include the heart, liver, kidneys, bladder and brain. During pregnancy, the fetus can also be examined – see *PRENATAL DIAGNOSIS*.

To take a scan, the child is asked to lie on a bed and an instrument is placed lightly on the skin. A jelly is used to make contact with the skin. The procedure is painless.

Ultrasound waves do not cause damage to the body. If necessary, scans can be repeated without worry.

UMBILICUS
The place where the umbilical cord was attached to the baby while in the womb; also called the navel or belly button. The umbilical cord is clamped at birth, and the remaining stump kept clean and dry to prevent INFECTION. If the skin around the ubilicus becomes red or the cord becomes moist, this in-

dicates an infection. If neglected, this can become dangerous: if in doubt get medical help. The stump drops off within ten to 14 days. The technique used to cut and clamp the cord does not affect the final size and shape of the child's umbilicus.

UNCONSCIOUS CHILD

An unconscious child is unresponsive, and the level of unconsciousness can be graded according to how well the child responds to different stimuli, such as talking or touching. A deeply unconscious child will not respond to any stimulus; a less unconscious child may withdraw his arm or speak in response to, say, a painful injection.

▓ ACTION **1** Call for immediate help and summon an ambulance. **2** Assess the situation, remembering the possibility of neck injury (see *EMERGENCY RESUSCITA-TION*). If breathing and pulse are absent, follow steps A, B and C of emergency resuscitation. If breathing and pulse are present, put the child in the RECOVERY POSITION. **3** Keep the child warm and continue to check his pulse and breathing while waiting for the ambulance.

▓ ACTION AT HOSPITAL If necessary, the child will be resuscitated. The reasons for the unconsciousness will then be investigated and treated. Possible causes will include:

  – POISONING;
  – INFECTION of the nervous system (for example, MENINGITIS);
  – HEAD INJURY;
  – severe trauma leading to blood loss (see *SHOCK*);
  – anaphylaxis (see *ALLERGY*);
  – EPILEPSY;
  – DIABETIC coma.

UNDESCENDED TESTICLE

A testicle that does not descend into the scrotum. Normally the testicle forms in the abdominal cavity of the fetus, and migrates down into the scrotum by the time the baby is born. However, in 2 percent of new-born boys, this migration is only completed over the first year of life. In a smaller number, the descent remains incomplete.

▓ TREATMENT The baby's scrotum is examined shortly after birth. If a testicle is undescended, regular checks are made. If it has not descended by the time the boy is one year old, then surgery is advisable and will usually be performed between the ages of one and three years. The operation involves bringing the testicle into the scrotum, and securing (suturing) it in place. The operation is advisable for various reasons: appearance – this is especially important as the boy grows older; fertility, which will decrease if the testicle remains undescended; and there is an increased risk of cancer occurring in the testicle, and ofTORSION OF THE TESTICLE or accidental trauma if the testicle is left undescended.

▓ OUTLOOK There are usually no problems following the operation, and fertility is normally unaffected.

URINARY TRACT INFECTION (UTI)

INFECTION of the urinary tract, caused by BACTERIA commonly originating from the bowel. It is commoner in girls than in boys.

▓ SYMPTOMS Older children will have pain on passing urine, and a feeling of urgently needing to pass urine. They may also have ABDOMI-

NAL PAIN, FEVER and blood in the urine. Babies' symptoms may be more non-specific: CRYING, feeding poorly, VOMITING, DIARRHEA and fever.

▦ ACTION If you suspect your child has a UTI, take him to the doctor, who will obtain a urine specimen to test for infection. See *URINE TESTS*.

▦ TREATMENT is with ANTIBIOT-ICS, usually given by mouth for a period of 14 days.

▦ FURTHER TESTS Special X-rays, ultrasounds and other newer forms of imaging may be indicated to investigate whether there is an underlying abnormality of the kidneys or of the urinary tract. A common problem associated with recurrent or chronic urinary infection in children is ureteral reflux – urine is forced up the ureters towards the kidneys when the bladder contracts. This in turn results in urine stagnating in the bladder and ureters where it becomes infected. Furthermore, if the urine is infected this can cause infection and scarring of the kidneys. Fortunately this usually ceases as the child gets older and, providing the urine is kept clear with antibiotics, no further treatment is necessary.

URINE TESTS

A urine test is required to diagnose or confirm a URINARY TRACT INFECTION or a kidney disease. The urine sample must be free from contamination and sent fresh to a laboratory. Easier to obtain from boys than girls – a small sterile plastic bag taped around the penis in boys or perineum in girls if often used in babies. Unfortunately, these specimens may be contaminated.

It may then be necessary to puncture the bladder with a needle to collect an uncontaminated sample. Alternatively, a clean specimen may be 'caught' from the free stream of urine as the child urinates.

Other urine tests, for protein and for glucose (sugar), can be carried out on ordinary nonsterile specimens'. Dipsticks' can provide an instant result concerning glucose or protein. Protein is present in the urine if the child has NEPHRITIS; also in NEPHROTIC SYNDROME. Glucose in the urine suggests DIABETES.

URICARIA

Commonly known as hives, this is an intermittent, very itchy rash, usually on the body, consisting of either small raised lumps or large patches (giant urticaria).

▦ CAUSES Broadly speaking, urticaria represents an ALLERGIC reaction of the skin. Children can become allergic to foods, dyes, drugs (such as penicillin), or plants. Other drugs, including aspirin, can cause urticaria by directly stimulating the release of histamine in the skin. Often the cause of the urticaria is unknown.

▦ SYMPTOMS The intensely itchy lumps come and go over a few hours, and clear to leave normal skin. In severe cases swelling may occur inside the mouth or in the airways, leading to wheezing and difficulty in breathing (angio-edema).

▦ ACTION Most episodes of urticaria will subside without any treatment. It is useful to try to identify the cause by considering what food, drink or medicines have been taken in the previous 24 hours. In this way recurrence may be avoided. Often, however, the cause remains elusive.

■ GET URGENT MEDICAL ADVICE if the more severe symptoms of wheezing or swelling of the mouth develop, or the child becomes distressed.

■ TESTS For severe cases, some dermatologists recommend skin or BLOOD TESTS to try to identify the irritating agent.

■ TREATMENT Avoiding known cause(s) is the first line of defense. Antihistamine drugs, such as chlorpheniramine or terfenadine, will relieve the symptoms, and may be given until the rash has cleared. Angio-edema is treated by the injection of adrenalin (which should always be available when skin testing is carried out).

■ OUTLOOK Urticaria is seldom a major problem in childhood.

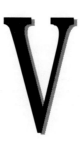

VAGINAL DISCHARGE

Many girls develop a white discharge from the vagina from time to time during childhood. It may cause itching and is sometimes bloodstained. There are many possible causes which include:
– Infections due to CANDIDIASIS (sometimes following a course of ANTIBIOTICS or the irritation of the vagina by PINWORMS.
– If the vulval skin is also red and itchy, the discharge may be part of a DERMATITIS caused by bubble-bath soaps, bath oils or nylon underpants.
– In a new-born baby girl, a clear vaginal discharge is normal, and results from the action of the mother's hormones on the baby's vagina.
– In adolescence it may, as in adults, be a sign of sexually transmitted disease

or, in children, a possible sign of abuse.
– A bloodstained discharge is much less common and may be the result of the child pushing an object, such as a bead, into her vagina.

■ ACTION If your child has a vaginal discharge that is foul smelling, profuse, itchy or bloodstained, take her to the doctor for investigation. A swab of the discharge may be taken, and other tests performed.

■ TREATMENT usually involves an externally applied cream or a drug taken by mouth. If the discharge is foul smelling, creamy or bloodstained, the child may have to be given an anesthetic in order to make it possible to look for, and remove, the foreign object.

VALVE DISEASE OF THE HEART
See *CONGENITAL HEART-DISEASE*.

VARICELLA
See *CHICKEN POX*.

VENTRICULAR SEPTAL DEFECT
See *CONGENITAL HEART-DISEASE*.

VERRUCA
See *WARTS*.

VIRUSES
Viruses are smaller than BACTERIA, and can only survive within living cells. The body produces ANTIBODIES when exposed to a virus, resulting in IMMUNITY to that virus. This usually occurs within a few days, and most viral INFECTIONS are mild and self-limiting. Immunity can also be induced by IMMUNIZATION.

Treatment of viral infections is usually symptomatic: rest, sleep, acetamenophen, and fluids and food as the child wishes. ANTIBIOTICS have no effect against viruses. Some ANTIVIRAL DRUGS are now becoming available, but as yet are used only for certain specific and serious infections. There is no specific treatment as yet for the commonest of the viral infections, the COMMON COLD.

VITAMIN DEFICIENCY
See VITAMINS. Vitamin deficiency is highly unusual in the United States, occurring mainly in certain high-risk groups, such as children with MALNUTRITION, unusual or inadequate diets, disorders such as liver or renal disease or, rarely, in PREMATURE babies.

Vitamin deficiency may occur singly or more than one may occur simultaneously in relation to malnutrition.

■ VITAMIN A DEFICIENCY will affect the clear part (cornea) of the eye and the outer lining of the eye (conjunctiva), causing dryness and thickening. Night vision may also be reduced. In severe cases, daytime sight may eventually be diminished.

The skin tends to be dry and scaly and there may be poor growth and intellectual impairment.

Treatment is by simple replacement of the deficient vitamin. Prevention is by adequate intake of dairy products and vegetables.

■ VITAMIN B DEFICIENCY There are several types associated with various clinical disorders.

Thiamine (vitamin B1) deficiency causes beriberi, mostly in Asian babies. Symptoms include heart failure, nerve dysfunction and psychological disturbances. Unless treated with thiamine injections, this is a rapidly fatal condition.

Riboflavine (vitamin · B2) deficiency is characterized by severe cracking at the corners of the mouth, a sore red tongue and lips, and excess blood vessel formation in the cornea. These clear quickly when daily doses of riboflavin are given.

Niacin (nicotinic acid) deficiency (pellagra) occurs particularly where corn is the main food in the diet. There is redness, swelling and dryness of skin exposed to sunlight. Thickening and infection also occur. The symptoms may arise in association with other vitamin B deficiencies, and will probably be associated with malnutrition including protein deficiency (kwashiorkor).

Treatment involves doses of all the B group of vitamins and an adequate protein intake.

Deficiency of pyridoxine (vitamin B6) may lead to ANEMIA and CON-

VULSIONS. A new-born baby who has had prolonged convulsions with no obvious cause might be pyridoxine deficient.

Pyridoxine injections will cure the illness. The vitamin is present in milk but is inactivated if heated.

Cyanocobalamin (vitamin B12) deficiency is also rare. The substance is necessary for red blood cell production by the bone marrow, and is also involved in the biochemical processes of the nervous system. The child becomes tired, has a poor appetite and develops anemia. The tongue may be sore, and neurological symptoms include ataxia (unsteadiness), paraesthesia (numbness) and poor tendon reflexes.

Injections of vitamin B12 several times a week will cure the illness.

Folic acid deficiency: some small PREMATURE infants with low folate levels develop anemia at about eight weeks. Children with MALABSORPTION such as CELIAC DISEASE can also develop mild folate deficiency and anemia. This can also occur when certain anti-convulsant drugs are used. Folate deficiency may also arise as part of a general vitamin deficiency state in malnutrition.

Symptoms include ANOREXIA (loss of appetite), FAILURE TO THRIVE, and increased susceptibility to infections and gastro-intestinal disturbances.

Treatment consists of giving folic acid daily.

Prevention of vitamin B deficiency is accomplished by a diet rich in milk, vegetables, cereals, fruits and eggs.

■ VITAMIN C (ascorbic acid) DEFICIENCY SCURVY is the main consequence, but this is rare in developed countries except in children on unusual diets. If fruit and vegetables are entirely lacking, there is a risk.

The main symptoms are bleeding gums, pain in the bones and BRUISING in the skin.

Treatment is vitamin C pills daily. Prevention is by adequate intake of fruit and vegetables.

■ VITAMIN D DEFICIENCY Most infants in developed countries are fed on commercially prepared cow's milk fortified with sufficient vitamin D. Those lacking the vitamin may get RICKETS.

■ VITAMIN E DEFICIENCY may occur in malabsorption, especially in diseases such as CYSTIC FIBROSIS and BILIARY ATRESIA. Premature infants will become anemic.

Treatment is vitamin E pills daily.

■ VITAMIN K DEFICIENCY leads to BLEEDING disorders. Bleeding in the first week of life at the umbilical cord site, or into the stomach, which is associated with VOMITING of blood, or into the intestine, which may produce SHOCK. Vitamin K deficiency may also occur in older children who have malabsorption.

New-born babies receive an injection of vitamin K to prevent bleeding problems.

Vitamin K needs to be given regularly to children with malabsorption, usually as a tablet.

In normal children, vitamin K is synthesized by BACTERIA in the intestines in sufficient amounts to avoid any deficiency.

VITAMINS

Organic substances occurring in minute quantities in plant and animal tissues. Vitamins are essential for specific functions of the tissues to proceed normally, and must be supplied in the diet or made in the body from dietary products. Deficiency of vitamins leads

VITAMINS

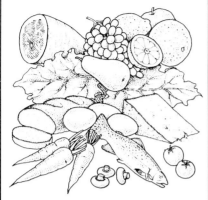

Food products containing vitamins.

to particular disorders and disease including RICKETS, SCURVY and BLINDNESS – see *VITAMIN DEFICIENCY*.

The important vitamins are vitamins A, B, C, D, E and K.

▨ VITAMIN A occurs naturally in dairy products, and can be made in the body from pigments occurring in vegetables. Impairment of this process may arise in liver disease or HYPOTHYROIDISM. The vitamin is necessary for the health of the epithelium (skin or tissue lining cavities), particularly that of the eye.

▨ VITAMIN B is concerned with the body's use and production (metabolism) of carbohydrate, lipids (fat) and amino-acids (protein products). It occurs as several different, interrelated chemical compounds including thiamine (vitamin B1); riboflavine and niacin (B2); pyridoxine (B6); cyanocobalamin (B12) and folic acid.

Thiamine, present in liver, kidney and eggs, is important in carbohydrate (sugar) metabolism. Riboflavine and niacin are necessary parts of enzymes involved in the metabolism of carbohydrates, proteins and fats. They occur in dairy products, meat, eggs and vegetables. Pyridoxine is present in milk. Cyanocobalamin needs to be bound to a protein produced by the stomach lining in order to be absorbed properly.

Folic acid, necessary for growth and normal red blood cell production, is present in most milks but in low concentrations in goat's milk.

▨ VITAMIN C (ascorbic acid) is essential for the formation of the protein structure of body tissues. It is present in human milk, fruit and vegetables, and commercially prepared food.

▨ VITAMIN D is present in milk, fish oils, animal fat and in some commercially prepared foods such as margarine. Sunlight acting on the skin can also provide vitamin D naturally. The vitamin increases the absorption of calcium and phosphate from the intestine, which in turn are important for bone calcification and growth.

▨ VITAMIN E occurs in milk, vegetables and many foods. It is necessary for the metabolism of fats, and for building muscle tissue.

▨ VITAMIN K occurs in milk and green plants, and is necessary for the production of certain clotting factors in the blood.

Excesses of vitamins can cause serious problems, particularly excesses of vitamins A and D. Given in great excess in a young child, even vitamin C (because it is an acid) can overwhelm the kidneys' ability to excrete it. Before giving vitamin supplements to your child, discuss the type and amounts with your doctor.

VOLVULUS

An acute obstruction of the bowel, caused by the twisting of a portion of it on its attachment to the back of the abdomen.

■ SYMPTOMS VOMITING, acute ABDOMINAL PAIN, and sometimes passage of blood through the anus. The child may be very ill and develop PERITONITIS.

■ INVESTIGATION An abdominal X-ray shows a large distended loop of bowel and evidence of INTESTINAL OBSTRUCTION.

■ TREATMENT Surgical correction of the twisting through an abdominal operation is required, occasionally the twisted portion of the bowel has become gangrenous and must be removed. There is a risk of death if the diagnosis is delayed and peritonitis and shock occur before there is the chance to operate.

VOMITING

More common, and fortunately less distressing, in children than in adults – see also *SPITTING UP*. Vomiting in young babies that is severe, very forceful and projectile may be a sign of PYLORIC STENOSIS. Vomiting also occurs in infants and young children in association with a variety of illnesses and INFECTIONS. When associated with a sudden onset of DIARRHEA, it usually indicates GASTROENTERITIS. Occasionally vomiting is indicative of more serious disease, as in MENINGITIS or APPENDICITIS.

■ ACTION Observe the child, noting whether the vomiting is followed by other symptoms. Let the child have sips of water and clear fluids, but don't force him to eat. If there is a FEVER, try acetamenophen. Get medical advice if there is no improvement, or if the child becomes generally ill, DEHYDRATED, develops a bad HEADACHE, is unduly drowsy or has a high fever.

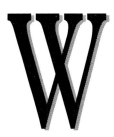

WARTS

Common warts are small, brownish, round lesions several millimeters in diameter, which usually occur on the hands; plantar warts are flattened warts on the soles of the feet; genital warts occur around the genital area.

■ CAUSE All warts are caused by VIRUSES known as human papilloma viruses. They are caught from other people with warts. The types of papilloma viruses causing skin warts are different from those that usually cause genital warts.

■ SYMPTOMS Pain occurs if the warts are in a sensitive place, such as under a finger nail, or on the sole of the foot. Many children find warts embarrassing. Genital warts can become sore because of their position. Since genital warts can be transmitted sexually, in children they may give rise to suspicions of sexual abuse.

■ ACTION Most warts regress spontaneously within a few months. If they persist, common warts can be treated at home with a simple wart paint (see under treatment) obtained from the drugstore. If this fails, and they are troublesome, seek advice from your doctor. Genital warts should only be treated by a doctor.

■ TREATMENT 1 Wart-removing solution usually contains salicylic acid, which works by softening the hard skin of the wart, allowing gentle rubbing with an emery board or pumice-stone to gradually remove the wart. Follow the instructions carefully. 2 If wart-removing solution fails, your doctor may try freezing with liquid nitrogen or carbon dioxide snow. The wart and the skin around it are frozen solid and then allowed to thaw. This kills the wart virus; the wart then separates from the surrounding skin and drops out, or off. Some children find the process painful; it is certainly uncomfortable. 3 Podophyllin is used for genital warts. It is applied by a nurse or doctor at a specialist clinic. It should not be used by patients themselves and is not recommended for young children. Laser surgery may be used.

■ LONG-TERM MANAGEMENT Since warts are so common, and relatively harmless, parents can usually deal with them themselves. Solution and ointments are easily obtainable from the drugstore. If the treatment causes pain, it should be stopped for a few days, then resumed. Covering the wart with waterproof plaster helps to soften the skin, and also prevents spread. Children with plantar warts need not be banned from swimming.

■ OUTLOOK Warts eventually go away. The body develops resistance to the virus, and kills it. But, of course, a different papilloma virus can still cause new warts.

WATER IN EARS

There is no danger to a child's ears from water, unless the child has a perforated eardrum – See *MIDDLE EAR INFECTION*. EXTERNAL EAR INFECTIONS can result from too frequent swimming. If avoiding swimming is a problem, your child cay try using ear plugs.

WAX IN EARS

It is usual for ears to produce wax, which serves to protect the delicate skin lining the ear canal from irritation by water and dirt. Excess wax normally moves to the outer opening of the ear canal where it can be easily removed with a piece of soft tissue paper. It is not necessary to remove wax that you cannot see, and it can be harmful to try to do so. The ear canals only become blocked with wax after it has been pushed into the ears by well-meaning parents wielding Q-tips.

■ ACTION If the ear canal becomes blocked with wax and the child hears less well than usual, get medical advice. Your doctor can easily remove soft wax with a syringe or, when the wax is very hard, he may advise the use of wax-softening drops for a few days.

WEANING

The transition from the initial milk diet of a baby to the mixed diet of the older child. Weaning also means the process of discontinuing breast or bottle feedings in favor of milk from a cup.

'Solids' are usually introduced to a baby between four and six months in response to a baby who is no longer drowsy and satisfied with milk feeds.

A spoonful of rice-based cereal is a useful starter. Sugary foods and foods with added salt should be avoided for as long as possible.

The baby will soon, if hungry, take an interest in other foods. Over the next few months fruits, vegetables and cereals can be pured and used in slowly increasing amounts to give variety.

At eight or nine months, hard foods and finger foods such as baby biscuits or crackers are welcomed as teething progresses. Eggs are usually not introduced into the diet until nine months or so, along with meats. When introducing new foods it is best to proceed one at a time so any reactions can be noted. As the child learns to chew, chunks of food can be managed and the toddler can be fed some of the normal family diet, cut into small pieces.

The toddler may wish to continue to drink large amounts of fluid from a bottle or a cup, but the amount taken is slowly reduced during the second year.

The health risks of this dietary transition are mainly due to INFECTION and are thus related to hygiene and environment. As with BOTTLE FEEDING, parents must be aware of the risks of infection and multiplication of BACTERIA when food is handled, or left out of the refrigerator in a warm place.

Weaning is a tricky stage for parent-child interactions, and outside advice may appear to aggravate matters instead of helping. Parents may feel under pressure if their child is not proceeding easily through the stages outlined above. However, each child is different and finding the right pattern takes time. It may help to remember that feeding-time battles are very common – see *FEEDING PROBLEMS*.

WEIGHT LOSS

See *FAILURE TO THRIVE, ANOREXIA NERVOSA, ULCERATIVE COLITIS*.

WELL-BABY CARE

In the United States, well-baby care is primarily carried out by private family doctors, pediatricians or through hospital or health department well-baby clinics. As the name implies, this is not intended as a service for sick children, but to provide preventive medicine: screening tests (for anemia, kidney disease, tuberculosis, and so on); IMMUNIZATIONS; development checkups (see *GROWTH PATTERNS* and *DEVELOPMENTAL DELAY*); and advice about NUTRITION, FEEDING PROBLEMS, SLEEP PROBLEMS and any other matters of concern to parents.

WETTING

It is common for children, in the early school years, to have occasional 'accidents' (involuntary passing of urine) during the day, often because they cannot find a bathroom in time. However, wetting can also be a sign of stress in a normally dry child. URINARY TRACT INFECTIONS and other medical complaints can also cause wetting. See also *BEDWETTING, TOILET TRAINING*.

▨ ACTION Do not over-react to the incident: all children are embarrassed by wetting accidents, and an angry response may only make the situation worse. Check whether there are any particular difficulties for your child, for example in using the school bathrooms, or whether your child is under any obvious stress. If the problem persists or occurs frequently, get medical advice. Your doctor may check for a urinary tract infection; or may suggest seeking the advice of a psychologist or child psychiatrist.

WHITLOW

See *PARONYCHIA*.

WHOOPING COUGH (PERTUSSIS)

A highly INFECTIOUS disease, caused by BACTERIA and spread through exhaled and coughed droplets. It is commonest in pre-school children and most serious in babies under six months of age. The INCUBATION PERIOD is seven to 14 days. A child is infectious from a week before the onset of symptoms to three weeks after the start of the spasmodic cough: sometimes for a total of about six weeks. The incidence of whooping cough has declined in the United States in areas with high IMMUNIZATION rates.

▨ SYMPTOMS are in three phases, each lasting about two weeks.

First phase: sneezing, a runny nose and slight FEVER. The cough develops gradually, mainly at night to begin with, then becoming worse during the day. During this time the child is most infectious, but because the symptoms are so like those of a COMMON COLD, the diagnosis is unlikely to be made unless the child is known to have been in contact with another child with the disease.

Second phase: the cough grows even worse, and comes in spasms lasting half a minute or more. The child's face turns red, and he may even become blue. Intake of breath after the cough produces the characteristic whoop. The cough may be set off by the slightest movement, crying or even eating. VOMITING often occurs after coughing and the child may have NOSEBLEEDS and small hemorrhages in his eyes. His APPETITE may be very poor, and together with the vomiting this can lead to DEHYDRATION and WEIGHT LOSS. CONVULSIONS can occur, particularly in babies who don't have the typical whoop, but who appear to choke and become blue.

In severe cases this second phase may last about four weeks. PNEUMO-

NIA may develop and chronic lung infections occasionally follow the illness. Lack of oxygen to the brain during the coughing spasms can lead to BRAIN DAMAGE.

Third phase: the cough gradually becomes less frequent and prolonged and the appetite improves. However, relapses can occur and the whooping can re-establish itself alarmingly.

▦ TESTS A nasal swab can indentify the bacteria.

A BLOOD TEST will show an increased number of lymphocytes (white blood cells) and characteristic ANTIBODIES.

▦ ACTION If you suspect whooping cough, get urgent medical advice. Milder cases can be treated at home.

Feedings should be small and frequent. Easily digestible, nutritious food helps to prevent weight loss.

Try to keep the child quiet, as exertion and crying can set off a spasm of coughing.

During a coughing spell, sit the child up, leaning him forwards to prevent inhalation of vomit.

The cough can be frightening for the child, who has difficulty catching his breath. Hold him on your lap and soothe him to minimize his anxiety, which can aggravate the cough.

Fever, which returns during the second phase of the illness, often indicates a lung infection (pneumonia or bronchitis). If this occurs, get medical advice. Your doctor may prescribe an ANTIBIOTIC.

▦ TREATMENT Admission to the hospital may be necessary if the cough is associated with breathing problems. This is especially import-ant in very young babies. Oxygen can be given, and the mucus in the nose and the back of the throat can be removed with a tube attached to a suction machine.

Antibiotics may reduce the severity of the disease if given in its early stages, but are not particularly effective once the cough has started. However, they can be used to treat bacterial pneumonia if this is a complication, and are often used to prevent spread of the disease to others.

Anticonvulsants may be necessary to treat convulsions.

▦ PREVENTION IMMUNIZATION is effective. It is given as part of the triple vaccine with DIPHTHERIA and TETANUS starting when the baby is two months old.

The risks from the disease are much greater than the risk of whooping cough immunization. Whooping cough immunization is recommended for all infants except those who are neurologically unstable and those who have had a serious reaction to a previous pertussis-containing vaccine.

Whooping cough can occur before two months of age and if an older child gets it, an unimmunized baby in the family is at risk. Mass immunization is tending to prevent this problem from arising, but if you find yourself in this situation, get urgent medical advice. Whooping cough in a baby under six months can be very serious indeed, even fatal.

▦ OUTLOOK Whooping cough remains potentially fatal, particularly in children under a year. Younger children are at risk of permanent brain damage, or long-term lung damage after the infection clears.

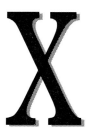

X-RAYS

These have more uses than many people suspect. An X-ray of the chest will show abnormalities within the lungs, the size and shape of the heart, and the bones of the chest and upper back. An X-ray of the bones will detect fractures or other abnormalities. X-rays of the abdomen will indicate blockages (obstructions) of the bowel, the position of the stomach and liver, and objects that have been swallowed, such as pins or coins.

Specialized X-ray techniques may involve: injection into a vein in the arm of a dye that shows up on X-ray to detect abnormalities of the kidneys, the blood vessels or the heart; or swallowing a solution that highlights abnormalities of the bowel when an X-ray is taken.

X-rays don't always provide a definite answer to a problem, but they help in the overall assessment.

■ PROCEDURE Simple X-rays cause no more discomfort than having a photograph taken; the child needs to remain still momentarily as the X-ray is being taken. The child should wear a protective lead apron over the genitalia when X-rays of the hips or abdomen are being taken. Reassure your child: the machinery is quite scarey. If you remain in the room while the X-ray is being taken, you should also wear a protective lead apron. If there is any chance that you could be pregnant, it is especially important that you are not exposed to X-rays.

■ SIDE-EFFECTS The radiation risk from a single X-ray is very slight, but small amounts add up. These risks are weighed against the benefit of successful diagnosis. X-rays of children are not taken without careful consideration.

Editorial panel

Professor Robert Hoekelman
Dr Noni MacDonald

(UK)

Professor David Baum
Dr Susanna Graham-Jones

Consulting editor

The consulting editor of *The New American Encyclopedia of Child Health* is Robert A. Hoekelman, M.D., Professor and Chairman of the Department of Pediatrics at the University of Rochester School of Medicine and Dentistry and Pediatrician-in-Chief at the Strong Memorial Hospital in Rochester, New York.

Dr. Hoekelman is a graduate of Dartmouth College and Columbia University College of Physicians and Surgeons. Upon completion of his pediatric training at Babies Hospital in New York City, he served two years in the U.S. Navy Medical Corps and practiced pediatrics in Canandaigua, New York, for 12 years, before joining the faculty of the University of Rochester in 1967.

He has edited or co-edited 20 medical textbooks and journals and has authored or co-authored over 100 book chapters and scientific papers. Most notable among these accomplishments are his editorship of *Primary Pediatric Care* (C.V. Mosby, 1987), a major textbook for medical and nursing students and practitioners; his editorship of the pediatrics section of the *Merck Manual of Diagnosis and Therapy* (Merck, Sharp, and Dohme, 15th Edition, 1987); and his co-authorship of *A Guide to Physical Examination* (J.B. Lippincott, 4th Edition, 1987). The latter two books have been the best sellers, world wide, among medical texts for years; all three books are currently being revised for new editions to be published in 1991.

Dr. Hoekelman has been a consultant on teaching, research and patient care programs to 17 university medical centers in the United States and has been a visiting professor at 26 others throughout the United States, Canada, and Australia. He is the father of four daughters and has two grandsons and one granddaughter.

American text editor

The American text editor, Dr. Noni E. MacDonald, is Associate Professor of Pediatrics and Microbiology at the University of Ottawa, Head of the Infectious Disease Service at the University of Ottawa and Director of the University's Cystic Fibrosis Clinic. She is on the editorial board of the *Pediatric Infectious Diseases* journal and a contributor to the American Society of Pediatrics's *Redbook*. Her research interests are viral infection in children with chronic disease; sexually transmitted disease in children and adolescents and cystic fibrosis. Formerly a colleague of Professor Hoekelman, she is married with two children and lives in Canada.

The contributors

Denise Kitchener (who also made a major contribution to shaping the content and approach of the book) studied medicine at the University of Witwatersrand, qualifying in 1970. She trained as a paediatrician at the Red Cross Children's Hospital in Cape Town, has worked in general practice, and as a consultant in paediatric cardiology. Since 1986 she has lived in the U.K. She has two children.

Dr Peter Campion, Senior Lecturer in General Practice at the University of Liverpool and a partner in an inner city general practice in Toxteth, Liverpool. Qualified 1970 at the London Hospital, worked in paediatrics at the Queen Elizabeth Hospital for Children, Hackney, M.R.C.P, 1973; family doctor 1974 to 1980; Lecturer in General Practice at Dundee University before moving to Liverpool in 1985.

Chrissie Verduyn, principal clinical psychologist for children's services, Bolton; formerly member of a multi-disciplinary team in child and adolescent psychiatry in Oxford.

Dr Elizabeth Didcock, neonatal registrar in Birmingham.

Dr Mary Eminson, child psychiatrist in Manchester.

Dr Karen Baker, registrar in Child and Family Therapy, Birmingham.

Ian McKinley, Senior Lecturer in Community Child Health at Manchester University; consultant paediatric neurologist to the Manchester Children's Hospitals 1978-86.

Dr Geoffrey Frost, consultant paediatrician, Kidderminster General Hospital.

The editors and publishers also acknowledge, with thanks, contributions from Dr Tony Costello and Brian Tongue.

Editorial
Editorial director
Andrew Duncan
Editors
Esther Caplan, Stella Maidment
Proofreading
Linda Hart, Laura Harper
Editorial assistant
Rosemary Dawe

Design
Art director
Mel Petersen
Design assistance
Beverley Stewart, Chris Foley
Artwork
Sandra Ponds and Will Giles